Women's Health in Primary Care

Women's Health in Primary Care

Edited by

Anne Connolly
GPSI Gynae, Bradford

Amanda Britton
GP Principal, Basingstoke

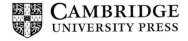

CAMBRIDGE
UNIVERSITY PRESS

CAMBRIDGE
UNIVERSITY PRESS

University Printing House, Cambridge CB2 8BS, United Kingdom

One Liberty Plaza, 20th Floor, New York, NY 10006, USA

477 Williamstown Road, Port Melbourne, VIC 3207, Australia

4843/24, 2nd Floor, Ansari Road, Daryaganj, Delhi - 110002, India

79 Anson Road, #06-04/06, Singapore 079906

Cambridge University Press is part of the University of Cambridge.

It furthers the University's mission by disseminating knowledge in the pursuit of education, learning and research at the highest international levels of excellence.

www.cambridge.org
Information on this title: www.cambridge.org/9781316509920

First published 2017

Printed in the United Kingdom by TJ International Ltd. Padstow, Cornwall

A catalogue record for this publication is available from the British Library

Library of Congress Cataloguing in Publication data
Names: Connolly, Anne, 1959– editor. | Britton, Amanda, 1957– editor.
Title: Women's health in primary care / edited by Anne Connolly and Amanda Britton.
Other titles: Women's health in primary care (Connolly)
Description: Cambridge, United Kingdom ; New York : Cambridge University Press, 2017. | Includes bibliographical references and index.
Identifiers: LCCN 2016059381 | ISBN 9781316509920 (alk. paper)
Subjects: | MESH: Women's Health | Primary Health Care | Great Britain | Case Reports
Classification: LCC RA778 | NLM WA 309 FA1 | DDC 613/.04244 – dc23
LC record available at https://lccn.loc.gov/2016059381

ISBN 978-1-316-50992-0 Paperback

Contents

Contents

Colour plates are to be found between pages 178 and 179

Contributors

Catherine Armitage, MBBCh DipGUM DRCOG MFSRH MRCGP
General Practitioner, Leeds Student Medical Practice, Leeds, UK

Najia Aziz, MBBS MFSRH Dip GUM PG Certificate in Healthcare Leadership Diploma in Psychosexual Medicine DRCOG
Consultant Community Sexual and Reproductive Health, Solent NHS Trust, Sexual Health Services, Winchester, UK

Helen Barnes
Lead GPSI, Guildford & Waverley Community Gynaecology Service, Guildford, UK

Dr Virginia A. Beckett, BSc (Hons) MBBS FRCOG
Consultant Obstetrician and Gynaecologist, Bradford Teaching Hospitals NHS Foundation Trust, UK

Jenny Blackman, MBChB MRCOG
Locum Consultant, Royal Devon and Exeter Hospital, Exeter, UK

Paula Briggs, FFSRH
Consultant in Sexual and Reproductive Health, Southport and Ormskirk Hospital NHS Trust, UK

Amanda Britton, MBChB DRCOG DCH FFSRH MRCGP
GP Principal, Basingstoke, UK

Pam Brown, MBChB FRCGP
General Practitioner, SA1 Medical Practice, Swansea, Wales

Elizabeth Burt BM BSc MRCOG
Obstetrics and Gynaecology Specialist Registrar, University College London Hospital, UK

Anne Connolly, MBChB DRCOG DFSRH MRCGP Dip GPSI gynae (hons)
GPSI gynae, Bevan Healthcare, Bradford and Chair of the Primary Care Women's Health Forum, UK

Victoria Corkhill, MRCOG MBChB BSc (hons) DFFP ST7 O&G
St. James' University Hospital, Leeds, West Yorkshire, UK

Christine Corrin, MBBS DRCOG MRCGP
Hospital Practitioner, St. James' University Hospital, Leeds, West Yorkshire, UK

Jane Dickson, MA MFSRH
Consultant in Sexual and Reproductive Healthcare, Oxleas NHS Foundation Trust, London, UK

Leila Frodsham, MRCOG MIPM
Consultant Obstetrician and Gynaecologist and Psychosexual Medicine Lead at Guy's and St Thomas' Hospital, London

Sarah Gray, BSc MBBS MRCGP DRCOG DFSRH FHEA
GP Specialist in Women's Health, Cornwall, UK

Amanda Hillard, RGN
Clinical Nurse Specialist, Harbourside Gynaecology Unit, Poole Hospital NHS Foundation Trust, Poole, Dorset, UK

Timothy Hillard, DM FFSRH FRCOG
Consultant Obstetrician and Gynaecologist, Poole Hospital NHS Foundation Trust, Poole, Dorset, UK

Charlotte Hutchings, BMedSci BM MRCGP
General Practitioner, Hartley Witney Practice, UK

Sian Jones, MBBCh FRCOG
Honorary Professor, University of Bradford, Bradford, UK; Fellow BSGE

Sally Kidsley, MBBCh PhD MRCOG MFSRH
Clinical Director at Solent Sexual Health Service, Royal South Hants Hospital, Southampton, UK

Kate London, MBChB DRCOG
Consultant Dermatologist St Lukes Hospital, Bradford, UK, Fellow of ISSVD and Member of BSSVD

Keith A. Louden, DM FRCOG
Consultant Obstetrician and Gynaecologist, Hampshire Hospitals NHS Foundation Trust, Winchester, UK

Sally Louden, MRCGP DRCOG Cert Gynae Imaging
General Practitioner in Alton, Hampshire, UK

Henny Lukman, MRCOG
Consultant Obstetrician and Gynaecologist, Princess Anne Hospital, Southampton, UK

Richard Ma, MBChB DCH DRCOG DFSRH Dip GUM MRCGP MSc PG Cert MedEd
General Practitioner, The Village Practice, Isledon Road, London, UK

Diana Mansour, FRCOG FFSRH
Consultant in Community Gynaecology and Reproductive Healthcare, New Croft Centre, Newcastle upon Tyne, UK

Jo Marsden, MBBS MD FRCS (Lond)
Consultant Breast Surgeon, King's College Hospital NHS Foundation Trust, London, UK

Ken S. Metcalf, MD FRCSEd FRCOG
Consultant Gynaecologist and Gynaecological Oncologist, University Hospital Southampton, UK

Christian Phillips, BM BSc (hons) DM FRCOG
Consultant Gynaecologist, Hampshire Hospitals, Basingstoke, Hampshire, UK and visiting Professor, University of Winchester

Robert A. Reichert, MD FACS
Consultant Surgeon, London North West Healthcare NHS Trust, London, UK

Carolyn Sadler, BMedSci BMBS MSc in Research Methods in Health
General Practitioner with a special interest in Gynaecology, and trustee for the National Association for Premenstrual Syndrome, Clifton Road Surgery, Ashbourne, Derbyshire, UK

Ertan Saridogan, PhD FRCOG
Consultant in Gynaecology, Reproductive Medicine and Minimal Access Surgery, University College London Hospital, London, UK

Tim Sayer, MBChB MD FRCOG
Consultant Gynaecologist, Hampshire Hospitals, Basingstoke, UK

Clare Searle MBChB MSc
General Practitioner, Park End Surgery, Community Gynaecology and Reproductive Health Care, Hertfordshire, UK

Judy Shakespeare, MA BM BCh FRCGP
Retired General Practitioner, Oxford, UK

Chantal Simonis, MB ChB MRCOG DM
Consultant in Sexual and Reproductive Health, Wessex Fertility Ltd, Southampton, UK

Fiona Sizmur, MBChB MRCOG FFSRH
Consultant Gynaecologist, Wessex Fertility Ltd, Southampton, UK

Joanna Speedie, MBChB MFSRH
Registrar in Community Sexual and Reproductive Healthcare, Newcastle upon Tyne Hospitals NHS Foundation Trust, Newcastle upon Tyne, UK

Clare Spencer, MA MB BChir (CANTAB) DM MRCOG MRCGP
General Practitioner with a special interest in gynaecology, Leeds

Jackie Tay, MD FRCOG
Consultant Obstetrician and Gynaecologist Leeds Teaching Hospital Trust

Susan Towers, MBChB MRCGP DRCOG DCH
Diploma in Practical Dermatology Cardiff, GPwSI Dermatology and GP Partner, The Ridge Medical Practice, Bradford, UK

Jacqui Tuckey, MBChB MRCOG
Consultant in Sexual and Reproductive Health,
Wessex Fertility Ltd, Southampton, UK

Alison Vaughan, MBChB FFSRH MIPM MRCGP DRCOG PGcert (Med Ed)
Associate Specialist Psychosexual Medicine, Park
Centre, Weymouth Community Hospital, Weymouth
and Salaried GP, Alma Clinic, Winton, Bournemouth,
UK

Dileep Wijeratne, MRCOG MBChB(Hons) BSc(Hons)
Senior Registrar in Obstetrics & Gynaecology,
Bradford Royal Infirmary, UK

Foreword

Knowledge is everywhere. It's accessible, in varying forms and its immediacy can sometimes be challenging in the clinical encounter. Here is a book covering all aspects of women's health that a clinician is likely to come across in everyday practice with practical advice on management.

We talk about 'end of life care' yet rarely of 'start of life', where the contribution of health to pregnancy, not only for the mother but also her baby, have such ramifications for the future life of both that this window of opportunity for maximizing health gain is sometimes forgotten.

If the outcome for both is good, the longer-term consequences are also improved and the life course approach to health care, which is bandied about frequently, becomes a reality. The focus of the NHS must be more about education and shared learning. It must be about proactive care where prevention rather than reactive disease intervention is the norm and where there is then shared ownership and responsibility.

This may be at school or in the adolescent years, with advice about normal physiological changes and the difference with pathology. It may also be when contraception and family spacing become relevant or through pregnancy success and mishap to the postnatal period, often the 'Cinderella' of pregnancy care. Equally, it may be in the postpregnancy era when a family is complete or the postreproductive period and beyond when there are opportunities for health care improvement. Sometimes just simple advice and reassurance is all that is required.

This superb book edited by two respected champions of community care have harnessed the knowledge and expertise of national experts to share their experience in an extremely comprehensive manner. It will be of immense value to practising clinicians, doctors and nurses alike, in primary and community care settings at a time when there is increasing demand for services more locally, often out of the traditional hospital outpatient environment.

For me personally this fills the gap which I think has inadvertently developed over the last 10 years between primary and secondary care colleagues in the management of women's health issues and it beautifully covers the ground from cradle to grave. The book is a must read and I strongly recommend it to you.

David Richmond
FRCOG President, Royal College of Obstetricians and Gynaecologists

Preface

This book was conceived to address the need to help primary and community care clinicians keep up to date with developments in the field of women's health, including chapters on vaginal discharge, maternal medicine, incontinence, pelvic pain and breast disease.

There has been a change of emphasis over recent years in women's health care. The traditional reliance on mainly reactive, consultant-led, hospital-based care has been transformed into a more holistic, proactive, primary-care-led approach, which aims to involve and educate women throughout their lives and help them to make healthier lifestyle choices.

The editors, both nationally respected educators and innovators in community gynaecology, have welcomed the contributions from leading experts from across the country, who have generously shared their enthusiasm and time to provide case-based chapters on topics as diverse as adolescent gynaecology to ovarian cancer.

Whether reading from start to finish or dipping into the chapters as needed, the book will be a valuable resource for all clinicians caring for women of all ages and also those studying for extra qualifications including DRCOG, DFSRH or MRCGP.

Women want and need care which is both accessible and evidence-based, but also takes a life course approach. They deserve care which helps them avoid hospitalization and intervention whenever possible and is provided by community-based carers who understand their needs and aspirations, and are supported with the resources presented in this book.

Chapter

1

The Physiology of the Menstrual Cycle and its Impact on Menstrual Cycle Disorders
Practical Implications for Primary Care

Paula Briggs

Key Points

- An understanding of the menstrual cycle enables a basic logical approach to investigation and management of menstrual disorders.
- Ovarian physiology is the basis of understanding normal and abnormal menstrual bleeding.
- The physiology of the normal menstrual cycle is disrupted in polycystic ovarian syndrome and the peri-menopause.
- Anovulation is associated with infrequent menstruation, but bleeding when it does occur can be heavy.
- This chapter explains the control, mechanism and hormonal changes during the menstrual cycle, making treatment of abnormalities logical.
- Progestins are the mainstay of treatment for dysfunctional uterine bleeding.
- Progestins provide endometrial protection in addition to control of abnormal uterine bleeding.
- Prior to providing treatment, baseline investigations should be undertaken, particularly for women over the age of 45. These include the use of transvaginal ultrasound and endometrial sampling.
- Use of an intrauterine system is recommended first line by the National Institute of Clinical Excellence (NICE) in the UK.
- Other treatment options exist for women who either decline or have a contraindication to use of intrauterine contraception.

Case Scenario

Esme is a 47-year-old social worker with two adopted children, aged 20 and 18. She has been married for 24 years and has never used contraception, as her husband is azoospermic. She has always had irregular, infrequent periods, but over the last few years they have become heavier, with clots and flooding to the extent that she has had to stay off work. Her last menstrual period (LMP) was six weeks ago. She has also gained weight, and her body mass index is now 41 kg/m².

On examination, no clinical abnormality is detected.

Her haemoglobin is 90 g/l.

A transvaginal ultrasound shows multiple small peripheral follicles on both ovaries, which have a polycystic pattern (PCO). It also shows an anteverted uterus with a thickened endometrium, suspicious of hyperplasia.

This chapter will describe the physiology of the menstrual cycle and the changes responsible for abnormal uterine bleeding (AUB) [1].

Hormonal Control of the Menstrual Cycle

The menstrual cycle is controlled by the hypothalamo-pituitary-ovarian axis (Figure 1.1). Gonadotrophin releasing hormone (GnRH), a ten amino acid protein hormone, is secreted in a pulsatile manner from the hypothalamus, via venous channels, stimulating the anterior pituitary. The anterior pituitary releases two gonadotrophins, follicle-stimulating hormone (FSH) and luteinizing hormone (LH), in a dose dependent upon the pulse pattern of GnRH release. FSH is responsible for stimulating the growth and development of the Graafian follicles in the ovary, and levels are higher early in the follicular phase of the menstrual cycle, when it initiates follicular development. There is also a small peak of FSH, just prior to ovulation, accompanying the LH peak. LH is also secreted by the

Women's Health in Primary Care, edited by Anne Connolly and Amanda Britton. Published by Cambridge University Press
© Cambridge University Press 2017

Hypothalamus

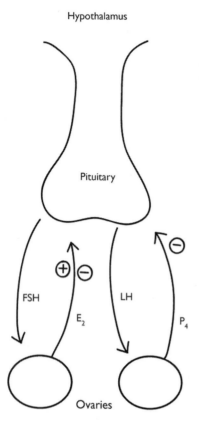

Figure 1.1 The hypothalamo-pituitary-ovarian axis. Reproduced with permission from reference [1].

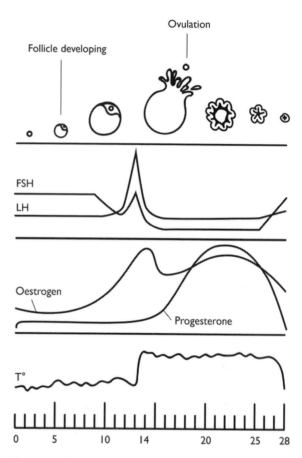

Figure 1.2 The menstrual cycle. Reproduced with permission from reference [1].

anterior pituitary and is at basal levels throughout the cycle, except for the very important LH peak, which occurs 24 hours before ovulation.

Development of the Graafian Follicle and Ovulation

At the beginning of every menstrual cycle (Figure 1.2), under the influence of the rising level of FSH, a number of primordial follicles start to mature. As these follicles grow, the granulosa cells, surrounding the oocyte, secrete oestrogen. This hormone circulates throughout the body and affects many organs. It also acts on the hypothalamo-pituitary-ovarian axis, and as the level of oestrogen rises, FSH secretion is suppressed. This is a negative feedback. Only one of the developing follicles generally will continue to mature, under the influence of FSH, and is destined to ovulate (dominant follicle).

When the follicle is mature, as indicated by a critical level of oestrogen secretion, the LH peak is triggered from the hypothalamo-pituitary axis. This is a

positive feedback. In response to the LH peak, the ripe Graafian follicle (16–22 mm in diameter) situated on the surface of the ovary ruptures, and the ovum is released surrounded by cumulus cells, to be swept up by the fimbriae of the fallopian tube. The oocyte-cumulus mass then travels down the fallopian tube, where it may be fertilized by spermatozoa. In the meantime, the remains of the follicle on the surface of the ovary forms the corpus luteum (yellow body). The colour is due to the deposition of carotene in the theca cells. The corpus luteum secretes progesterone in addition to oestrogen. In the absence of a pregnancy, the corpus luteum has an inherent lifespan of 12–14 days. If the oocyte is fertilized in the fallopian tube, the early embryo secretes beta human chorionic gonadotrophin (beta HCG) within days, maintaining the corpus luteum, which continues to secrete progesterone and oestrogen.

The Effect of Oestrogen and Progesterone on the Endometrium

As the oestrogen secreted by the developing follicles circulates throughout the body, its most overt effect is on the endometrium. Prior to ovulation in the follicular phase, the oestrogen causes both the glands and the stroma in the endometrium to proliferate (proliferative endometrium). This is also referred to as the proliferative phase. After ovulation has occurred, in the luteal phase, progesterone is secreted by the corpus luteum in addition to oestrogen. These two hormones in combination are responsible for the development of many tortuous glands with cells rich in glycogen (secretory endometrium). This is also referred to as the secretory phase of the menstrual cycle. This explains why physiologists divide the menstrual cycle into *follicular and luteal phases* and histologists refer to *proliferative and secretory phases*. The terms are totally interchangeable.

If conception does not occur, the corpus luteum succumbs and both oestrogen and progesterone levels fall. Consequently the endometrium sloughs off (menstruation).

Therefore, the menstrual cycle can be used as an indication as to whether ovulation is occurring. Regular menstrual cycles suggest that ovulation is occurring, whereas an absence of menstruation suggests the absence of ovulation or follicular development. A woman can have bleeding without ovulation, as follicular development can occur in the absence of ovulation. During follicular growth, oestrogen is secreted, which results in endometrial proliferation. When the follicle fails to ovulate and ceases to develop, oestrogen levels fall resulting in endometrial shedding, distinct from the menstrual cycle as described above.

Bioassays of the Menstrual Cycle: Mucus and Temperature Changes

Mucus Changes

The changes in oestrogen and progesterone levels during the menstrual cycle are responsible for the characteristic changes in the cervical mucus. The quantity and quality of cervical mucus is dependent upon the salt and water content, which is regulated by the relative systemic levels of oestrogen and progesterone.

Oestrogen has the effect of stimulating copious amounts of watery/slippery mucus, which is often described as being similar to egg white. The effect of progesterone, after ovulation, is to rapidly change the mucus into a 'gluey' consistency. If you study the cervical mucus changes of a woman through her menstrual cycle, in the days after menstruation, she has low levels of oestrogen and little mucus is secreted. In the mid-follicular phase, as the levels of oestrogen rise, there is a corresponding increase in watery/slippery mucus, until just prior to ovulation, when there is a maximal level of unopposed oestrogen, with a corresponding increase in slippery mucus. This enhances the passage of sperm if sexual intercourse takes place in this fertile phase (basic fertile pattern) [2]. As soon as ovulation occurs and progesterone is secreted, the mucus changes to a 'gluey' consistency, impermeable to sperm (basic infertile pattern). These physiological changes act as a bioassay to pinpoint various stages of the menstrual cycle and are the basis for natural family planning using the Billings method.

Basal Body Temperature

The effect of the progesterone secreted in the luteal phase is to elevate body temperature. One can measure a woman's temperature on waking each morning (basal body temperature) and in the presence of ovulation, this will show an increase of about 0.5 degrees centigrade during the luteal phase. This can also be used retrospectively as a bioassay, to determine the timing of ovulation and the efficiency of the luteal phase.

Polycystic Ovaries/Polycystic Ovary Syndrome

This is the most common endocrine condition to affect women and is complex, with multisystemic repercussions. The finding of polycystic ovaries (PCO) is an ultrasound diagnosis with 12 or more, small peripheral follicles in either ovary [3]. Approximately 20% of women will have this appearance on ultrasound scan. Polycystic ovary syndrome (PCOS) is diagnosed in the presence of the above ultrasound findings together with the symptoms of hyperandrogenism. The most common symptom of increased free androgen levels is oligo/amenorrhoea. Approximately half of the women found to have PCO on ultrasound scan will have PCOS at some time during their lifetime. Gaining weight increases this risk as a result of a decrease in sex hormone binding globulin (SHBG) levels, resulting in an increase in circulating free androgens. In addition, obesity causes insulin resistance, which augments hyperandrogenism. High levels of free androgens can also cause hirsuitism and acne. Many women with irregular menstruation are likely to have PCOS [4].

Esme's case history illustrates two common pathologies, which relate to a disturbance of normal menstrual physiology; PCOS and perimenopausal abnormal uterine bleeding, specifically infrequent heavy menstrual bleeding (HMB).

PCOS and the Menstrual Cycle

Esme illustrates the typical woman with this condition. She has never had a regular cycle, due to irregular and sporadic ovulation. If her husband had not had fertility issues, then ovulation could have been induced using oral anti-oestrogens such as clomiphene citrate and if that failed, FSH injections.

In women with PCOS and infrequent ovulation, there are long periods of unopposed oestrogen secretion, due to the small follicles all producing this hormone. In the absence of ovulation and without a corpus luteum forming, there is no progesterone produced to induce the secretory change in the endometrium, nor is there regular endometrial shedding. Consequently the endometrium becomes hyperplastic, sometimes developing atypical changes, a precursor to endometrial cancer.

Esme's BMI is in the morbidly obese range. This carries a risk of insulin resistance, potentially leading to impaired glucose tolerance, predisposing to type 2 diabetes mellitus. She should have a glucose tolerance test.

Esme has a number of risk factors for endometrial cancer, including being significantly overweight, nulliparous and having PCOS with infrequent ovulation and menstruation.

She should be engaged in a weight management program, with a focus on regular small meals, not skipping meals, reducing refined carbohydrate and (increasing) exercise.

Management should include endometrial sampling to exclude cancer and the provision of a treatment, in the form of progestogen, to reduce endometrial hyperplasia, which will have the added benefit of reducing HMB. The most effective route of administration is an intrauterine system as this delivers the progestogen directly to the endometrium. Alternative treatment options include oral progestogens.

Perimenopausal Heavy Menstrual Bleeding

In Esme's case HMB is likely to be exacerbated by her perimenopausal state. As women approach the menopause transition, anovulatory cycles become more common and in the absence of progesterone secretion, the endometrium continues to proliferate without secretory change or regular shedding. This results in a situation whereby unopposed oestrogen has a similar effect to that seen in women with PCOS.

Obesity is associated with an increase in conversion of cholesterol to oestrogen and in addition to the changes to the menstrual cycle, is an additional risk factor for endometrial cancer.

The investigation and treatment of HMB is similar to that described for PCOS above and in the case of a woman with a BMI greater than 40, treatment using a progestogen would be recommended.

Progesterone, Progestogens and Progestins

There is sometimes confusion in the terminology used to describe progestogens. A progestogen is any hormone with progesterone-like activity on the endometrium, meaning that it induces secretory change. Following ovulation, the ovary secretes natural progesterone. Pharmacologically prepared progesterone is not active if taken orally, but can be administered parenterally, either by injection or by pessary delivered vaginally or rectally. Synthetically produced progesterone-like hormones, such as those found in oral contraceptives or for therapeutic use, are called progestins.

References

1. Kovacs G, Briggs P, Basic Physiology: The Menstrual Cycle. *Lectures in Obstetrics, Gynaecology and Women's Health*, Springer, 2015, pp 3–7.

2. Billings EL, Brown JB, Billings JJ, Burger HG, Symptoms and hormonal changes accompanying ovulation. *Lancet* 1972;1:282–284.

3. The Rotterdam ESHRE/ASRM-Sponsored PCOS Consensus Workshop Group. Revised 2003 consensus on diagnostic criteria and long-term health risks related to polycystic ovary syndrome (PCOS). *Hum Reprod* 2003;19:41–47.

4. Duncan WC, A guide to understanding polycystic ovary syndrome (PCOS). *J Fam Plann Reprod Health Care* 2014;40:217–225.

Management of Children and Adolescents with Gynaecological Problems in Primary Care

Jane Dickson

Key Points

- The commonest gynaecological symptom in prepubertal girls is vaginal discharge, usually caused by vulvovaginitis.
- Examination under anaesthetic is indicated for blood-stained vaginal discharge in children.
- Safeguarding processes should be implemented if there is any suspicion of sexual abuse, e.g. diagnosis of sexually transmitted infection.
- Vaginal examinations are rarely necessary for menstrual symptoms in adolescents.
- Treatment of precocious puberty and primary amenorrhoea/delayed puberty should be undertaken by a specialist, e.g. paediatric endocrinologist/adolescent gynaecologist.
- Pregnancy may be the cause of menstrual dysfunction and a thoughtful enquiry should be made about sexual activity.
- Gynaecological symptoms may be 'functional', i.e. presentation for other causes of anxiety, e.g. abuse, bullying.
- Dysmenorrhoea in adolescents may be the first presenting sign of endometriosis.
- A risk assessment must be undertaken in sexually active young people.
- Female genital mutilation must be reported to the police in an under 18-year-old girl.

Table 2.1 Causes of vaginal discharge in girls

Hormonal	Oestrogen related, e.g. newborn female
Bacterial	Non-specific mixed vaginal flora, e.g. coliforms, staphylococci Group A beta-haemolytic streptococci *Haemophilus influenzae*
Viral	Varicella Measles Rubella
Fungal	*Candida*
Other infections	Threadworms Sexually transmitted infections, e.g. chlamydia, gonorrhoea, trichomoniasis
Foreign bodies	
Vulval dermatitis	Soap Bubble bath Sand Prolonged contact of urine/faeces with skin Irritants, e.g. perfume, dye
Urological problems	Urethral prolapse Ectopic ureter
Vaginal tumours	Embryonal rhabdomyosarcoma Mesonephric carcinoma Clear cell adenocarcinoma

- The anus is anatomically very close to the vagina, predisposing to cross contamination of flora.
- The vulval and vaginal skin is thin and delicate because of low oestrogen levels.
- The vaginal pH is neutral so predisposes to infectious colonization.

A child with discharge should be examined. This needs to be done sensitively either sitting on a parent's lap or on a couch in a 'frog-leg' position. The labia should be parted and a swab can be taken (however, conventional swabs may be too large so a small wire

Vaginal Discharge

Vaginal discharge is the most common gynaecological symptom for a prepubertal girl (Table 2.1). Non-specific bacterial vulvovaginitis is the most frequent cause of symptoms and may be very distressing, particularly if the symptoms are recurrent. Itching and soreness may be associated [1,2]. Prepubertal girls are predisposed to vaginal discharge because:

Women's Health in Primary Care, edited by Anne Connolly and Amanda Britton. Published by Cambridge University Press
© Cambridge University Press 2017

swab should be used). If this would cause too much distress or a foreign body is suspected then this should be undertaken under general anaesthetic.

In vulvovaginitis, the discharge may be clear, yellow or green and rarely there is associated vaginal bleeding. Discharge may be foul smelling and there may be accompanying itch, soreness or dysuria. If bleeding is present, other more serious conditions must be excluded, e.g. sexual abuse, foreign body, tumours and precocious puberty. Non-specific mixed bacterial vulvovaginitis is the commonest cause of discharge and this may relate to poor hygiene, particularly contamination from the anus on wiping. Treatment of this and other bacterial causes is with an antibiotic to which the organism(s) is sensitive. *Candida* is a rare cause of prepubertal discharge, unless there is a precipitating factor e.g. wearing nappies, antibiotics, diabetes mellitus. If the symptom is predominantly itch, especially at night, a diagnosis of threadworms should be considered. History may be enough to lead to the diagnosis; otherwise a piece of sticky tape placed at the anus may identify worms or eggs.

Vulval skin conditions may rarely present with discharge – itch and soreness are more usual features. Atopic eczema and lichen sclerosis may be present in children and the management of these conditions would include emollients and topical steroids.

Management of Vulvovaginitis and Vaginal Discharge

- Antibiotics can be used when a specific pathogen is identified or mebendazole is the treatment of choice if threadworms are identified.
- If there is a sexually transmitted organism present or there is any suspicion of abuse then safeguarding procedures should be implemented.
- Simple hygiene, e.g. front to back wiping.
- Avoid perfumed soap, bubble bath, lotions and shampoo.
- Emollients may be helpful.
- Loose fitting underwear and no pants at night.
- Avoid constipation, soiling and bedwetting.
- Examination under anaesthetic for unexplained vaginal bleeding or suspicion of a retained foreign body.

Case Scenario: Ellie

Ellie is a happy and chatty child. On direct questioning she says that her 'front bottom' is sore. Her mother has noticed yellow discharge for about a week. On examination, in 'frog-leg' position, she has vulval erythema and yellow discharge. A swab shows mixed organisms including coliforms. Treatment would be with a broad-spectrum antibiotic with advice about appropriate soap products, hygiene and front to back wiping.

Puberty and Amenorrhoea

Charlotte

Charlotte is a 15-year-old who has not yet had a period. She has small breasts and no pubic hair. She has not been sexually active. She is very clever and is thriving at school.

Normal Puberty and Menarche

Normal puberty follows a very set pattern. Tanner described physical features in the 1960s and 1970s (Table 2.2 and Figure 2.1) [2].

Normally breast development begins at around age 10, followed by pubic hair six months later. There is then an increase in height. Following this, Tanner stage 4 pubic hair and stage 3–4 breast development occurs, and these usually immediately precede menstruation. Menstruation is closely related to bone age and the average age for the menarche is between 12 years 10 months and 13 years.

Factors which influence the timing of puberty and menstruation include:

Table 2.2 Tanner staging

Stage	Pubic hair	Breast development
1.	Prepuberty	Prepuberty
2.	Narrow border along the labia majora	Small mound and areolar starts to grow
3.	Becoming darker and more curly – spreading to mons	Further increase and loss of contour of separation between breast and areolar
4.	Increasing, but still just at mons	Areolar and nipple form secondary mound
5.	Spreads to adult female triangle pattern	Adult breast appearance

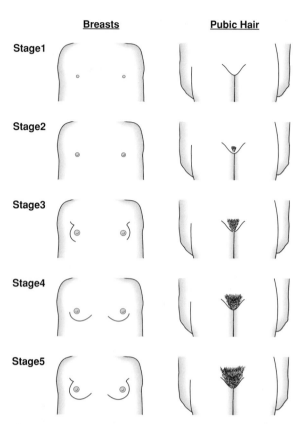

Figure 2.1 Tanner staging of puberty.

- Genetic factors
- Nutrition
- Exercise
- General health
- Racial differences, e.g. it is normal for African girls to have an earlier onset.

Amenorrhoea

Amenorrhoea is the absence of periods. It is *primary* amenorrhoea if there have never been any periods and it is *secondary* amenorrhoea if periods were present, but have stopped for six months.

Primary Amenorrhoea

Primary amenorrhoea with absence of development of secondary sexual characteristics should be investigated at 13 years old. In the presence of secondary sexual characteristics, it should be investigated at 15 years old (Table 2.3) [3]

Table 2.3 Causes of primary amenorrhoea [3,4]

Constitutional	• Constitutional delay
Systemic	• Chronic disease, e.g. cystic fibrosis • Weight loss • Endocrine, e.g. thyroid disease
Hypothalamic-pituitary dysfunction	• Hypothalamic (hypogonadotrophic hypogonadism), e.g. intense exercise, idiopathic • Intracranial pathology, e.g. brain tumours, head injury, hydrocephalus • Pituitary, e.g. hypopituitarism, hyperprolactinaemia • Laurence–Moon–Biedl syndrome • Prader–Willi syndrome • Kallman syndrome
Gonadal dysfunction	• Premature ovarian failure • Turner syndrome • Gonadal dysgenesis, e.g. Swyer syndrome • Polycystic ovarian syndrome
Anatomical abnormalities	• Mullerian agenesis, e.g. Rokitansky syndrome • Complete androgen insensitivity syndrome • Absent or imperforate vagina

Constitutional Delay

Constitutional delay is often familial and occurs when bone age is less than chronological age. Menstruation will occur when bone age catches up with chronological age. Patients should be followed up and careful consideration should be given to the social consequences of this problem, e.g. difficulties with peers.

Chronic Disease

Any systemic disease can impair development and delay menstruation. Treatment of the disease will usually resolve the situation. Conditions associated include diabetes mellitus, hypothyroidism, chronic renal disease, cystic fibrosis, congenital cardiac disease and coeliac disease.

Hypothalamic-Pituitary Dysfunction

The commonest hypothalamic-pituitary causes are idiopathic or related to extreme exercise/weight loss. Conditions that compress the pituitary or hypothalamus will lead to reduced LH and FSH production.

Some rare syndromes, which may lead to dysfunction, include:

- *Laurence–Moon–Biedel* – Autosomal recessive condition associated with obesity, retinitis pigmentosa, learning disability, polydactyly and hypogonadism.

- *Prader–Willi* – hypotonia, learning disability, characteristic facies, obesity.
- *Kallman* – agenesis of olfactory bulbs and anatomical defects of hypothalamus which leads to anosmia and lack of secondary sexual development.

Ovarian Dysfunction and Failure

Ovarian dysfunction may present as primary or secondary amenorrhoea. Premature ovarian failure is an extremely distressing diagnosis as it confers loss of fertility.

Causes of Premature Ovarian Failure

- Idiopathic
- Chemotherapy
- Radiotherapy
- Metabolic disease, e.g. galactosaemia
- Autoimmune conditions, e.g. Addison's disease
- Infections, e.g. mumps
- Chromosomal anomalies, e.g. Turner syndrome.

Turner Syndrome

The premature ovarian failure associated with Turner syndrome relates to gonadal dysgenesis. Turner syndrome occurs in 1 in 2000–3000 live female births and is related either to the classic karyotype 45X0 or a mosaic form e.g. 45X/46XX or 45X/46XY. The ovaries have a 'streak' appearance – it is thought that normal numbers of oocytes develop until the fifth month *in utero*, but they then degenerate rapidly so that very few are present by birth. Spontaneous menstruation may occur especially when there is mosaicism, but premature ovarian failure usually results.

The physical appearance of those with Turner syndrome may vary markedly, but there are typical features more generally associated with the X0 karyotype.

Those features may include:

- Short stature
- Webbing of the neck
- Cubitus valgus
- Lymphoedema of hands or feet
- Widely spaced nipples
- Cardiac or renal abnormalities
- Coarctation of the aorta
- Autoimmune hypothyroidism.

Diagnosis may be made in infancy if there are typical features or as a result of investigation of short stature in childhood. Amenorrhoea is often the presentation in adolescence. LH and FSH levels are high and oestradiol levels are low. Chromosomal analysis should be performed. Presence of a Y chromosome or fragment means that the gonads should be removed because there is a high risk of malignancy.

Swyer Syndrome

Swyer syndrome is 46XY gonadal dysgenesis. It is due to a gene mutation, usually of the SRY gene. The external physical appearance is often of a tall female. There is no testosterone so the internal female genitalia develop, but there are intra-abdominal dysgenetic testes present rather than ovaries. These testes have up to a 40% chance of malignancy so should be removed as soon as the condition is discovered. As in Turner syndrome, the FSH and LH levels are high. Because a uterus is present, childbearing may be possible with egg donation and fertility treatment.

Anatomical Abnormalities

Anatomical abnormalities may account for primary amenorrhoea when secondary sexual characteristics are present. The uterus may be absent when the müllerian duct has failed to develop, such as is the case in complete androgen insensitivity syndrome and Rokitansky–Kuster–Hauser syndrome. Absent or imperforate vagina may also present as primary amenorrhoea, but is actually cryptomenorrhoea (i.e. menstruation is occurring but not being seen).

Complete Androgen Insensitivity Syndrome (CAIS)

In CAIS a girl has the karyotype 46XY. It is an X-linked recessive condition. The appearance is female, often with normal breasts, but sparse pubic and axillary hair, and they may be taller than average. *In utero*, there are normal testes producing testosterone and müllerian inhibitory factor – this means that the structures derived from the müllerian duct, i.e. uterus and upper vagina, degenerate and so are not present, and the external female genitalia are normal.

Diagnosis may be made in infancy due to the presence of gonads in the inguinal area or later as a consequence of primary amenorrhoea. Investigation will reveal normal LH and FSH levels, high testosterone and low oestradiol. Some testosterone is converted into

Table 2.4 Investigations for amenorrhoea in primary care

Clinical examination	Body mass index Pubertal staging Indications of endocrine disease e.g. hirsuitism Signs of Turner syndrome
Investigations	Pregnancy test Follicle-stimulating hormone Luteinizing hormone Estradiol Prolactin Thyroid function tests Testosterone Sex hormone binding globulin Karyotype

oestradiol, the presence of which allows breast development. Treatment involves gonadectomy (best performed after puberty to allow for normal breast development), vaginal reconstruction surgery and long-term oestrogen replacement therapy.

Rokitansky–Kuster–Hauser Syndrome

This syndrome occurs in 1 in 5000 female births and there is a 46XX genotype and normal female appearance. There is failure of development of the müllerian duct, which means there is no uterus or upper vagina, but normal ovaries are present. There is usually a short blind-ending vagina and there may be associated renal, skeletal and auditory abnormalities. LH, FSH and oestradiol levels will all be normal.

The most important aspects of treatment are psychological support and the creation of a vagina so that penetrative sexual intercourse may be achieved. This would initially be with vaginal dilators, but surgical treatment may be necessary where this fails. It is feasible for these women to have their own genetic children using their ova and a surrogate mother, and currently significant research is being undertaken to develop uterine transplant techniques.

Cryptomenorrhoea

There is cyclical pain in association with amenorrhoea and this is due to an obstruction, usually in the vagina. The commonest cause for this is an imperforate hymen – there may be an abdominal mass with pressure symptoms, such as urinary retention. A blue bulging membrane can be seen on parting the labia. This is treated with a simple incision. Other rare causes include a transverse vaginal septum and cervical agenesis.

It may be necessary to refer for imaging, e.g. ultrasound scan of pelvis, MRI pelvis/pituitary/hypothalamus or X-ray of wrist if constitutional delay is suspected.

Treatment of Delayed Puberty/Menarche

Treatment is best undertaken by a specialist, e.g. paediatric endocrinologist or adolescent gynaecologist. Usually very low-dose oestrogen is given initially. Later, treatment will usually involve either combined hormonal contraception (as hormone replacement) or conventional hormone replacement therapy.

Secondary Amenorrhoea

Secondary amenorrhoea may occur in adolescents and the most likely causes are:

- Pregnancy
- Premature ovarian failure
- Polycystic ovarian syndrome
- Pituitary disorders
- Hypothalamic disorders.

Polycystic Ovarian Syndrome (PCOS) (See Chapter 14)

PCOS is classically related to obesity and there may be signs of raised androgens, e.g. acne, hirsuitism. There may be oligoamenorrhoea or secondary amenorrhoea (very rarely primary amenorrhoea). Initial management is with weight loss and exercise and combined hormonal contraception (CHC) is often very effective. CHC causes sex hormone binding globulin levels to increase and this 'mops up' androgens. This leads to cycle regulation and reduction in androgen-related side effects. Any CHC may be used, e.g. pills, patch or vaginal ring, but some preparations may be particularly helpful. These include co-cyprindiol (e.g. Dianette®) which contains the anti-androgen cyproterone and the drosperinone-containing combined pill, Yasmin®. There is a link with insulin resistance and metformin may have a beneficial effect on menstrual regulation, but this would be part of specialist rather than primary care management [4,5].

Precocious Puberty [2,3]

This is puberty occurring before the age of 8 in girls and 9 in boys. In 74% of girls it is idiopathic. It may be gonadotrophin dependent, i.e. when the hypothalamic-pituitary-gonadal axis is prematurely activated, e.g. brain tumours, hypothyroidism. It may also be gonadotrophin independent, where there are raised sex steroids, e.g. congenital adrenal hyperplasia, adrenal or ovarian tumours and McCune–Albright syndrome. These children should be referred to a paediatric endocrinologist.

In premature adrenarche, there is an isolated raised androgen level leading to pubic hair, body odour and acne. It is important to rule out other causes of raised androgens, e.g. congenital adrenal hyperplasia, tumours, but otherwise it does not cause long-term problems. It may be related to insulin resistance and a later development of polycystic ovarian syndrome.

Case Scenario: Charlotte

Charlotte needs to be investigated as she has primary amenorrhoea and is 15 years old. She has a normal body mass index and minimal androgen-dependant secondary sexual characteristics, e.g. pubic and axillary hair. Investigations show her to have a very high testosterone level and normal LH and FSH levels. Her chromosomes demonstrate a 46XY pattern and she has no internal female genitalia on ultrasound scan. She has a diagnosis of complete androgen insufficiency syndrome and treatment will involve gonadectomy, oestrogen replacement therapy and vaginal treatment, e.g. dilation or surgery.

Period Problems

Case Scenario: Safia

Safia is 14 years old. Her periods began when she was 11. She has extremely painful periods, which are often associated with diarrhoea. She misses at least two days of school every month because of her pain.

Heavy Menstrual Bleeding

Heavy or painful menstruation is the commonest reason for an adolescent to be referred to a gynaecologist. Adolescents may have irregular cycles for the first years following menarche. Cycles in this situation are often anovulatory, which results in heavy dysfunctional bleeding – the endometrium becomes thick and unstable under the influence of unopposed oestrogen. Girls with regular periods are more likely to be ovulating and increased fibrinolysis and prostaglandins are thought to be responsible for heavy bleeding in these situations.

Approximately one in ten adolescent girls will require treatment for heavy menstrual bleeding. Despite the fact that different management options may be preferred, the NICE heavy menstrual bleeding guidance still applies [6]. Initial assessment should include a full blood count and when simple treatment is not effective, consider conditions such as von Willebrand disease and idiopathic thrombocytopenic purpura. Vaginal examination is not usually required, as it is unlikely to add value to the assessment.

Periods may present additional problems to young women with learning disabilities as there may be problems related to the use of sanitary wear, e.g. soiling, hiding used sanitary products. Also, if epileptic, their fits may heighten either premenstrually or during periods. In these situations menstrual control may be even more important to quality of life.

Treatment Options

- The Mirena® intrauterine system is the first-line treatment, but this may not be practical in young women who have never been sexually active. The uterine cavity length needs to be at least 5 cm, but if it is felt that this is the best treatment option, e.g. young woman with special needs, insertion could be considered under general anaesthetic [7]. The Jaydess® intrauterine device is smaller, lasts for three years and is not currently licenced for the management of heavy menstrual bleeding, but may well have some benefits in this area [8].
- Antifibrinolytics, e.g. tranexamic acid 1 g tds, are helpful to reduce menstrual flow and these may be used in conjunction with non-steroidal anti-inflammatory drugs, e.g. mefenamic acid 500 mg tds, which are also helpful in reducing menstrual pain because of anti-prostaglandin action.
- Combined hormonal contraception (CHC) is a safe treatment option provided there are no absolute contraindications, e.g. thrombophilia. Options include the combined oral contraceptive pill and the combined contraceptive patch (Evra®). The patch is particularly useful for young women with learning disabilities as it can be placed on parts of the body where it is difficult to remove, e.g. shoulder. CHC can be used either cyclically or continuously in a tailored manner. This means using pills or patches continuously and taking a break of 4–7 days when there have

been three consecutive days of breakthrough bleeding.

- Progestogen containing injectables may be considered in this group, e.g. Depo-Provera® or Sayana Press®. These are given every 13 weeks and have a high likelihood of resulting in amenorrhoea. However, careful consideration needs to be given before use because of potential risk to bone mineral density in those who have not achieved peak bone mass. When there are considerable risk factors for osteoporosis, e.g. immobility, oral steroid uses, low body mass index, depot is best avoided. If it is the only option 'addback oestrogen', e.g. an oestrogen patch could be used. Sayana Press® has been licensed for self-administration.
- The progestogen-containing contraceptive implant, e.g. Nexplanon® may sometimes be tried, but bleeding irregularity is a common side effect.
- Cyclical progestogen, e.g. norethisterone 5 mg tds given 21 days each cycle (D5–26), is an option, but may cause considerable androgenic side effects, e.g. acne, hirsuitism.

Acute Heavy Bleeding

Very rarely an adolescent may a have a very acute heavy bleed that requires hospital admission, resuscitation and transfusion. Treatment would be high-dose progestogens, e.g. norethisterone 5–10 mg tds or high-dose COC could be used, e.g. 3–4 pills per day until bleeding stops.

Dysmenorrhoea

Menstrual pain may be disabling in adolescents and is more usually associated with ovulatory rather than anovulatory cycles. It often develops 6–12 months after the onset of menstruation and is known as primary dysmenorrhoea as it is not related to pathology. Prostaglandins are responsible and cause uterine spasms and other related symptoms, e.g. diarrhoea, pain radiating to thighs, nausea. Non-steroidal anti-inflammatory agents, e.g. mefenamic acid 500 mg tds, are helpful for this type of pain. Alternatively, some of the agents used for heavy menstrual bleeding, e.g. combined hormonal contraception, can be useful.

In adolescents where pain does not resolve with simple measures, pathology should be considered.

Endometriosis is the commonest cause of secondary dysmenorrhoea and it has been estimated that it may be responsible for chronic pelvic pain in as many as 73% of adolescents, where pain is unresponsive to treatment. In these situations laparoscopy may be necessary and endometriosis may be seen as clear vesicles rather than the typical brown lesions of older women. Treatment options are the same as those for older women.

Rarely, dysmenorrhoea may be caused by anatomical anomalies of the uterus. Menstrual flow is partly obstructed, causing pain because of accumulated blood. Treatment would be surgical.

Adolescent girls might be sexually active, so problems related to sexually activity should not be neglected. Both pregnancy and sexually transmitted infections can lead to problems with pain and bleeding, so a sexual history should be taken. It may be necessary to ask a parent to leave in order to make these inquiries.

Case Scenario: Safia

Safia's periods have been heavy and painful since they became regular. She has no problems when she is not menstruating and has never been sexually active. She has no other symptoms of note and has no family history of bleeding problems. The most likely problem is primary dysmenorrhoea. She does not require other investigation initially and treatment options include mefenamic acid and combined hormonal contraception.

Legal and Ethical Issues

Sexual Abuse

Sexual abuse should be considered in many gynaecological presentations, e.g. genital soreness, genitourinary injuries, vaginal discharge, recurrent dysuria, sexually transmitted infections and pregnancy. Additionally there are non-gynaecological symptoms where abuse should be considered, e.g. faecal soiling, rectal bleeding, enuresis and generalized abdominal pain. A young person's behaviour may change to indicate distress or anxiety, e.g. self-harm, an eating disorder or there may be inappropriate sexualized behaviour when abuse has occurred. Where there are any concerns, local safeguarding processes must be implemented.

Normal

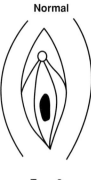

Type 1
Partial/total removal of clitoris

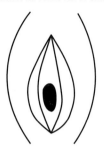

Type 2
Partial/total removal of clitoris and labia minora

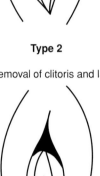

Type 3
'Infibulation' cutting labia minora and/or labia majora and sealing vaginal orifice

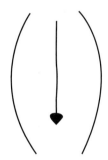

Type 4 – Other harmful procedures e.g. pricking, cutting, piercing

Figure 2.2 World Health Organisation female genital mutilation classification.

Consent and Child Sexual Exploitation

Approximately 30% of young people have sexual intercourse before the age of 16. Many relationships are consensual, but a risk assessment should be undertaken to ensure that there is no child sexual exploitation. Firstly, there should be assessment of competency (Fraser ruling when applied to contraception and Gillick competence when applied to wider aspects of care and consent) [9,10,11].

Child sexual exploitation involves those under 18 in exploitative situations, contexts and relationships where young people receive something, e.g. money, gifts, as a result of engaging in sexual activity. It is an abuse of power by those exploiting by virtue of their age, gender, intellect, strength and/or economic or other resources.

Risk factors include vulnerabilities, e.g. learning or physical disability, living in care, mental health problems and addictions, lack of support networks, e.g. family/friends, and past history of abuse or exploitation. Concerns should trigger safeguarding processes.

Female Genital Mutilation (FGM)

Female genital mutilation is defined as partial or total removal of the female genitalia for non-medical reasons (Figure 2.2). It is illegal in the UK and it is also illegal to take a girl out of the country to have it performed. If suspected or confirmed in a girl under the age of 18, it must be reported to the police (most local safeguarding structures now interact specifically with the police). It is also mandatory for FGM to be recorded in medical records [12,13].

FGM is practised in 29 African countries and also some areas outside Africa, e.g. Yemen, Indonesia and Malaysia. Very high incidence areas (>90%) in Africa are Somalia, Guinea, Djibouti and Egypt. The age at which FGM is carried out is variable, but the majority will occur before the age of 15 and in about half the countries will occur before the age of 5. In many countries it is practised by traditional practitioners using crude instruments, but in some countries, e.g. Egypt, more is undertaken by health care professionals. The reasons given for the procedure are complex and vary from region to region, but include 'custom', 'rite of passage', 'cleansing' and 'status'. Short-term complications include haemorrhage, urinary retention, infection and death. Long-term complications include scarring, urinary and gynaecological problems, and sexual and psychological problems.

If FGM is identified in an adult, it is important to record that advice has been given that the procedure is illegal and make inquiry about intentions for female children. Risk factors include status of family, family history of FGM, family from high prevalence area and any talk of a 'special holiday' – the long summer holidays are the most high-risk time. If there are any concerns, then safeguarding procedures should be followed.

Increasingly, young women present with concerns about their labial appearance. Female genital cosmetic surgery may be prohibited under the FGM act, unless it is necessary for physical or mental health. It is very important for primary care physicians to provide reassurance.

References

1. Hayes L, Creighton SM, Prepubertal vaginal discharge. *Obstetr Gynaecol* 2007;9:159–163.

2. Garden AS, Hernon M, Topping J, *Paediatric and Adolescent Gynaecology for the MRCOG and Beyond*, 2nd edn. London: RCOGPress, 2008.

3. Michala L, Creighton S, Adolescent gynaecology. *Obstetr Gynaecol Reprod Med* 2014;24(3):74–79.

4. Hickey M, Balen A, Menstrual disorders in adolescence: investigation and management. *Hum Reprod Update* 2003;9(5):493–504.

5. Hoeger K, Davidson K, Kochman L *et al.* The impact of metformin, oral contraceptives, and lifestyle modification on polycystic ovary syndrome in obese adolescent women in two randomised, placebo-controlled clinical trials. *J Clin Endocrinol Metab* 2008;93(11):4299–4306.

6. NICE. Heavy menstrual bleeding: assessment and management. January 2007. www.nice.org.uk/guidance/cg44 (accessed September 2016).

7. Bayer L, Hillard P, Use of Levonorgestrel Intrauterine System for medical indications in adolescents. *J Adolesc Health* 2013;52:S54–S58.

8. Clinical Effectiveness Unit FSRH. Intrauterine contraception. April 2015. http://www.fsrh.org/standards-and-guidance/documents/ceuguidanceintrauterinecontraception/ (accessed September 2016).

9. The Third National Survey of Sexual Attitudes and Lifestyles. *Lancet* 2013;382:1757–1856.

10. Clinical Effectiveness Unit, BASHH. UK National Guideline on the management of sexually transmitted infections and related conditions in children and young people 2010. www.bashh.org/documents/2674.pdf (accessed September 2016).

11. BASHH and Brook. Spotting the signs. April 2014. http://www.bashh.org/BASHH/News/BASHH/News/News_Items/Spotting_the_Signs_-_CSE_Proforma.aspx (accessed September 2016).

12. HM Government. Multi-Agency Practice Guidelines. Female genital mutilation 2011. https://www.gov.uk/government/uploads/system/uploads/attachment_data/file/512906/Multi_Agency_Statutory_Guidance_on_FGM__-_FINAL.pdf (accessed September 2016).

13. RCOG Green-top Guideline No. 53 July 2015. Female Genital Mutilation and its Management.

Chapter 3

Contraceptive Choices in Primary Care

Joanna Speedie and Diana Mansour

Key Points

- The majority of women attend primary care for their contraception. Offering information about all methods of contraception increases uptake of the long-acting reversible methods.
- The long-acting reversible methods of contraception are more reliable as they are non-user dependent.
- Many contraceptive methods have non-contraceptive benefits.
- Use of the UKMEC reduces risk when prescribing contraception. Refer to http://www.fsrh.org/documents/ukmec-2016/.
- There are very few contraindications to use of progestogenic methods of contraception.
- Erratic menstrual bleeding is common in the first few months of using a progestogenic method of contraception and in some women continues with ongoing use.
- The LNG-IUS (Mirena®) is licensed for contraception, management of HMB and the progestogenic component of HRT.
- The CuIUD is the most effective method of emergency contraception and should be offered to all women.
- Condoms have a high contraceptive failure rate, but prevent the acquisition and transmission of STIs.
- Sterilization is a permanent procedure and reversal is not funded by the NHS.

Introduction

The third UK National Survey of Sexual Attitudes and Lifestyles recently reported that 16% of British pregnancies are unplanned and a further 29% of women are ambivalent about being pregnant. This is difficult to explain as contraceptive methods are provided free of charge by primary, community and acute hospital services.

Over 80% of couples rely on their general practitioner or practice nurse for birth control information, therefore keeping up to date in this field is important. This has been highlighted by two projects in the US. Health care professionals (HCPs) who are well educated in modern long-lasting reversible options are more likely to discuss them, women are more likely to use them and unplanned pregnancies fall [1,2].

This chapter will examine the 16 contraceptive methods available in the UK, reviewing their advantages and associated challenges.

Combined Hormonal Contraception (CHC) [3]

Case Scenario

Rebecca is 21 years old and has been seeing her current boyfriend for one year. They use condoms but she has had to take oral emergency contraception twice recently. She has come to see you to discuss contraception and thinks 'the pill' would be a good choice. Her friend takes Yasmin® and likes it, so Rebecca would like to take it too.

Composition

Combined hormonal contraceptives (CHCs) contain synthetic oestrogen and progestogen and can be

---

Women's Health in Primary Care, edited by Anne Connolly and Amanda Britton. Published by Cambridge University Press

Table 3.1 Types of progestogen in CHCs

Generation	Progestogen type	Example of CHC
First	Norethisterone	Loestrin®
Second	Levonorgestrel Norgestimate	Microgynon 30® Cilest®
Third	Desogestrel Gestodene	Marvelon® Femodene®
Fourth	Cyproterone acetate Drosperinone	Dianette® Yasmin®
Non-oral progestogens	Norelgestromin Etonogestrel	Evra patch® Nuvaring®
Unclassified	Dienogest Nomegestrol acetate	Qlaira® Zoely®

administered as pills, patches or in a vaginal ring. Most available CHCs contain ethinylestradiol at varying dosages, although some newer combined oral contraceptives (COCs) contain estradiol, which is thought to have less metabolic impact. Since the launch of COCs 50 years ago, the oestrogen dose has gradually decreased and most pills now contain less than 35 micrograms of ethinylestradiol. This has reduced oestrogenic side effects and lower associated cardiovascular risks.

CHCs contain different progestogens, which are frequently grouped into 'generations' depending on the decade in which they were launched, the route of administration and the estimated venous thromboembolism risk (Table 3.1).

Mode of Action

CHCs work by:
- Inhibiting ovulation
- Thickening cervico-uterine mucus
- Causing endometrial atrophy
- Altering tubal motility and secretions.

Effectiveness

All forms of CHC have similar failure rates – 0.3% in the first year of use with perfect use and 9% with typical use. Contraceptive efficacy is not affected by broad-spectrum antibiotics, but may be reduced by taking enzyme-inducing drugs.

Advantages Including Non-Contraceptive Benefits

- Withdrawal bleeds become regular, lighter and less painful in CHC users and CHCs are recommended by the National Institute of Health and Care Excellence (NICE) [4] for women with heavy menstrual bleeding. CHCs can treat pain associated with endometriosis.
- Women can choose when to have a bleed. Pills, patches and vaginal rings can be used 'back to back', thus decreasing the frequency of bleeds. When problematic bleeding occurs for four or more days, a hormone break of four to seven days can be taken.
- CHCs result in a decreased risk of ovarian, endometrial and colorectal cancer.
- CHCs improve acne, especially preparations containing cyproterone acetate or drosperinone. Maximum benefit is seen after 12 months of use.
- CHCs improve premenstrual symptoms, particularly in those containing drosperinone.

Disadvantages and Risks

- Women may experience temporary hormonal side effects on starting CHCs, such as breast tenderness, nausea and bloating. The vaginal ring may increase vaginal discharge. About 10% of patch users report a local skin reaction.
- Menstrual headaches/migraines can occur during the hormone-free interval when circulating synthetic hormones fall.
- The vaginal ring requires a cold chain delivery system and can only be kept at room temperature for four months.
- CHC users may have a small increased risk of myocardial infarction and stroke.
- CHC use approximately doubles the risk of VTE, however the absolute risk is still very low. It is highest in the first 3 months of use and when CHC is restarted after a hormone-free break of at least one month (see Table 3.2).
- There may be a small increased risk of breast cancer – this most likely depends on the oestrogen dose and type of progestogen used, and the duration of CHC use. At 10 years after stopping a CHC the risk will be similar to that of a woman who has never used a CHC. Women with BRCA mutations have an increased risk of breast cancer,

Table 3.2 VTE risk with CHCs

Exposure	Risk per 10,000 women per year
Background risk in women of reproductive age	2
CHC containing levonorgestrel, norethisterone, norgestimate	5–7
Vaginal ring or patch	6–12
CHC containing drospirenone, desogestrel, gestodene, cyproterone acetate	9–12
Pregnancy	29
Postpartum	300–400

but it is not known whether CHC use increases this risk further.

• CHCs may increase the risk of cervical cancer after five years of use, but it will be back to that of a non-user 10 years after discontinuation.

Contraindications to Use

For a full list of contraindications please refer to the Faculty of Sexual and Reproductive Health (FSRH) UK Medical Eligibility Criteria (UK MEC) [5]. UK MEC summarizes various conditions and assigns them a category to define the risk associated with using that method of contraception (Table 3.3).

CHCs have more contraindications to use than any other form of contraception, yet they are safe for the majority of women. Absolute contraindications include smoking more than 15 cigarettes a day and age over 35 years, migraine with aura, current breast cancer, cardiovascular disease, VTE or severe liver disease.

Starting and Switching

Please refer to Table 3.7 at the end of the chapter.

A first-line pill is one that contains 30 micrograms ethinylestradiol combined with either levonorgestrel or norethisterone.

Diarrhoea and Vomiting

If vomiting occurs within two hours of taking a COC then another pill should be taken as soon as possible with the next pill taken at its normal time.

For those with severe diarrhoea lasting more than 24 hours the COC should be continued with extra precautions used while the woman has diarrhoea and for a further seven days. If vomiting or diarrhoea occurs in the last week of the pill packet the seven-day gap should be omitted.

Table 3.3 UK MEC Criteria

UK MEC category	Definition
UK MEC 1	A condition for which there is no restriction for the use of the contraceptive method
UK MEC 2	A condition for which the advantages of using the method generally outweigh the theoretical or proven risks
UK MEC 3	A condition where the theoretical or proven risks usually outweigh the advantages of using the method. The provision of a method requires expert clinical judgement and/or referral to a specialist contraceptive provider, since use of the method is not usually recommended unless other more appropriate methods are not available or not acceptable
UK MEC 4	A condition which represents an unacceptable health risk if the contraceptive method is used

As the vaginal ring and patch avoid first-pass metabolism they are both unaffected by diarrhoea and vomiting.

Missed COC Rules [6]

During the hormone-free interval, follicular development returns, with 20% of women having ovarian follicles larger than 10 mm diameter on the seventh day. During the first week of pill-taking these follicles are suppressed and ovarian quiescence returns. For further details, see Figure 3.1.

Incorrect Use of Patch and Ring

Table 3.4 Incorrect use of patch and ring

Circumstance	Timeframe	Are extra precautions needed i.e. abstinence or condoms?
Extended patch/ring-free interval	≤48 hours	No
	>48 hours	7 days (consider emergency contraception if unprotected sex in patch/ring-free interval)
Patch detachment/ring removal	≤48 hours	No if method used correctly for 7 days prior
	>48 hours	7 days (consider emergency contraception if detachment/removal in Week 1 and unprotected sex in Week 1 or hormone-free interval)
Extended use of patch	≤9 days	No
	>9 days	7 days
Extended use of ring	≤4 weeks	No
	>4 weeks	7 days

If one pill has been missed (more than 24 hours and up to 48 hours late)	If two or more pills have been missed (more than 48 hours late)

Continuing contraceptive cover

• The missed pill should be taken as soon as it is remembered.

• The remaining pills should be continued at the usual time.

Continuing contraceptive cover

• The most recent missed pill should be taken as soon as possible.

• The remaining pills should be continued at the usual time.

• Condoms should be used or sex avoided until seven consecutive active pills have been taken. This advice may be overcautious in the second and third weeks, but the advice is a backup in the event that further pills are missed.

Minimizing the risk of pregnancy

Emergency contraception (EC) is not usually required but may need to be considered if pills have been missed earlier in the packet or in the last week of the previous packet.

Minimizing the risk of pregnancy		
If pills are missed in the first week (Pills 1–7)	If pills are missed in the second week (Pills 8–14)	If pills are missed in the third week (Pills 15–21)
EC should be considered if unprotected sex occurred in the pill-free interval or in the first week of pill-taking.	No indication for EC if the pills in the preceding 7 days have been taken consistently and correctly (assuming the pills thereafter are taken correctly and additional contraceptive precautions are used).	OMIT THE PILL-FREE INTERVAL by finishing the pills in the current pack (or discarding any placebo tablets) and starting a new pack the next day.

Figure 3.1 Missed COC rules. Reproduced with permission of the FSRH.

Follow-Up

Initially a three-month supply of CHC should be given, after which 6–12-month supplies can be issued. At every visit BP and BMI should be checked. CHCs should be discontinued immediately if the woman develops any contraindication to their use. Only 3 months' supply of the ring can be supplied at any one time due to its shelf life.

Progestogen-Only Pill (POP) [7]

Case Scenario

Tara has been using a COC for six months. At a follow-up visit she reports having several migraines with visual aura. You explain that she can no longer take the COC. Tara wants to continue taking an oral method.

Composition

Traditional POPs contain either norethisterone, levonorgestrel or etynodiol diacetate. Newer POPs contain desogestrel (DSG).

Mode of Action

POPs work by:

- Thickening cervical mucus
- Causing endometrial atrophy
- Inhibiting ovulation in about 50% of women taking traditional POPs and 97% in those using a desogestrel POP.

Effectiveness

The failure rate is 0.3% in the first year of use with perfect use and 9% with typical use. Contraceptive efficacy is not affected by broad-spectrum antibiotics, but may be reduced by taking enzyme-inducing drugs.

Advantages

- POPs can be used by most women, even those with contraindications to CHCs, with little effect on coagulation or metabolic parameters.
- No associated increased risk of developing any malignancies.
- POPs can be taken up until menopause and do not mask menopausal symptoms.

Disadvantages

- POPs cause irregular bleeding patterns. At 12 months, about 50% of women taking a desogestrel POP will be amenorrhoeic or have infrequent bleeding, 40% will have 3–5 bleeding episodes every three months and 10% prolonged and/or frequent bleeds. About 40% of those taking a traditional POP at one year will have regular bleeds, 40% irregular bleeds and 20% amenorrhoea.
- Women may experience temporary hormonal side effects when starting POP, including acne, breast tenderness and headaches.

Contraindications to Use

There are very few contraindications to use of POPs. The only absolute contraindication is current breast cancer.

When to Start

Please refer to Table 3.7 at the end of the chapter. The POP should be taken at the same time every day with no hormone-free interval.

Diarrhoea and Vomiting

The instructions are similar to those for COCs except when severe diarrhoea lasts more than 24 hours, the POP should be continued with extra precautions used while the woman has diarrhoea and for a further 48 hours afterwards.

Missed POP Rules

Traditional POPs have a 3-hour window period, whilst a desogestrel POP has a 12-hour window period.

If a woman is >3 or 12 hours late taking POP, she should take the missed pill as soon as possible, continue the pill packet as normal and use extra protection for the next 48 hours.

Emergency contraception will be needed if there has been any unprotected sex occurring after the time of the missed pill.

Progestogen-Only Injectable Contraception [8]

Case Scenario

Laura is 18 years old and is requesting contraception. She can't remember to take a pill every day. Her periods are heavy and painful, therefore she would be happy if she had no periods or lighter bleeding.

Composition

There are two injectable contraceptives available in the UK. The most frequently used injection contains depo medroxyprogesterone acetate (DMPA), which is available as either intramuscular Depo-Provera® or subcutaneous Sayana Press®. The other injection contains norethisterone enanthate (NET-EN), however this is rarely used in clinical practice and is only licensed for short-term contraception following a vasectomy or rubella immunization.

Mode of Action

Injectable contraception works by:

- Inhibiting ovulation
- Altering the cervical mucus
- Inducing endometrial atrophy.

Effectiveness

Failure rate in the first year of use is 0.2% with perfect use and 6% with typical use. Contraceptive efficacy is not affected by diarrhoea/vomiting/broad-spectrum antibiotics or enzyme-inducing drugs.

Advantages

- The injection is long-acting, effective and non-user dependent.
- It helps heavy painful periods, with most users having infrequent or no periods at 1 year. NICE list DMPA as a treatment option for heavy menstrual bleeding [4].
- It may decrease the risk of developing endometrial and ovarian cancer.
- It decreases the formation of functional ovarian cysts.
- It reduces fibroid formation and growth.

Disadvantages and Risks

- Almost 70% of users have no periods by one year of use and 10% report frequent and/or prolonged bleeding but it is rarely heavy.
- There is associated weight gain for some women, particularly if their starting BMI is 30 kg/m^2 or more.
- Ovulation inhibition decreases oestradiol levels, resulting in a 4–6% loss of bone mineral density (BMD). This is largely recovered when the injection is stopped and is not clinically important for many women. Injectables, however, should be avoided in women who have, or who develop, osteoporotic risk factors. In young women who have not yet reached their peak BMD and in women aged over 45 years, use of the injection is UK MEC 2. It is advised that women over 50 years switch to alternative contraception.
- On cessation of DMPA it can take up to one year for fertility and a normal pattern of menstruation to return.
- Injection site reactions can occur in up to 20% of subcutaneous DMPA users.
- Some women experience hormonal side effects such as headaches, mood changes and bloating.

- Injectables may induce adverse effects on lipid profiles (see below).
- There is a weak link between DMPA use of more than five years and cervical cancer. This risk diminishes with time on cessation of DMPA.
- Potential increased risk of HIV acquisition and transmission. There is no clear link and it is unclear what the cause of this may be. Women who are at increased risk of HIV can use the injection without any limitations [UK MEC 1].

Contraindications to Use

For a full list of contraindications please refer to FSRH UK MEC guidelines. The only absolute contraindication to use of DMPA is current breast cancer. Injectable contraception should be used with caution in those with multiple cardiovascular risk factors, CVD or history of a stroke, as DMPA decreases HDL-cholesterol and increases LDL-cholesterol.

Unlike oral contraceptives, DMPA is safe to use in women taking liver enzyme-inducing drugs.

When to Start

Please refer to Table 3.7 at the end of the chapter.

Administration

- Intramuscular DMPA is given every 13 weeks into the gluteus maximus. The deltoid should be used if the woman is obese to ensure intramuscular administration.
- Subcutaneous DMPA is injected every 13 weeks into the subcutaneous fat of the anterior thigh or abdomen over five to seven seconds. It now can be self-administered following training.
- Intramuscular NET-EN is injected slowly into the gluteus maximus every eight weeks using a large-bore needle.

Overdue DMPA Injections

A DMPA injection is only overdue when the injection interval is more than 14 weeks. In this situation, if the woman has not had unprotected sex since the injection expired, a further dose can be administered, but she should use additional protection for the next seven days.

If she is three days overdue for her injection and has had unprotected sex in this time levonorgestrel 1.5 mg should be given along with the injection, and extra protection used for the next seven days.

If she is up to five days overdue for her injection and has had unprotected sex in this time she can be offered ulipristal acetate (UPA) 30 mg and advised to return in five days for her next injection. She also needs to use extra protection for these five plus the subsequent seven days, meaning 12 days in total.

If she is more than 14+5 days overdue for her injection and has had unprotected sex more than five days ago, the injection should not be administered until pregnancy can safely be excluded. Alternative contraception should be provided until this can be confirmed.

Follow-Up

Women should be asked about their general health and any nuisance side-effects at each visit. An assessment of any osteoporotic risk factors should be undertaken at least every two years.

Progestogen-Only Subdermal Implant [9]

> **Case Scenario**
>
> Jane is 18 years old. She gave birth six weeks ago and is using condoms for contraception. She had a 'pill failure' so wants to use the most reliable form of contraception.

Composition

There is one implant available in the UK called Nexplanon containing 68 mg etonogestrel.

Mode of Action

Implants work by:
- Inhibiting ovulation
- Altering the cervical mucus
- Inducing endometrial atrophy.

Effectiveness

Implants are the most effective reversible method of contraception with a failure rate of less than 0.1%

over three years of use. Contraceptive efficacy is not affected by diarrhoea/vomiting/broad-spectrum antibiotics, but may be reduced by taking enzyme-inducing drugs.

Advantages

- The implant is long-acting, effective and non-user dependent.
- It is safe to use when breastfeeding.
- There is no effect on lipid or carbohydrate metabolism.
- There is no effect on bone mineral density.
- There is no increased risk of breast cancer.

Disadvantages and Risks

- Menstrual bleeding can be erratic, with about 25% of women experiencing a regular bleeding pattern, 30% infrequent bleeding, 20% no periods and 25% prolonged or frequent bleeding.
- Some women may experience hormonal side effects such as acne, headaches and bloating.
- Insertion and removal risks include:
  - Bruising
  - Bleeding
  - Infection
  - Non-insertion
  - Deep insertion
  - Scarring
  - Damage to blood vessels or nerves
  - Breakage or bending of the implant (note that the implant will still be effective).

Contraindications to Use

For a full list of contraindications please refer to FSRH UK MEC guidelines. The only absolute contraindication to use of the implant is current breast cancer.

When to Start

Please refer to Table 3.7 at the end of the chapter.

Follow-Up

Follow-up is not routinely organized. Women should be advised to return if they experience any problems, for example bleeding problems, or if they cannot feel their implant.

Table 3.5 Key differences between Mirena® and Jaydess® IUS

	Mirena® IUS	Jaydess® IUS
Composition	52 mg levonorgestrel	13.5 mg levonorgestrel
Licenced indications	Contraception Heavy menstrual bleeding Provide the progestogen component of hormone replacement therapy (HRT)	Contraception
Licensed duration of use for contraception	5 years	3 years
Device dimensions	32 mm × 32 mm	28 mm × 30 mm
Inserter tube diameter	4.4 mm	3.8 mm

Intrauterine System [10]

Case Scenario

Samira is 42 years old, has four children and has completed her family. She and her husband have been using condoms for contraception. Recently her periods have become heavier.

Composition

There are two intrauterine systems (IUSs) that are now available in the UK – Mirena® IUS and Jaydess® IUS (see Table 3.5).

Mode of Action

IUS works by:
- Inducing endometrial atrophy
- Altering the cervico-uterine mucus.

Effectiveness

The five-year failure rate for Mirena® is 0.8% and three-year failure rate for Jaydess® is 0.9%. Contraceptive efficacy is not affected by diarrhoea/vomiting/broad-spectrum antibiotics or enzyme-inducing drugs.

Advantages

- Mirena® decreases menstrual blood loss by over 90% and reduces period pain. After three years

23.6% of women have no periods compared with 12.7% of Jaydess® users.
- Mirena® is the most effective medical treatment for heavy menstrual bleeding, as recommended by NICE [4] and can relieve pain associated with endometriosis.
- Mirena® may reduce the size of small fibroids.
- Mirena® can be used to treat endometrial hyperplasia and decrease the risk of endometrial cancer.
- When used alongside oestrogen, Mirena® can treat premenstrual syndrome and be the progestogen component of HRT.

Disadvantages

- Erratic vaginal bleeding is common in the first six months of use.
- Some women may experience hormonal side effects such as breast tenderness, mood swings and bloating in the first few months following fitting.
- When the IUS fails up to 50% of pregnancies are ectopic.
- Small persistent follicular cysts may occur in Mirena® users but rarely cause problems. The risk is less with Jaydess®.
- Perforation risk is <2 per 1000 insertions. This risk increases to 6 per 1000 insertions in lactating women.
- About 1 in 20 devices are expelled, usually in the first three months following fitting.
- Pelvic infection is increased in first 20 days postinsertion, usually due to an undetected sexually transmitted infection.
- Non-visible threads can occur following cervical treatment, if threads are cut too short, if the device moves in the uterine cavity, or if the IUS fails and the woman is pregnant.

Contraindications to Use

For a full list of contraindications please refer to FSRH UK MEC guidelines. Absolute contraindications to IUS use include current breast cancer, cervical cancer awaiting treatment, endometrial cancer, postpartum or postabortion sepsis, current symptomatic pelvic infection, unexplained vaginal bleeding and gestational trophoblastic disease with elevated βHCG levels.

When to Start

Please refer to Table 3.7 at the end of the chapter.

When to Replace/Stop

- If pregnancy is not desired then women should be advised to avoid sex or use a barrier method for seven days before removal with alternative contraception started immediately. Alternatively, the new method can be started seven days before the IUS is removed.
- Mirena®, fitted after the age of 45 years, will be effective for seven years. At the end of seven years, if the woman is amenorrhoeic it can remain in until she is 55 years, as long as she continues to be amenorrhoeic during this time.
- Women under 45 years presenting with a Mirena® that has been *in situ* for between five and seven years can have this replaced immediately as long as a pregnancy test is negative. She will need to use extra protection for seven days following the fit. A repeat pregnancy test should be done three weeks after the last episode of unprotected sex prior to the IUS change.
- If Mirena® has been in place for more than seven years, delay replacement until pregnancy can be excluded.
- If Jaydess® has been *in situ* for more than three years, delay replacement until pregnancy can be excluded.

Follow-Up

All women should be reviewed at three to six weeks postinsertion to exclude perforation, infection and expulsion. After this the woman should be advised to reattend if she is experiencing any problems.

Copper Intrauterine Devices [10]

Case Scenario

Samantha is 32 years old. She has tried various pills, the injection and implant, but discontinued all of them because of 'hormonal side effects'. She is wondering what effective, non-hormonal contraceptive options are available.

Composition

Copper intrauterine devices (Cu-IUDs) contain copper and come in different shapes and sizes. The most effective IUDs contain more than 300 mm^2 of copper.

Mode of Action

Cu-IUDs work by:

- Their toxic effect on eggs and sperm
- Inhibiting sperm motility
- Causing a foreign body reaction in the endometrium
- Altering uterine and tubal fluid.

Effectiveness

There is an overall failure rate of less than 2% after five years of use. Contraceptive efficacy is not affected by diarrhoea/vomiting/broad-spectrum antibiotics or enzyme-inducing drugs.

Advantages

- Effective and immediately reversible
- Works immediately after fitting
- Non-hormonal contraceptive
- Cu-IUDs are the most effective emergency contraception method
- Inexpensive
- Cu-IUDs do not increase cancer risks.

Disadvantages and Risks

- Cu-IUDs can increase menstrual blood loss by 25% and worsen period pain.
- Cu-IUDs increase the length of menstruation by one to two days.
- Cu-IUD users are more prone to bacterial vaginosis.
- Risks of perforation, expulsion, infection and non-visible threads are similar to IUS users.

Contraindications to Use

For a full list of contraindications please refer to FSRH UK MEC guidelines. Absolute contraindications include cervical cancer awaiting treatment, endometrial cancer, postpartum or postabortion sepsis, current symptomatic pelvic infection, unexplained vaginal bleeding and gestational trophoblastic disease with elevated βHCG levels.

When to Start

Please refer to Table 3.7 at the end of the chapter.

When to Stop

- If pregnancy is not desired, unprotected sex should be avoided for seven days prior to removal and alternative contraception started immediately.
- When a Cu-IUD is fitted over the age of 40 it can be left in until after the menopause.
  - If the last menstrual period (LMP) occurs before 50, Cu-IUDs should remain for a further two years.
  - If LMP was after 50, Cu-IUD can be removed after a further one year.

Follow-Up

All women should be reviewed at three to six weeks postinsertion to exclude perforation, infection and expulsion. After this the woman should be advised to reattend if she is experiencing any problems.

Condoms, Caps, Diaphragms and Fertility Awareness [11,12]

Barrier methods are associated with increased failure rates, but may suit some women spacing their family or, in the case of condoms, require protection against STIs. Male condoms are associated with high contraceptive failure rates (2% with perfect use, 20% with typical use), but are effective at decreasing the transmission of bacterial and viral STIs. Latex, non-latex and polyisoprene condoms are widely available in the UK. Couples need to be educated on how to use condoms properly, and what lubricants are appropriate, as oil-based lubricants can damage latex condoms.

Cervical caps have failure rates of 13.5% with typical use and 4% for perfect use, whilst diaphragms are associated with failure rates of 12% with typical use and 6% with perfect use. Caps and diaphragms should be used with spermicide and inserted into the vagina prior to sex. They should remain in place for at least six hours following sex, but should be removed no later than 48 hours. Both devices should be fitted by a heath professional and the woman may need a different size if, for example, she has a baby or changes weight.

Fertility awareness is only appropriate for women having regular cycles. There are several indicators which predict ovulation, including working out the fertile phase after keeping a menstrual calendar for at least three months, measuring basal body temperature at the beginning of each day to detect a rise of 0.2–0.4 °C after ovulation and examining the cervical mucus daily to identify the changes over the month. Using all three methods perfectly can result in less than 1 in 100 women becoming pregnant each year. Other options such as fertility monitors can detect concentrations of oestrogen metabolites and luteinizing hormone in the urine – the monitor will advise the woman when it is and is not safe to have sex.

Emergency Contraception [13]

Case History

Leanne is 36 years old and has a new partner. She is currently on day 13 of her cycle and admits to several episodes of unprotected sex this month. Her menstrual cycles range from 27 to 31 days. She is requesting emergency contraception and would like to discuss STI screening and ongoing contraception.

Copper IUD

A Cu-IUD can be inserted up to five days after the first episode of unprotected sex in the cycle or up to five days after the earliest expected date of ovulation. It is the most effective method of emergency contraception with associated success rates of over 99%.

Levonorgestrel

One dose of levonorgestrel 1.5 mg can be taken up to 72 hours after unprotected sex and used multiple times per cycle, if necessary. Women taking liver-enzyme-inducing drugs need to take 3 mg as a stat dose although a Cu-IUD is preferred.

This is a very safe option with no absolute contraindications. It works by delaying or stopping ovulation prior to the luteinizing hormone surge, but is less effective when taken close to the time of ovulation. This method is 58–95% effective at preventing pregnancy. Side effects include nausea and vomiting. If menstruation is delayed then a pregnancy test should be performed three weeks after the last episode of unprotected sex.

Contraception can be 'quickstarted' immediately after taking levonorgestrel and additional precautions taken until the method is effective.

Ulipristal Acetate (UPA)

UPA (30 mg) can be taken up to 120 hours after unprotected sex and can be used more than once in a cycle. UPA should be avoided in women with liver problems, severe asthma and those using liver-enzyme inducers (for a full list of contraindications, please refer to FSRH UKMEC guidelines).

UPA is a progesterone receptor modulator which stops or delays ovulation, but is less effective after the LH surge. It is over 95% effective at preventing pregnancy, but its action may be altered by hormonal contraception. Therefore, initiation of a new hormonal method should be delayed for five days after taking UPA and additional contraception used for 48 hours to seven days, depending on the method. UPA is also excreted in breast milk, so breastfeeding should be avoided for seven days following its ingestion. The side-effect profile is similar to levonorgestrel 1.5 mg.

Male Sterilization [14]

> **Case History**
>
> David is 41 years old, married with three children. Both he and his wife feel their family is complete and he is requesting a vasectomy.

Preprocedure

Before a vasectomy is carried out the health care professional must be confident that the man understands that this is a permanent procedure and reversal is not funded by the NHS. Special caution should be taken with men who are young, who have not fathered children or who suffer from mental health issues.

The Procedure

Generally, vasectomies are carried out under local anaesthesia in an outpatient setting. The procedure interrupts the vas deferens with most surgeons using the 'no scalpel' technique. This is minimally invasive and involves making a puncture wound in the scrotum through which the vas deferens can be identified and divided.

Postprocedure

Men should be advised to rest, wear supportive pants and avoid sex for 48 hours. Simple analgesia is advised.

Postvasectomy semen analysis should be performed 12 weeks postprocedure to confirm that there are no sperm present. If at 12 weeks azoospermia is found, then no further semen samples are needed. If sperm continue to be identified, repeat semen samples will be needed. If motile sperm are still noted seven months postprocedure, a repeat procedure is advised. Alternative contraception should be continued until a semen sample reveals no sperm.

Complications

- Bleeding (<20%)
- Haematoma formation
- Infection (<2%)
- Failure (1 per 2300 procedures)
- Chronic scrotal pain at three months postprocedure (~10%).

Female Sterilization [14]

> **Case History**
>
> Jill is 29 years old and pregnant with her fifth baby. She is struggling to cope financially and mentally. All of her children have been born by caesarean section. She wants to be sterilized at the time of her caesarean as she is adamant she does not want any more children.

Preprocedure

Women should be counselled that sterilization is a permanent procedure and its reversal involves major surgery, which is not funded by the NHS. Some may complain of menstrual problems following surgery as hormonal contraceptives have been stopped. Women frequently seek help in this situation and restart hormonal contraception or proceed to endometrial ablation or even hysterectomy.

Effective contraception is advised up until the day of surgery and a pregnancy test performed on that day. If unprotected sex has occurred in the prior three weeks the procedure should be delayed until a pregnancy can confidently be excluded.

The Procedure

Traditionally, sterilization has been performed via laparotomy or laparoscopy with the fallopian tubes occluded using rings, clips or by excising part of the tube. Risks include damage to the bladder, bowel and blood vessels, along with any complications associated with general anaesthesia. The failure rate is between 1 in 200 and 1 in 400 procedures.

More recently, hysteroscopic sterilization (Essure®) has become popular. Micro-inserts are placed into the fallopian tubes via a hysteroscope leading to tubal fibrosis over the next three months. During this time alternate contraception should be used until tubal occlusion can be confirmed by radiological imaging – normally an ultrasound scan. The main complications associated with this procedure include failure to place the micro-inserts, pain, uterine perforation and tubal spasm. The failure rate is thought to be 1 in 500 after five years.

Stopping Contraception at the Time of Sterilization

Table 3.6 When to stop contraception poststerilization

Method of contraception used	When to stop following female sterilization	Special instructions
CHC	After 7 days	If sterilization performed on day 1 following the hormone-free interval, continue CHC for another 7 days or omit the hormone-free interval and continue CHC for 7 days
POP	After 7 days	
Implant	At any time	
IUS	After 7 days	
IUD	After 7 days	

Table 3.7 Switching methods of contraception

	Switching to CHC	Switching to POP	Switching to implant	Switching to injection	Switching to IUS	Switching to IUD
Having menstrual cycles	Day 1–5 of cycle – no ep needed Anytime in the cycle if reasonably certain she is not pregnant – 7 days ep needed	Day 1–5 of cycle – no ep needed Anytime in the cycle if reasonably certain she is not pregnant – 48 h ep needed	Day 1–5 of cycle – no ep needed Anytime in the cycle if reasonably certain she is not pregnant – 7 days ep needed	Day 1–5 of cycle – no ep needed Anytime in the cycle if reasonably certain she is not pregnant – 7 days ep needed	Day 1–7 of cycle – no ep needed Anytime in the cycle if reasonably certain she is not pregnant – 7 days ep needed	Anytime if reasonably certain she is not pregnant – no ep needed
Women who are amenorrhoeic	Anytime in the cycle if reasonably certain she is not pregnant – 7 days ep needed	Anytime in the cycle if reasonably certain she is not pregnant – 48 h ep needed	Anytime in the cycle if reasonably certain she is not pregnant – 7 days ep needed	Anytime in the cycle if reasonably certain she is not pregnant – 7 days ep needed	Anytime in the cycle if reasonably certain she is not pregnant – 7 days ep needed	Anytime in the cycle if reasonably certain she is not pregnant – no ep needed
Postpartum (breastfeeding or not breastfeeding)	*This guidance only applies to women who are not breastfeeding* Day 21 postpartum – no ep needed After day 21 follow the above advice depending on whether she is menstruating again or not	Up to day 21 – no ep needed After day 21 48 h ep needed	Up to day 21 – no ep needed After day 21 follow the above advice depending on whether she is menstruating again or not	Up to day 21 – no ep needed After day 21 follow the above advice depending on whether she is menstruating again or not	Anytime after 4 weeks if reasonably certain she is not pregnant – 7 days ep needed	Anytime after 4 weeks if reasonably certain she is not pregnant – no ep needed

Table 3.7 (*cont.*)

	Switching to CHC	Switching to POP	Switching to implant	Switching to injection	Switching to IUS	Switching to IUD
Following 1st or 2nd trimester termination of pregnancy	Day 1–5 – no ep needed. After day 5 if reasonably certain she is not pregnant – 7 days ep needed	Day 1–5 – no ep needed. After day 5 if reasonably certain she is not pregnant – 48 h ep needed	Day 1–5 – no ep needed. After day 5 if reasonably certain she is not pregnant – 7 days ep needed	Day 1–5 – no ep needed. After day 5 if reasonably certain she is not pregnant – 7 days ep needed	If surgical termination – insert IUS at time and no ep needed. If medical termination if inserted more than 7 days postprocedure ensure all products of conception have been passed then use 7 days ep	If surgical termination – insert IUD at time and no ep needed. If medical termination ensure all products of conception have been passed pre IUD fit – no ep needed
Switching from CHC	Day after last active tablet/ patch/ ring – no ep needed	During hormone free interval – no ep needed. During Week 1 of CHC use – 48 h ep needed. Week 2–3 of CHC use – no ep needed as long as CHC used properly in last 7 days	Day 1 of hormone free interval – no ep needed. From Day 2 of hormone free interval and during week 1 of CHC use – 7 days ep needed (if any unprotected sex after day 3 of the hormone free interval continue CHC for another 7 days). Week 2–3 of CHC use – no ep needed as long as CHC used properly in last 7 days	During hormone free interval – no ep needed. During Week 1 of CHC use – 7 days ep needed (if any unprotected sex during hormone free interval or Week 1 continue CHC for another 7 days). Week 2–3 of CHC use – no ep needed	Day 1 of hormone free interval – no ep needed. From day 2 of hormone free interval and during Week 1 of CHC use – 7 days ep needed (or continue CHC for 7 days). Week 2–3 of CHC use – no ep needed	Day after last active tablet/ patch/ ring – no ep needed
Switching from POP	Switching from POP with 3 h window period – 7 days ep needed. Switching from POP with 12 h window period – no ep needed	Switch immediately – no ep needed	Switch anytime – 7 days ep needed	Switch anytime – 7 days ep needed	Switch anytime – 7 days ep needed	Day after last tablet – no ep needed
Switching from implant	Anytime pre expiry of method – no ep needed	Anytime pre expiry of method – no ep needed		Anytime pre expiry of method – no ep needed	Anytime pre expiry of method – no ep needed	Anytime pre expiry of method – no ep needed
Switching from injection	Anytime pre expiry of method – no ep needed	Anytime pre expiry of method – no ep needed	Anytime pre expiry of method – no ep needed		Anytime pre expiry of method – no ep needed	Anytime pre expiry of method – no ep needed

(cont.)

Table 3.7 (cont.)

	Switching to CHC	Switching to POP	Switching to implant	Switching to injection	Switching to IUS	Switching to IUD
Switching from IUS	Immediately postremoval – 7 days ep needed (or leave IUS in for 7 days then remove)	Immediately postremoval – 48 h ep needed (or leave IUS in for 48 h then remove)	Immediately postremoval – 7 days ep needed (or leave IUS in for 7 days then remove)	Immediately postremoval – 7 days ep needed (or leave IUS in for 7 days then remove)		Immediately postremoval – no ep needed (avoid unprotected sex for 7 days pre change)
Switching from IUD	Day 1–5 of cycle remove IUD and start CHC immediately – no ep needed After day 5 immediately postremoval – 7 days ep needed (or leave IUD in for 7 days then remove) – only do this if the woman has had no unprotected sex in last 7 days	Day 1–5 of cycle remove IUD and start POP immediately – no ep needed After day 5 immediately postremoval – 48 h ep needed (or leave IUD in for 48 h then remove) – only do this if the woman has had no unprotected sex in last 7 days	Day 1-5 of cycle remove IUD and start implant immediately – no ep needed After day 5 immediately postremoval – 7 days ep needed (or leave IUD in for 7 days then remove) – only do this if the woman has had no unprotected sex in last 7 days	Day 1-5 of cycle remove IUD and start injection immediately – no ep needed After day 5 immediately postremoval – 7 days ep needed – only do this if the woman has had no unprotected sex in last 7 days	Day 1-5 of cycle remove IUD and start IUS immediately After day 5 – no ep needed immediately postremoval – 7 days ep needed (or leave IUD in for 7 days then remove) – only do this if the woman has had no unprotected sex in last 7 days	

ep = extra protection.

References

1. Harper CC, Rocca CH, Thompson KM *et al.* Reductions in pregnancy rates in the USA with long-acting reversible contraception: a cluster randomised trial. *The Lancet* 2015;386:562–568.

2. Peipert JF, Madden T, Allsworth JE *et al.* Preventing unintended pregnancies by providing no-cost contraception. *Obstet Gynaecol* 2012;120(Suppl. 6):1291–1297.

3. Faculty of Sexual and Reproductive Healthcare. Combined hormonal contraception. 2011. http://www.fsrh.org/pdfs/CEUGuidanceCombinedHormonalContraception.pdf (accessed October 2015).

4. National Institute of Clinical Excellence. Heavy menstrual bleeding. 2007. https://www.nice.org.uk/guidance/cg44 (accessed October 2015).

5. Faculty of Sexual and Reproductive Healthcare. The UK medical eligibility criteria for contraceptive use. 2016. http://www.fsrh.org/documents/ukmec-2016/ (accessed July 2016).

6. Faculty of Sexual and Reproductive Healthcare. Missed pill recommendations. 2011. http://www.fsrh.org/pdfs/CEUStatementMissedPills.pdf (accessed October 2015).

7. Faculty of Sexual and Reproductive Healthcare. Progestogen-only pills. 2015. http://www.fsrh.org/pdfs/CEUGuidanceProgestogenOnlyPills.pdf (accessed October 2015).

8. Faculty of Sexual and Reproductive Healthcare. Progestogen-only injectable contraception. 2014. http://www.fsrh.org/pdfs/CEUGuidanceProgestogenOnlyInjectables.pdf (accessed October 2015).

9. Faculty of Sexual and Reproductive Healthcare. Progestogen-only implants. 2014. http://www.fsrh.org/pdfs/CEUGuidanceProgestogenOnlyImplants.pdf (accessed October 2015).

10. Faculty of Sexual and Reproductive Healthcare. Intrauterine contraception. 2015. http://www.fsrh.org/pdfs/CEUGuidanceIntrauterineContraception.pdf (accessed October 2015).

11. Faculty of Sexual and Reproductive Healthcare. Barrier methods for contraception and STI prevention. 2012. http://www.fsrh.org/pdfs/CEUGuidanceIntrauterineContraception.pdf (accessed October 2015).

12. Faculty of Sexual and Reproductive Healthcare. Fertility awareness methods. 2015. http://www.fsrh.org/pdfs/CEUGuidanceFertilityAwarenessMethods.pdf (accessed October 2015).

13. Faculty of Sexual and Reproductive Healthcare. Emergency contraception guidance. 2012. http://www.fsrh.org/pdfs/CEUguidanceEmergencyContraception11.pdf (accessed October 2015).

14. Faculty of Sexual and Reproductive Healthcare. Male and female sterilisation. 2014. http://www.fsrh.org/pdfs/MaleFemaleSterilisation.pdf (accessed October 2015).

Managing Contraception Problems in Primary Care

Fiona Sizmur

Key Points

- Stopping and switching methods of contraception is common, but leaves women at risk of pregnancy.
- All women starting contraception should be offered easy access to advice if they experience any problems and be encouraged to maintain their current method until starting an alternative.
- Acceptable bleeding patterns vary between women and influence their expectation and tolerance of unscheduled bleeding as a side effect of their contraceptive method. Establishing this is important to inform appropriate contraceptive choice.
- Investigation and exclusion of other causes is an essential first step in the management of unscheduled bleeding.
- It is important to question at each visit any change in nature or new onset of headache, particularly for women using combined hormonal methods.
- Headache in the hormone-free interval can be managed effectively without needing to discontinue the method.
- All combined hormonal contraceptives reduce acne.

Contraception is primarily used for the prevention of pregnancy. However, increasingly women are making their choices not solely based on the effectiveness of the method, but also on the non-contraceptive benefits as a lifestyle choice.

Experience of unacceptable side effects, concerns over media reports, change in lifestyle or the need for greater reliability may all prompt a desire to switch methods. This is not infrequently preceded by a period of stopping the current method, and during this time

many will be exposed to the risk of conception. These so-called 'stoppers and switchers' are one of the biggest challenges to preventing unplanned pregnancies [1].

Women should be made aware when they start a new method what side effects might be experienced and be offered ready access to support and advice on how to manage these. Reinforcing the importance of continuing with the current method until such advice is sought will hopefully reduce the numbers of women who discontinue prematurely. This chapter aims to cover the management of some of the more frequent problems encountered using the most common contraceptive methods.

Case Scenario

Lucy is a 17-year-old college student. She competes in athletics at a national level and came to see you eight months ago because of problems with frequent, heavy periods, which were interfering with her studies and sport. At that time she was started on a desogestrel progesterone-only pill (POP). She had attended surgery in the past for her acne and is currently using a topical preparation, Duac® gel (benzoyl peroxide 5%, clindamycin 1%). She takes no other regular medications, but was prescribed sumatriptan during her GCSEs in case she experienced recurrence of migraines.

The POP had been very effective in making her amenorrhoiec until 2 months ago when she started experiencing painful bleeds every 2–3 weeks.

Unscheduled Bleeding

Progestogens (P) and oestrogens (E), used alone or in combination, affect ovarian sex steroid production via central mechanisms, have a direct action on the ovary and may also directly affect the endometrium.

Prolonged exposure to a low-dose progestogen such as is used in POP, etonogestrel implant (ENG implant), levonorgestrel intrauterine system (LNG IUS) and medroxyprogesterone acetate injection (DMPA) appears to cause an overall increase in superficial vascular fragility within the endometrium. Different progestogens appear to have differing effects on the local mediators of endometrial function causing dysregulation of the endometrial breakdown and repair cycles, thereby increasing endometrial instability.

In contrast, high-dose progestogen, used therapeutically in the management of menorrhagia, leads to pseudo-decidualization of the endometrium and reduced bleeding.

The exact mechanisms of breakthrough bleeding are not fully understood, so predicting the endometrial response to different contraceptive hormones in different women remains elusive.

Unscheduled bleeding (UB) is a common problem in any progesterone-only method, particularly during the first three months after initiation, and will usually settle without treatment. Any woman reporting symptoms should be assessed for the risk of sexually transmitted infections (STIs). One small study of combined oral contraceptive (COC) users suggested chlamydia infection to be three times more likely in the presence of unscheduled bleeding, compared to a control group without bleeding, but who had either recently changed sexual partners or reported vaginitis [2]. Gonorrhoea is also a rare cause of UB. It would be important to establish if Lucy has been, or is currently, sexually active. This will allow appropriate sexual health screening as well as assessment of contraceptive needs.

Consideration should also be given to other causes, such as missed pills, pregnancy, gynaecological pathology and interactions with concurrent prescribed or over-the-counter medications. Non-compliance with pill-taking or recent illness preventing absorption or ingestion of pills may predispose to unscheduled bleeding, as well as identify a risk of pregnancy.

Clinical options to treat problematic UB in contraceptive users are currently limited and there are few studies supporting the long-term benefits of any regime. However, there are pragmatic measures, which may assist some women [3].

Progesterone-Only Pill (POP)

Whilst using POP, 50% of women will be amenorrhoeic or have infrequent bleeding, 40% will bleed regularly and 10% will have erratic bleeding with some experiencing frequent bleeding/spotting episodes.

- There is some evidence that variable bleeding patterns are initially more common in users of desogestrel pills than users of the more traditional levonorgestrel (LNG) or norethisterone (NET) pills, although infrequent bleeding or amenorrhoea is more common in the longer term (50% compared to 10%) [4].
- Many women become concerned that the effectiveness of the pill is reduced with breakthrough bleeding, but they can be reassured that there is no evidence of this, provided there have been no concerns regarding compliance or absorption.
- Since the type and dose of progestogen used, route of administration, endogenous circulating estradiol levels and ovulation can affect bleeding patterns, some may consider changing the progestogen-only method, although there is little evidence to support this approach.
- There is no evidence to support the use of higher doses in the form of multiple pills.

Combined Hormonal Contraception (CHC)

Oestrogen has a beneficial effect, producing a more stable endometrium by stimulating stromal proliferation, and therefore UB is less common using CHC (20% of users in first three months). Any UB usually settles with time and therefore changing the method in the first three months is often unhelpful. However, it remains one of the commonest reasons for discontinuation.

Suggestions for managing this UB include:

- Change the E dose – 20 mcg pills have reportedly higher rates of bleeding disturbances compared to 30 and 35 mcg preparations. However, comparative studies are difficult due to the differing progestogens used. There appears to be no proven added benefit to increasing the ethinylestradiol dose from 30 to 35 mcg.
- Change the P dose – there are many new novel progestogens now available in combined contraceptive pills. Comparative trials have been small or of poor quality and systemic reviews have

been unable to demonstrate any one to be superior in terms of bleeding patterns [5]. However, new progestogens such as nomegestrel acetate with high receptor selectivity, produce a thin decidualized endometrium with atrophied glands and report an absence of withdrawal bleeds in some cycles. Since this is neither consistent nor predictable it may still be unacceptable to some women.

- Change the regime:

  - One study showed a reduction in unscheduled bleeding with triphasic compared to monophasic regime, using the same E and P [6].
  - When compared to the standard monthly regimes, extended CHC use has been shown to decrease the number of bleeding days in the longer term, although women commonly discontinue in the early months due to initially higher rates of UB. Such extended regimes include scheduled extended pill-taking (including tricycling) for a predetermined number of days followed by a hormone-free interval of seven or fewer days, as well as unscheduled extended pill-taking or patient tailored regimes. In the latter, COC is taken continuously for a minimum of 28 days, for as long as the patient desires, until the occurrence of persistent breakthrough bleeding signals the need for a short (less than seven day) break before restarting again [7,8].
  - There is some evidence that the combined vaginal ring may offer better cycle control than oral methods.

DMPA, IUS, IUCD and Implant

Alteration in bleeding pattern is common in DMPA users and may cause up to 50% of women to discontinue the method. However, 70% of women experience amenorrhoea by 12 months. Similar bleeding patterns are seen in the equivalent subcutaneous preparation.

Frequent bleeding or spotting is common in the first few months after insertion of LNG-IUS devices, but decreases over time with all doses; 24% of those using a 52 mg device are amenorrhoeic compared to 13% of those using a 13.5 mg device, at 3 years; 20% of women experience UB in the first few months of IUCD use, which usually settles.

The bleeding pattern in the first three months of implant use is broadly predictive of future bleeding patterns, although 50% of women with prolonged or frequent bleeding at three months may still improve [9].

- Addition of E either alone or in combination as a CHC for short-term (up to three months) use, has been shown to be beneficial in controlling UB in both implant users and DMPA. However, once discontinued, it does not appear to confer any benefits in the long term.
- NSAIDs, e.g. mefenamic acid 500 mg tds, appear to be effective at reducing bleeding through inhibition of inflammatory prostaglandins in the endometrium. Some benefit has been shown for DMPA, implant and Cu-IUD users, although little benefit was seen compared to placebo for IUS users.

Although good practice is to counsel patients regarding side effects of their chosen method, studies comparing intensive to routine counselling prior to etonogestrel implant insertion and other long-acting reversible contraception (LARC) methods, have shown little or no benefit in continuation rates [10,11]. Awareness of women's preferences and tolerances of bleeding patterns is, however, useful when offering contraceptive choices and it is worth exploring these at initial consultation. Surveys have shown almost equal numbers of women expressing preference for monthly bleeds or less frequent bleeds, as well as no bleeding [12].

Case Scenario

Lucy explains that she has not become sexually active. On examining her records you note that her migraines were preceded by aura, and therefore oestrogen is contraindicated. After considering her options, she decides to try the etonogestrel implant Nexplanon®. However, she is concerned that it doesn't make her acne or headaches any worse.

Acne

Hormones undoubtedly influence acne. Oestrogens suppress luteinizing-hormone-driven androgen production and increase sex-hormone-binding globulin, both of which will decrease levels of free androgens and improve acne, as well as reduce excess hair growth.

The effect of progestogens is less clear. Older-generation levonorgestrel and norethisterone may activate the androgen receptor, worsening acne, desogestrel and norgestimate are less active, and drospirenone blocks androgens from binding to the receptor altogether. It might therefore be expected that combined pills with differing progestogens would have variable effects on acne. Some studies have shown cyproterone acetate and drospirenone-containing COCs to be superior, but overall few differences in effect have been noted, and a large Cochrane review showed that *all* COCs reduced acne lesions with the effects of the oestrogen outweighing the effects of the progestogen [13]. Beneficial effects may not be apparent until at least three to four months and during this period adjuvant therapies such as topical retinoids and antibiotics may help.

Acne has been reported as a transient side effect of IUS in the first few months after fitting, but only 2% of women discontinue this method as a result. In a recent study of DMPA use, acne was not reported as an undesirable side effect [14].

Lucy should be advised that acne can occur as a new side effect, but in patients with pre-existing acne, improvement is much more commonly experienced than deterioration [15].

Headache

Headache is a common event in all women, with or without the addition of contraceptive hormones; an important consideration when assessing studies looking at the effect of hormones on frequency of headache. Migraine with aura, but not migraine without aura, is associated with a twofold increased risk of ischaemic stroke, although the absolute risk is very low in healthy, non-smoking women.

- Women using CHC should be questioned at each visit regarding any change in nature or new onset of headache [16].
- Initial exacerbation of headache in early months of using both CHC and progesterone-only methods appears to resolve with continued use, although two studies have reported an increase in headaches over time with DMPA.
- The incidence of headache does not appear to be altered by oestrogen dose, progestogen type or method of hormone delivery.
- Withdrawal headache – timing of headache is also important; the hormone-free interval is a key time

of increased headache triggered by the withdrawal of oestrogen, and can be managed without unnecessarily discontinuing the method. This can be achieved with continuous use of CHC in an extended or tailored regime, e.g. tricycling pill packets and reducing the hormone-free interval to three to four days, or by using oestrogen supplementation, e.g. 2 g oestrogen gel daily in the hormone-free interval [17].
- Switching women to a desogestrel pill has been found to improve oestrogen-related headache and migraine.

Case Scenario

Lucy explains that she has not had any migraines since she left school and wonders if she will be OK to have the combined pill now?

Evidence suggests that migraine with aura is a marker of an individual at an increased risk of ischaemic stroke, and even a distant past history or single episode is associated with an increased risk. Given the availability of alternative and effective, non-oestrogenic contraception it would be prudent to avoid combined methods, as per UK MEC guidelines [18]. The risk-to-benefit ratio becomes less certain for women using CHC for medical as well as contraceptive indications. Decisions to do so should be made on an individual basis, taking into account the woman's particular circumstances and with full discussion of all management options. By avoiding additional risk factors such as smoking and obesity it may help ensure the risk to benefit assessment stays in a favourable balance.

Case Scenario

Lucy is seen in surgery again two years later. The implant had been very successful in managing her periods and she had been amenorrhoeic since about three months after initial insertion. She is now in a relationship and sexually active, but has started to have frequent light periods again and feels that the implant is affecting her sex drive. She is also anxious because she thinks it feels 'different' in her arm.

Libido

Low sexual desire is the most common sexual problem amongst women, with prevalence rates ranging from

20–30%. Oestrogens in CHC can cause an overall drop in total and free testosterone levels to varying degrees amongst individuals exposed. Whilst it is known that androgen insufficiency contributes to decreased libido, sexual desire is also informed by a complex interaction of physical, emotional and environmental factors, and studies show that despite reduced levels of testosterone, sexual interest is not always affected.

Heterogeneity of studies and the complex nature of factors influencing sexual desire make comparison of effect of pill type on libido difficult. A more androgenic pill might theoretically be helpful for those with reduced sexual desire, but this hasn't been borne out in clinical practice.

- It is worth asking about specific symptoms, which may be influencing sexual enjoyment. Use of a lower dose pill ($<$ 20 mcg) has been reported to decrease desire as a result of vaginal dryness.
- Women experiencing breast tenderness may benefit from a less oestrogenic pill or one with a lower oestrogen dose, which may help reduce discomfort in a physical relationship.
- Estradiol valerate used in combination with dienogest has been demonstrated to improve desire. In addition, using a 24/4 pill regime may have a better effect than traditional 21/7 regimes.
- Most studies report no change in libido while taking hormonal contraception and indeed many studies suggest an increase [19]. For those experiencing problems it may be worth reflecting on the complex nature of sexual desire and other influencing factors aside from the hormonal ones.

Case Scenario

After excluding all other causes of bleeding you examine the implant and notice a 'dimple' mid-way along the implant.

Implants

Broken, Bent and Impalpable Implants

The *in-vitro* release rate from damaged implants is only slightly increased, compared to undamaged implants, and contraceptive efficacy is unlikely to be affected. The decision to replace the implant is therefore a matter of clinical judgement and personal preference for the woman. A trained remover should ensure that the entire length of the device is removed.

If the implant is impalpable, the woman should be referred to a specialist with experience in this field and with access to real time ultrasound, for removal. It is important to exclude any risk of pregnancy and provide ongoing contraception whilst this is arranged. Local sexual and reproductive health services should be able to provide information on specialist services.

Implant Site Reactions

Implant site reactions such as pain, bruising, slight irritation and itching are common and usually present in the first few days or weeks after insertion. Reassurance or mild antihistamines are usually sufficient to alleviate symptoms. Fibrosis at the implant site is rare, and there is a theoretical risk of skin atrophy if the same insertion site is used repeatedly. For this reason FSRH guidance [20] recommends switching arms after two insertions at one site. Infections are uncommon and although they should be treated with appropriate antibiotics, don't often settle spontaneously and usually require removal of the implant. Since the introduction of barium sulfate into the device, allergic type reactions presenting similarly to infection, have also been reported.

Case Scenario

Lucy requests that her implant is removed and decides to use an IUS instead to manage her periods and provide long-term contraception. She attends surgery for an uneventful fitting, but returns eight weeks later unable to feel the threads. She has been experiencing irregular bleeding along with cramping abdominal pain. Chlamydia screening taken at the time of fitting was negative. At pelvic examination the coil threads cannot be visualized.

IUS/IUD

Lost Threads

In a situation when the threads of an IUS or IUCD cannot be seen or palpated then either the threads have been drawn into the uterus/cervical canal or the device has migrated or been expelled. The options below should therefore be considered:

- Exclude pregnancy and refer for ultrasound.
- If a positive pregnancy test – removal of the device early in pregnancy (before 12 weeks) helps

to reduce, but not eliminate the risk of miscarriage. Although the SPC for 52 mg IUS recommends removal of the device and consideration of termination of the pregnancy, there have been no reports of birth defects to date in limited evidence of pregnancy outcome. While the absolute risk of ectopic pregnancy is reduced, the likelihood of any pregnancy being an ectopic pregnancy is greater than if the pregnancy were to occur without a device *in situ*. In some studies half the pregnancies that occurred were ectopic and therefore an early scan is essential.

- If a negative pregnancy test – advice regarding ongoing contraception and consideration for the need for emergency hormonal contraception is required.
- If pregnancy can be excluded, an experienced practitioner may attempt removal of the device with a thread retriever if removal is requested.
- If ultrasound confirms the device to be correctly within the uterus, the patient can be reassured and the device left *in situ* until due for removal.
- If an ultrasound scan cannot locate the intrauterine method and there is no definite evidence of expulsion, a plain abdominal X-ray to include pelvic views should be arranged to identify an extrauterine device. If this confirms an uncomplicated perforation the patient should be referred for elective laparoscopic removal of the device. Reinsertion may be offered following a minimum of four weeks after perforation. Additional contraception is required.
- If an adequate film does not identify the device, expulsion can be assumed and reinsertion offered.

Non-Fundally Placed Devices

The IUD and IUS may still provide contraceptive effect when displaced from their optimal position at the fundus, but there is no definitive evidence that this is the case, or that displacement reduces efficacy. Theoretically the efficacy of an IUS device may be less affected by position due to its primary effect of local progestogen release. Indeed a small trial looking at a type of IUS device placed in the cervix demonstrated no pregnancies.

There is also evidence that devices can move within the uterine cavity, both in an upward or a downward direction, particularly in the initial months after insertion.

In asymptomatic women a 'wait and see' approach can be adopted, rescanning at a later interval, whilst using alternative contraception.

Consensus opinion from the FSRH Guideline Group [21] is that contraceptive effect cannot be guaranteed for a non-fundally placed device, especially if more than 2 cm from the fundus on ultrasound measurement. However, the decision to remove or replace the device is a matter of individual clinical judgement following discussion with the woman and considering her individual circumstances.

Infection/Pelvic Inflammatory Disease (PID)

The overall risk of pelvic infection within the first three months after fitting is low (approximately 0.5%), with the risk being greatest in the first 21 days.

A diagnosis of PID, and empirical antibiotic treatment, should be considered and usually offered in any sexually active woman who has recent onset, bilateral lower abdominal pain associated with local tenderness on bimanual vaginal examination, after exclusion of pregnancy. Testing for gonorrhoea and chlamydia is recommended, since a positive result supports the diagnosis, however absence of infection does not exclude PID. Making a definitive diagnosis is difficult and therefore a low threshold for treatment is recommended, with broad-spectrum antibiotics covering STIs as well as aerobic and anaerobic bacteria isolated in the genital tract.

There is little evidence to recommend removal of the IUD as this does not appear to alter outcome and any decision to do so must be balanced against risk of pregnancy.

Actinomyces-Like Organisms (ALOs)

Actinomyces israelii is a commensal of the genital tract and actinomyces-like organisms (ALOs) are occasionally reported on cervical screening samples. The role of ALOs in women using IUDs is unclear, but in asymptomatic women when these are reported, colonization rather than infection is most likely and the device may be safely left in place. Although *Actinomyces* pelvic infection is rare, if a woman with known ALOs presents with pelvic pain symptoms, then removal of the device should be considered after liaising with microbiology regarding treatment.

References

1. Wellings K, Brima N, Sadler K, *et al*. Stopping and switching contraceptive methods: findings from Contessa, a prospective longitudinal study of women of reproductive age in England. *Contraception* 2015; 91(1):57–66.

2. Krettek JE, Arkin SI, Chaisilwattana P, Monif GR, Chlamydia trachomatis in patients who used oral contraceptives and had intermenstrual spotting. *Obstet Gynecol* 1993;81(5(Pt 1)):728–731.

3. Faculty of Sexual & Reproductive Healthcare (FSRH). Problematic bleeding with hormonal contraception. July 2015.

4. Collaborative Study Group on the Desogestrel-containing Progestogen-only Pill. A double-blind study comparing the contraceptive efficacy, acceptability and safety of two progestogen-only pills containing desogestrel 75 micrograms/day or levonorgestrel 30 micrograms/day. *Eur J Contracept Reprod Health Care* 1998;3(4):169–178.

5. Lawrie TA, Helmerhorst FM, Maitra NK, *et al*. Types of progestogens in combined oral contraception: effectiveness and side-effects. *Cochrane Database Syst Rev* 2011;(5):CD004861.

6. Kashanian M, Shahpourian F, Zare O, A comparison between monophasic levonorgestrel-ethinyl estradiol 150/30 and triphasic levonorgestrel-ethinyl estradiol 50–75–125/30–40–30 contraceptive pills for side effects and patient satisfaction: a study in Iran. *Eur J Obstet Gynecol Reprod Biol* 2010;150(1):47–51.

7. Jensen JT1, Garie SG, Trummer D, Elliesen J, Bleeding profile of a flexible extended regimen of ethinylestradiol/drospirenone in US women: an open-label, three-arm, active-controlled, multicenter study. *Contraception*. 2012;86(2):110–118.

8. Godfrey EM, Whiteman MK, Curtis KM, Treatment of unscheduled bleeding in women using extended- or continuous-use combined hormonal contraception: a systematic review. *Contraception*. 2013;87(5):567–575.

9. Mansour D, Bahamondes L, Critchley H, Darney P, Fraser IS, The management of unacceptable bleeding patterns in etenogestrel-releasing contraceptive implant users. *Contraception* 2011;83:202–210.

10. Modesto W, Bahamondes MV, Bahamondes L, A randomized clinical trial of the effect of intensive versus non-intensive counselling on discontinuation rates due to bleeding disturbances of three long-acting reversible contraceptives. *Hum Reprod* 2014;29(7):1393–1399.

11. Teunissen AM, Grimm B, Roumen FJ, Continuation rates of the subdermal contraceptive Implanon(®) and associated influencing factors. *Eur J Contracept Reprod Health Care* 2014;19(1):15–21.

12. Merki-Feld GS, Breitschmid N, Seifert B, Kreft M, A survey on Swiss women's preferred menstrual/withdrawal bleeding pattern over different phases of reproductive life and with use of hormonal contraception. *Eur J Contracept Reprod Health Care* 2014;19(4):266–275.

13. Arowojolu AO, Gallo MF, Lopez LM, *et al*. Combined oral contraceptive pills for treatment of acne. *Cochrane Database Syst Rev* 2009:CD004425.

14. Wanyonyi SZ, Stones WR, Sequeira E, Health-related quality of life changes among users of depot medroxyprogesterone acetate for contraception. *Contraception* 2011;84:e17–e22.

15. J Urbancsek, An integrated analysis of nonmenstrual adverse events with Implanon® *Contraception* 1998;58:109S-115S.

16. MacGregor EA, Contraception and headache. *Headache* 2013;53(2):247–276.

17. Faculty of Sexual and Reproductive Healthcare (FSRH). UK medical eligibility criteria for contraceptive use. 2016.

18. Z Pastor, K Holla, R Chmel, The influence of combined oral contraceptives on female sexual desire: A systemic review. *Eur J Contracept Reprod Health Care* 2013;18:27–43.

19. Faculty of Sexual and Reproductive Healthcare (FSRH). Clinical Effectiveness Unit (CEU) Progestogen-only Implants. Feb 2014.

20. Faculty of Sexual and Reproductive Healthcare (FSRH) Clinical Effectiveness Unit (CEU). Intrauterine Contraception. 2015 (Updated June 2015).

21. Clinical Effectiveness Group, British Association for Sexual Health and HIV, Guideline Development Group: Ross J (lead author) McCarthy G (lead editor on behalf of BASHH CEG). UK National Guideline for the Management of Pelvic Inflammatory Disease 2011 (updated June 2011).

Chapter 5

Management of Vaginal Discharge in Primary Care

Catherine Armitage

Key Points

- Physiological and infective (non-STI) are the most common causes of altered vaginal discharge in the reproductive years.
- Sexual history *must* be part of the assessment, irrespective of the age of the woman, as one cannot rely on symptoms as guide to risk of STIs.
- Explore symptomatology when a woman says she has 'thrush' – a woman's self-diagnosis of *Candida* or bacterial vaginosis (BV) is not proven to be reliable.
- Have a very low threshold for examining a symptomatic woman. Empirical treatment runs the risk of over-diagnosis of *Candida*.
- Narrow-range pH paper is a useful tool in near-patient assessment.
- Test for multiple possible diagnoses when undertaking genital examination, with low threshold for repeat examination/testing in recurring/persisting symptoms.
- Do not overlook *Trichomonas vaginalis* as a possible differential diagnosis.
- Caution with use of a label of 'recurring *Candida*'/ 'recurring BV'-ensure it is appropriately diagnosed on testing/according to national guidelines.
- Genital dermatoses, including contact dermatitis, and *Herpes simplex* viral infection are commonly and mistakenly attributed to vulvovaginal candidiasis. Consider a woman's vulval care routine during the assessment in case of exogenous triggers for symptoms.
- The vast majority of cases of vaginal discharge can be diagnosed and managed in primary care – establish if the local sexual health service has a clinician who has an interest in recurring *Candida*/ BV to use as a point of contact/referrals – this may be more appropriate than gynaecological referral, at least in the first instance.

Case scenario: Emma

Emma attends in the last booked appointment of your evening surgery. Emma is 19 and is a first-year student at the local university, having been registered with you since she started university the preceding September. She is complaining of having a vaginal discharge over the last four days. The discharge is white and sometimes thick. This is the third such episode since September – after speaking to her sister and also some internet searching during the last two episodes, she thought it was *Candida*, so used some over-the-counter treatments and the discharge resolved. She thinks this is a third episode and wants some treatment to deal with the symptoms *and* to stop the symptoms recurring, so is now seeing a clinician for the first time about it.

Introduction

A woman attending with vaginal discharge is an extremely common presentation in primary care settings. It is normal for women of reproductive age to have some degree of vaginal discharge [1]. The characteristics may vary, depending on the stage of the menstrual cycle. In the follicular phase, before ovulation, the mucus goes from thick (non-fertile) to thinner and more slippery (fertile). As oestrogen levels fall and progesterone levels increase after ovulation/in the luteal phase, the mucus becomes thicker once more, and is hostile to sperm.

From the onset of puberty, the increasing oestrogen levels lead to colonization of the vagina with lactobacilli. Lactobacilli metabolize glycogen and so produce lactic acid, making the vaginal environment acidic, associated with a pH of less than/equal to 4.5. Other commensals include anaerobic bacteria,

Women's Health in Primary Care, edited by Anne Connolly and Amanda Britton. Published by Cambridge University Press
© Cambridge University Press 2017

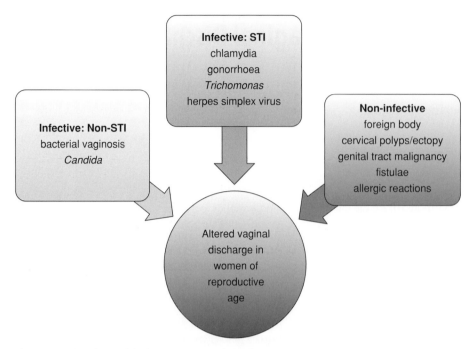

Figure 5.1 Altered vaginal discharge in women of reproductive age.

alpha-haemolytic streptococci and coagulase-negative staphylococci. Some commensal organisms result in altered discharge if they proliferate – including *Candida albicans*, *Staphylococcus aureus* and *Streptococcus agalactiae* (Figure 5.1.) [1].

What are the Commonest Causes of Altered Vaginal Discharge in Women of Reproductive Age?

The most common causes are physiological, bacterial vaginosis (BV) and *Candida*, but STIs and non-infective causes should be considered

Bacterial Vaginosis (BV)

BV is the commonest cause of abnormal discharge in women during the reproductive years [2]. The prevalence varies depending on the study group.

In BV, the pH of the vagina is above 4.5. Lactobacilli may be present, but the vaginal flora is altered, with the presence of anaerobic bacteria. *Gardnerella vaginalis*, *Prevotella* species, *Mycoplasma hominis* and *Mobiluncus* species have been cultured. There is debate

as to whether BV is an imbalance only in vaginal flora, or whether it is initiated as a sexually transmitted infection – the current position is that it is *not* a sexually transmitted infection, but has some characteristics of sexually transmitted infections, such as being associated with recent change of sexual partner, with the presence of an STI and with receiving oral sex. Other associations with BV include Afro-Caribbean race, vaginal douching, smoking and the presence of an intrauterine device. An increased incidence of BV has been described in women who have sex with women. BV has also been described in women who have never had sex.

Clinical features include the woman describing a malodorous vaginal discharge, *not* typically associated with itch or discomfort. Approximately 50% of women are asymptomatic. Genital examination reveals a white discharge, typically thin, coating the walls of the vagina and vestibule. Inflammation is not usually noted.

BV is not a sexually transmitted infection, but the prevalence of BV is high in women with pelvic inflammatory disease (PID). In pregnancy, BV is associated with second trimester miscarriage, premature rupture of membranes, preterm delivery and postpartum endometritis [2].

Diagnosis

Diagnosis of BV in sexual health services is made based on a combination of symptoms, signs and Gram-stained vaginal sampling.

Amsels criteria requires at least three of the following four to be present:

1. Thin white homogenous discharge
2. Clue cells on microscopic examination of sample from discharge (*not* Gram stained)
3. pH of vaginal fluid greater than 4.5
4. Release of fishy odour on addition of 10% potassium hydroxide (alkali).

In current practice, the 'whiff test' is less frequently used due to health and safety concerns.

Gram-stained microscope slides can be evaluated with the Hay/Ison criteria or the Nugent score. The Hay/Ison criteria are:

1) Normal – lactobacilli predominate
2) Intermediate – mixed flora
3) BV – predominant *Gardnerella/Mobiluncus.*

The British Association for Sexual Health and HIV (BASHH) recommend the Hay/Ison criteria for use in genito-urinary medicine services [2]. The Nugent score is based on the relative proportions of bacterial morphotypes to give a score between 0 and 10. Greater than 6 is BV.

Isolation of *Gardnerella vaginalis* on high vaginal swab is insufficient to diagnose BV, as it can be cultured from the vagina in 30–50% of asymptomatic women who do not meet all the diagnostic criteria. Using narrow-range pH paper along with history can guide immediate management whilst waiting for test results to come back.

Management

In managing a woman with BV, she should be advised to consider her vulval care routine – this may include avoidance of vaginal douching (intravaginal cleansing with liquids) along with avoiding perfumed products around the genitalia/in the bath. These can create an imbalance in pH and so encourage the development of BV.

Treatment

Treatment is indicated for symptomatic women and also may be indicated in women undergoing some surgical procedures, including instrumentation of the uterus.

Recommended regimens are:

1. Metronidazole 400 mg bd 5–7 days
2. Metronidazole 2 g single dose
3. Intravaginal metronidazole gel (0.75%) once daily for five days
4. Intravaginal clindamycin cream (2%) once daily for seven days.

All have clearance rates of about 70–80% at four weeks – the 2 g single dose may be slightly less effective. Advice on side effects with metronidazole, including interaction with alcohol, should be given, whatever the route of administration.

Non-antibiotic treatment with probiotics or with lactic acid preparations have not been shown to be effective so no recommendation on usage can be made at present.

BV in Pregnancy and Breastfeeding

Results of clinical trials investigating screening and treating BV in pregnancy have been conflicting. In conclusion, symptomatic women should be treated in the same way as non-pregnant women. There is insufficient evidence to recommend routine treatment for asymptomatic pregnant women, though women with additional risk factors for preterm birth may benefit from treatment before 20 weeks' gestation [2]. Metronidazole is present in breast milk and can alter taste – high doses should be avoided in breastfeeding.

Some studies support screening for, and treatment of, BV before surgical termination of pregnancy to reduce the incidence of subsequent endometritis or PID.

Recurring BV

Recurring BV has no formal definition. Studies looking at treatments have included administration of twice weekly metronidazole gel over a 16-week period, and use of probiotics. Lactic acid gel and acetic acid gel have not been adequately evaluated in well-designed RCTs. Assessment of a woman with recurring BV should include details of her vulval care routine, along with revisiting her sexual history. A symptom diary of up to three months may help to identify triggers, with a view to reduction/elimination where possible.

Appropriately detailed discussion of BV should occur, supported by written information. Dialogue should include treatments and risks of recurrence. Male partners do not need to be screened routinely. Testing for STIs is recommended for any woman with genital symptoms, and in women diagnosed with BV due to the links between BV and STIs.

Candida

Vulvo-vaginal candidiasis is common in the reproductive years – it is a symptomatic inflammation of the vagina and/or vulva caused by superficial fungal infection. The overgrowth of yeast is attributed to *Candida albicans* in 80–90% cases, with *C. glabrata* responsible for a further 5%. *C. tropicalis, C. krusei, C. parapsilosis, C. kefyr, C. guilliermondii* and *Saccharomyces cerevisiae* make up the remainder. The presence of *Candida* does not necessarily require treatment unless symptomatic, as between 20–50% of women will have vaginal colonization [3,4]. *Candida* occurs most commonly when there is oestrogen in the vagina, so is more common between puberty and the menopause, and during pregnancy. Overgrowth of *Candida* can be triggered by antibiotic use, immunosuppression and diabetes mellitus. The lifetime incidence of vulvovaginal candidiasis is estimated to be 50–75%. Prevalence of vulvovaginal candidiasis is not known, but it is diagnosed in 5–15% of women who attend sexual health/sexual and reproductive health clinics [4].

Symptoms could include vaginal discharge, discomfort/itch, dysuria and superficial dyspareunia. Signs on examination could include erythema, fissuring, oedema and excoriation, along with discharge.

No symptom or sign is pathognomonic for vulvovaginal candidiasis, so laboratory testing is useful, as many women might have other conditions such as allergy or genital dermatoses. Up to two-thirds of women who have self-diagnosed uncomplicated candidiasis do not actually have the condition [5].

There is limited and contradictory evidence on the risk of vulvo-vaginal candidiasis in users of combined hormonal contraceptives. Using the combined vaginal ring does not appear to have any effect on the number of pathogenic bacteria or inflammatory cells, although users have been reported to experience more vaginal discharge and irritation compared to other combined hormonal contraceptive users [4].

In genito-urinary medicine settings, sampling from the anterior fornix and vaginal walls is taken and assessed by Gram stain and plating on fungal media,

such as Sabourauds agar. Reporting of yeasts on high vaginal swabs used in primary care can vary locally, so it would be prudent to check availability with the microbiology department. The pH is not altered in *Candida* and so would be less than 4.5, therefore use of narrow-range pH paper is helpful in differentiating between *Candida* and BV.

Management

Once diagnosed on testing, management includes general advice on vulval care routines such as use of bland emollients as a soap substitute and skin conditioner, along with avoiding perfumed products/potential irritants [3]. As all topical and oral azole therapies give a clinical and mycological cure rate of over 80% in uncomplicated acutely symptomatic women, choice of regime is a matter of personal preference, availability and affordability. Commonly selected oral regimens include 150 mg fluconazole as single dose. Commonly selected topical regimens include 500 mg clotrimazole pessary. Topical treatments can damage latex condoms and diaphragms.

There is no evidence to support the treatment of male partners in either episodic or recurring vulvovaginal candidiasis. Test of cure is unnecessary.

Pregnancy

Asymptomatic colonization and symptomatic episodes are more common during pregnancy. Topical treatments are indicated, with no single optimal regimen. Longer courses may be needed and oral therapy is contraindicated. There is no association documented with adverse pregnancy outcomes.

Recurring Candida

Recurring *Candida* is diagnosed based on at least four documented episodes of symptomatic *Candida* in a year, with at least partial resolution between episodes. Positive microscopy, or a moderate/heavy growth of *C. albicans* should be documented on at least two occasions when symptomatic. Approximately 5% of women in the reproductive years with a primary episode of vulvo-vaginal candidiasis will develop this as a recurring condition [3]. Recurring *Candida* is usually due to *C. albicans*, but is attributed to host factors rather than a more virulent strain. As well as the triggers already outlined, such as immunosuppression, use of systemic corticosteroid treatment, diabetes mellitus, pregnancy and use of broad-spectrum antibiotics,

Table 5.1 Summary of the symptoms and signs of the commonest infective causes of vaginal discharge [1,7]

	Bacterial vaginosis	Vulvo-vaginal candidiasis	Trichomoniasis
Notes	Commonest cause of abnormal vaginal discharge. Not sexually transmitted	Perceived by women to be more common than it actually is. Not sexually transmitted	An STI – diagnosis should be made with a reliable method as there will be implications for partner(s)
Discharge	Homogeneous (thin and watery)	Variable but often thick, lumpy and white	Variable – may be frothy
Odour	Malodour	No malodour	Malodour
Associated symptoms (not all may be present)	Usually none (unless accompanied by *Candida*)	Itch/soreness, external dysuria, external dyspareunia	Itch/soreness, dysuria, lower abdominal pain
Typical signs (not all may be present)	Discharge coats the vagina and vestibule. No vaginal/vulval inflammation (unless accompanied by *Candida*)	May look normal or any of: vaginal inflammation, vulval inflammation, fissures, oedema, satellite lesions	May look normal or: frothy discharge, vulvitis, vaginitis, cervicitis – 'Strawberry cervix' often quoted but actually rare: < 2%
Vaginal pH (take from lateral wall) Normal = 3.5 to 4.5	> 4.5	≤4.5 (i.e. normal)	> 4.5

a link between recurring *Candida* and allergy has been observed.

Testing for *Candida* species may be useful, as non-*albicans* types are resistant to azole therapies. Checking a full blood count (anaemia of chronic disease/white cell count in relation to immunosuppression) and random blood glucose/glycosylated haemoglobin may be useful in recurring symptoms or florid symptoms. HIV testing may also be recommended, as recurring *Candida* is associated with immunosuppression. Currently available combined oral contraceptive pills have not been conclusively shown to be linked with recurring *Candida*, but as hyperoestrogenaemia has been linked with symptoms, it may be pragmatic to try alternative contraception in women with proven recurring *Candida*.

Treatment for recurring *Candida* involves an induction regimen followed by maintenance, lasting at least 6 months. The recommended regimen is fluconazole 150 mg every 72 hours for three doses as induction, followed by 150 mg fluconazole once weekly for 6 months. Approximately 90% of women will remain disease-free at 6 months, and 40% at 12 months. There are no trials addressing the optimal duration of suppressive therapy. There is no evidence to support the use of probiotics and insufficient evidence to make any recommendations on diet. Cetirizine 10 mg once daily for 6 months may lead to remission in women who fail to respond to the maintenance regimen with fluconazole. Zafirlukast 20 mg twice daily for 6 months may induce remission [3].

The majority of non-*albicans* types are *C. glabrata* – this is still susceptible to azoles, but has a higher minimum inhibitory concentration when being tested for sensitivity to treatment. Nystatin pessaries are the only licenced alternative to azole therapy. Other unlicensed treatments such as boric acid, amphotericin B and flucytosine have been suggested as alternatives – it would be advisable to seek advice from the local genito-urinary medicine service and the local pharmacy services if considering prescribing these alternatives.

It is possible that BV and *Candida* can be diagnosed simultaneously on both microscopy and on HVS.

Trichomonas Vaginalis (TV)

TV is associated with altered vaginal discharge and is often overlooked in testing in primary care. It is sexually transmitted via the intravaginal or intraurethral route. 10–50% of women are asymptomatic, though vaginal discharge can occur in up to 70% of women with symptoms. The discharge can be variable in consistency – the classical description of frothy yellow discharge occurs in 10–30% of women with discharge as a symptom. Only 2% of women have the 'strawberry cervix' appearance on naked eye assessment.

In genito-urinary medicine services, it is diagnosed on wet-mounted microscopy – the flagellated protozoa can be seen swimming in the saline mount. It can also be diagnosed on culture testing. The pH is greater than 4.5 in the presence of TV. The first-line treatment is metronidazole, either as 2 g single dose, or 400–500 mg twice daily for five to seven days. Checking the process and availability of testing for TV locally is advisable [6].

In the case of Emma, she should not be labelled as having recurring *Candida* as she does not meet the diagnostic criteria.

Assessment of a Woman with Altered Vaginal Discharge

History

Facts to establish in the history are duration of symptoms, consistency of discharge, triggers/relievers and patterns of symptoms, such as being cyclical/related to menses, along with the use of over-the-counter treatments. Presence of any malodour or itch is also important to ascertain. Past medical history should be routinely sought. Contraceptive use, current and past, should be discussed.

Questioning should also include/exclude symptoms such as altered bleeding, dysuria, abdominopelvic pain and superficial/deep dyspareunia – these symptoms may suggest sexually transmitted infections. Absence of these symptoms does not exclude sexually transmitted infections, so risk should be considered and sexual history should therefore form part of the assessment.

Examination

A woman should be offered genital examination when symptomatic. This is particularly relevant when she has symptoms affecting the upper reproductive tract, or is pregnant/postpartum/after termination of pregnancy or postinstrumentation of the uterus. She should also be examined if she is at a higher risk of STIs based on the sexual history, for example being under 25, or if she has bloody discharge, uncertain symptoms or recurring symptoms/symptoms that have not responded to treatment [7].

If a woman is at low risk of STIs and declines examination, she could be treated based on history, using the presence of itch or malodour as a guide. This is flawed as self-diagnosis is not reliable, and BV can co-exist with STIs – this should be discussed with the woman. Any woman who is managed in this way should be

Table 5.2 Core components of sexual history [8]

- Symptoms/reasons for attendance
- Last sexual intercourse/contact (LSI/LSC), partner gender, anatomic sites of exposure, condom use, symptoms/suspicion of infection in partner
- Previous sexual partner details (PSP) as for LSC
- Note total number of partners in past three months if more than two
- Past history of testing/diagnosis of STIs
- Last menstrual period (LMP) and menstrual pattern, contraceptive history and cervical cytology history (could include history of HPV vaccination)
- Pregnancy and gynaecology history
- Blood-borne virus risk assessment and vaccination history for those at risk
- Past medical and surgical history
- Medication history/drug allergies
- Agree method of giving results
- Establish competency
  Consider also:
- Gender based/intimate partner violence/safeguarding in relation to children and vulnerable adults
- Alcohol and recreational drug history

advised to return if symptoms persist/recur, with a view to examination at the next consultation.

Consent for examination, including assessment with Cusco/Wintertons speculae along with the types of tests taken, should be sought and received. As the age for first cervical cytology examination varies through the four nations of the United Kingdom, it would be helpful to check if a woman has had such an examination before. Offer of a chaperone should be included in the discussion and outcome documented. Examination of the external genitalia should include assessment of anatomy/architecture, along with any skin changes. Lichen sclerosus, lichen planus, eczema, lichen simplex, including contact dermatitis, psoriasis and vulval intraepithelial neoplasia can all give genital symptoms, including discomfort and itch. Presence of discharge/blood at introitus should be noted. Inspection of the vaginal walls and cervix should be noted during speculum examination, as well as establishing if a foreign body is present. Vaginal pH can be tested. Endocervical sampling for gonorrhoea and chlamydia can be taken, though some GUM clinics are moving over to clinician-taken vulvo-vaginal sampling in place of this. High vaginal swabs should be taken from the vaginal walls for *Candida*, and the posterior fornix for BV and TV. Bimanual examination is indicated in the presence of upper genital tract symptoms. Urine testing and pregnancy testing may be appropriate based on history.

HIV and syphilis testing completes the package of STI testing, with testing for hepatitis B and C in addition based on blood-borne virus risk assessment.

The newer tests for gonorrhoea and chlamydia, such as the nucleic acid amplification technique (NAAT) tests, do not need incubation and once taken, can last for 30 days. This means getting samples to the laboratory quickly is not an issue, and swabs can be taken on a Friday evening without any concern that a delay in getting to the lab will impact on results.

In the case of Emma, a sexual history must be part of the assessment, but as she is under 25, she already falls into a higher-risk group for STIs. Ideally she should be examined with tests taken for infective causes, both STI and non-STI. Use of narrow-range pH paper can guide the management at the time of the consultation whilst waiting for test results.

Management

Management depends on presentation. Treatment may be offered based on symptoms whilst waiting for test results. It is important to agree a method of results giving, based on clinical suspicion, and timeframes based on local laboratory turn-around times. Use of bland emollients as a soap substitute and moisturiser is useful advice for most women affecting by altered vaginal discharge. A woman's vulval care routine may be playing a part in her symptoms. She should avoid potential irritants in toiletries, antiseptics, wipes and products marketed for feminine hygiene and avoid washing underwear in biological washing powder and fabric conditioners. There is insufficient evidence to recommend the use of tea tree oil [4]. Written information to support discussion is a helpful guide to ongoing self-care.

Conclusion

The commonest causes of altered vaginal discharge in women of reproductive age are physiological, BV and *Candida* – but other causes must be considered.

Sexual history should form part of the assessment. Low threshold for examination is encouraged, especially in those at higher risk of STIs and those with recurring or persisting symptoms. The vast majority of cases can be managed in primary care, as careful history and genital examination help make the diagnosis in most cases.

Further Reading and Resources

British Association for Sexual Health and HIV. UK National Guideline on the management of vulval conditions. 2014 www.bashh.org/documents/Vulval%20conditions_2014%20IJSTDA.pdf (accessed August 2015).

FPA (formerly known as the Family Planning Association). Patient information leaflets. www.fpa.org.uk/sites/default/files/thrush-bacterial-vaginosis-information-and-advice.pdf (accessed 16 August 2015).

Training for Clinicians

Royal College of General Practitioners – *Introductory Certificate in Sexual Health*. Open to all generalists who would like to gain some knowledge in sexual and reproductive health. www.rcgp.org.uk (accessed September 2016).

Faculty of Sexual and Reproductive Health – *Diploma*. Open to doctors and nurses. Is a qualification with elements of training and assessment within the trainee journey. Anyone with an interest in sexual and reproductive health can aim for this, whether planning to work as a generalist or a specialist in the field. www.fsrh.org (accessed September 2016).

British Association for Sexual Health and HIV – *STI foundation* (STIF) courses and competency frameworks – with a focus on management of STIs. Theoretical courses with separate competency assessments, many of which are aimed at clinical staff either with an interest in sexual health or those working in specialist services. www.stif.org.uk (accessed September 2016).

References

1. Faculty of Sexual and Reproductive Health. Clinical guidance – Management of vaginal discharge in non-genitourinary medicine settings. February 2012. www.fsrh.org/pdfs/CEUGuidanceVaginalDischarge.pdf (accessed August 2015).

2. British Association for Sexual Health and HIV. UK National Guideline for the management of Bacterial Vaginosis. 2012. www.bashh.org/documents/4413.pdfAccessed (accessed August 2015).

3. British Association for Sexual Health and HIV. UK National Guideline on the management of Vulvovaginal Candidiasis. 2007. www.bashh.org/documents/1798.pdf (accessed August 2015).

4. NICE. Clinical Knowledge Summary: Candida-female genital. December 2013. http://cks.nice.org.uk/Candida-female-genital (accessed August 2015).

5. Ferris DG, Dekle C, Litaker MS, Women's use of over-the-counter antifungal medications for gynecologic symptoms. *J Family Pract* 1996;42(6): 595–600.

6. British Association for Sexual Health and HIV. UK national guideline on the management of Trichomonas Vaginitis. 2014. www.bashh.org.documents/TV_2014 %20IJSTDA.pdf (accessed August 2015).

7. Lazaro N on behalf of RCGP Sex, Drugs and Blood Borne Virus Group and British Association for Sexual Health and HIV. Sexually Transmitted Infections in Primary Care, 2nd edn. 2013. www.bashh.org/ documents/Sexually%20Transmitted%20Infections %20in%20Primary%20Care%202013.pdf (accessed August 2015).

8. British Association for Sexual Health and HIV. UK national guideline for consultations requiring sexual history taking. 2013. www.bashh.org/documents/ Sexual%20History%20Taking%20guidelines%202013 .pdf (accessed August 2015).

Chapter 6

Sexually Transmitted Infections Managed in Primary Care

Richard Ma

Key Points

- The latency, resistance patterns and human sexual behaviour are some of the reasons why sexually transmitted infections (STIs) are so prevalent.
- Newer technologies such as nuclear acid amplification tests (NAAT) have enabled STI testing to be more acceptable, less invasive and the tests are more sensitive and specific.
- STIs can be broadly divided into: bacterial, viral, protozoal and infestations.
- Diagnosis or suspicion of one STI should alert the clinician to the possibility of others – including blood-borne viruses such as HIV and hepatitis.
- STIs can be possible explanations for symptoms that commonly present in primary care such as dysuria, pruritus, rash and abnormal vaginal bleeding.
- A sexual history should help to ascertain if the patient is at risk of STIs and inform appropriate examination and investigations.
- Consider how to take a sexual history sensitively without sounding judgemental.
- Consider how sexual history-taking, STI and HIV testing could be part of routine clinical care in your setting.

Epidemiology of Sexually Transmitted Infections

The incidence of sexually transmitted infections (STIs) has been increasing. According to Public Health England, there were almost 440,000 diagnoses of STIs in 2014 in England; the most commonly diagnosed STI was chlamydia. Men who have sex with men (MSM) and young heterosexuals under the age of 25 were the groups that bore the most of the burden of STIs, although STIs can affect both men and women as long as they remain sexually active [1].

STIs cause anxieties and embarrassment for the individual, as well as risking onward transmission to their sexual partners. If left untreated they can have long-term complications such as: pelvic infections, joint problems, dementia, epididymo-orchitis, fertility problems and neonatal infections. Long-term untreated HIV and hepatitis infections can cause malignancies and can also be fatal.

STIs can be passed on horizontally (through sexual intercourse) and vertically (via maternal-foetal transmission). Most STIs do not survive for long *in vitro* and their inefficient transmission means they require close bodily contact to do so, and yet incidence of most STIs is increasing. The success of STI transmission could be explained by three factors: latency, resistance and human sexual behaviour.

Infections such as herpes, genital warts and HIV have long latency periods before symptoms develop, enabling them to be diagnosed and treated. The longer the latency, the longer the infectiousness, so early diagnosis and treatment could possibly reduce the infectiousness of STIs. It is important for people to be able to access STI testing and treatment quickly to reduce infectiousness. Concerns about confidentiality are a common reason given by people who feel unable to attend some health care settings to get tested and treated.

Some STIs are resistant to common treatment: HIV has different resistance patterns that respond to different anti-retroviral therapies (ARTs), a co-infection with more than one strain of HIV could make effective treatment difficult. Some parts of the UK are

---

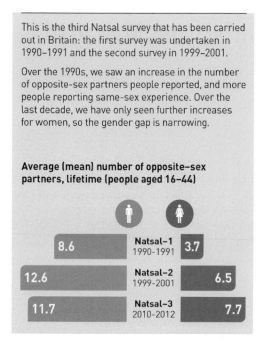

This is the third Natsal survey that has been carried out in Britain: the first survey was undertaken in 1990–1991 and the second survey in 1999–2001.

Over the 1990s, we saw an increase in the number of opposite-sex partners people reported, and more people reporting same-sex experience. Over the last decade, we have only seen further increases for women, so the gender gap is narrowing.

Average (mean) number of opposite–sex partners, lifetime (people aged 16–44)

8.6	Natsal–1 1990-1991	3.7
12.6	Natsal–2 1999-2001	6.5
11.7	Natsal–3 2010-2012	7.7

Figure 6.1 Results of the British National Survey of Sexual Attitudes and Lifestyles (NATSAL) surveys, 1–3.

Table 6.1 Classification of sexually transmitted infections

Organism	Infective agent	Condition
Bacterial	*Neisseria gonorrhoeae*	Gonorrhoea
	Chlamydia trachomatis	Chlamydia
	Treponema pallidum	Syphilis
Protozoal	*Trichomona vaginalis*	Trichomoniasis
Viral	Herpes simplex 1 and 2	Herpes
	Human immunodeficiency virus	HIV/AIDS
	Hepatitis A virus HAV, hepatitis B virus HBV, hepatitis C virus HCV	Hepatitis A, B and C respectively
	Human papilloma virus (types 6 & 11)	Genital warts
	Molluscum contagiosum virus	*Molluscum contagiosum*
Infestations	*Sarcoptes scabiei*	Scabies
	Phthirus pubis	Pubic lice

now seeing cases of gonorrhoea that are resistant to common first-line antibiotics. This demonstrates the importance of antibiotic stewardship in the treatment of some STIs.

STIs do not always present with genital symptoms; signs and symptoms at extragenital sites such as skin, eyes, brain and joints are possible. For example, syphilis can present with genital ulcers in the acute stage, but at later stages, with dermatological (rash), cardiovascular (aortitis) and cerebral manifestations (dementia). Reiter's syndrome – now known as reactive arthritis – presents with arthritis, conjunctivitis and urethritis, and can be preceded by infection with chlamydia.

Sexual Behaviour and STI Transmission

Human sexual behaviour facilitates transmission of STIs; this is the reason why opportunistic health promotion and prevention advice should be offered routinely in sexual health consultations. The increases in diagnoses through the decades might be explained by changes in sexual behaviour and partnerships, which result in more opportunities for sex. According to the third British National Survey of Sexual Attitudes and Lifestyles (NATSAL-3), young people aged

between 16 to 24 were most likely to report two or more sexual partners of the opposite sex in the past year; the average number of opposite-sex partners have increased amongst people aged 16 to 44 in the last three decades (Figure 6.1) [2–4].

Modern molecular technology has made it possible to test for many STIs using nuclear acid amplification tests (NAATs), which are much more sensitive and specific. Sampling can be less invasive and more acceptable for patients; for example, a urine test from men or self-taken vulvo-vaginal swabs from women. Other NAATs available include those for herpes virus, *Trichomonas* and syphilis (*Treponema pallidum*).

Managing STIs: Basic Principles

The principles of managing STIs depends on whether they are bacterial, protozoal, infestations or viral. For all STIs, prompt diagnosis and treatment (in practice, empirical treatment before microbiological results are available) are needed to reduce infectiousness. Partner notification and safer sex advice reduce onward transmission and reinfection.

Sexually transmitted infections (STIs) can be broadly divided into those caused by four types of infective agents: bacterial, protozoal, viral and infestations. Table 6.1 lists common STIs and their infective agents. Table 6.2 is a summary of their clinical manifestations, diagnosis and treatment and refers to clinical guidelines from the British Association for Sexual Health and HIV (BASHH, www.bashh.org).

Table 6.2 Summary of sexually transmitted infections

Infection	Symptoms and signs	Diagnosis	Treatment	Comments
Chlamydia	Asymptomatic in 80% of women Abnormal vaginal discharge, abnormal vaginal bleeding Dysuria, "cystitis" Pelvic pains Rectal and pharyngeal infections can be asymptomatic	First catch urine – sensitivity 65–100%. Vulvo-vaginal swab for chlamydia NAAT test – sensitivity 90–95%. Tests from extra-genital sites as indicated by sexual history – check with local laboratory what tests are available	Doxycycline 100BD 7/7 Azithromycin 1 g stat Erythromycin 500 BD 10–14/7 Ofloxacin 200 mg BD or 400 mg OD 7 days	Abstain from sex during treatment and until partner(s) treated Partner notification Rule out other STIs Follow-up HIV test in three months
Gonorrhoea	Abnormal vaginal discharge Pelvic pains	NAAT test as for chlamydia Many laboratories now offer dual testing for both chlamydia and gonorrhoea Rectal and pharyngeal infections can be asymptomatic – check with laboratory for tests	Ceftriaxone 500 mg IM + azithromycin 1 g stat Cefixime 400 mg po stat (as at October 2015)	As above Refer to GUM for treatment, sensitivities and partner notification
Trichomoniasis	Abnormal vaginal discharge Vulval soreness	Microscopy and culture using specific culture medium NOT CERVICAL CYTOLOGY Some laboratories now offer NAAT testing	Metronidazole 2 mg stat or 400 BD 7/7	Abstain from sex during treatment and until partner(s) treated Partner notification
Syphilis	Primary syphilis: Genital ulcer – can be sore or painless Inguinal lymphadenopathy Secondary syphilis: Palmar/plantar rash Tertiary syphilis: Aortitis, dementia	Dark ground microscopy of material from ulcer Some laboratories offer NAAT testing of ulcer swab Serology to diagnose other stages	Benzathine penicillin IM Doxycycline 100 mg BD 14–28 days	Refer to GUM for treatment and partner notification
Molluscum	Usually STI in adults Small papules with central umbilification	Clinical diagnosis	Expectant treatment	Rule out other STIs Partner notification unnecessary, but recommend check up
Genital warts	Caused by HPV types 6 and 11 NOT caused by types 16 and 18 which cause cervical cancers Perianal lesions common in both sexes even without history of anal sex	Clinical diagnosis	Cryotherapy Podophyllotoxin Imiquimod	Rule out other STIs Partner notification unnecessary, but recommend check up Partner notification might be useful to reassure about infectiousness and transmission
Genital herpes	Painful genital ulcer, blisters or fissures Febrile illness, dysuria and frequency Inguinal lymphadenopathy	Clinical diagnosis Swab ulcer for NAAT Serology not helpful	Aciclovir 200 mg 5 × a day Aciclovir 400 mg TDS Valaciclovir 500 mg B, famciclovir 250 mg TDS All five-day treatment	Rule out other STIs Partner notification useful to reassure about infectiousness and transmission Serology not helpful, does not indicate current infection

(cont.)

Table 6.2 *cont.*

Infection	Symptoms and signs	Diagnosis	Treatment	Comments
Scabies	Itching especially in finger webs Itching worse at night Itch due to sensitivity reaction to mite secretions	Clinical diagnosis Sometimes can see scabies burrows in finger webs and wrists	Permethrin 5% Malathion 0.5%	Rule out other STIs Partner notification to check if has same symptoms Itch can last several weeks Repeated treatment causes skin irritation
Pubic lice	Itching in pubic area Black spots in underwear (caused by lice faeces)	Clinical diagnosis Adult lice can be visible to naked eye	Permethrin 5% Malathion 0.5%	Rule out other STIs Partner notification to check if has same symptoms A repeat treatment a week later to kill any lice emerging from nits

Case History: Pelvic Pain

Annabelle is 24 years old and presents to you with lower abdominal pain, pain on having sex and abnormal vaginal discharge. She had an intrauterine device (IUD) fitted three weeks ago on day three of her normal menstrual cycle. She was using condoms until the IUD was fitted.

What differential diagnoses will you consider?

You might consider a range of differentials such as: malposition of IUD, pelvic inflammatory disease (PID), acute chlamydia infection, constipation and ectopic pregnancy. A sexual history would help you to determine the likely diagnosis.

She is unlikely to be pregnant, and therefore unlikely to have ectopic pregnancy, if she had a copper IUD fitted at day three of her normal menstrual cycle, but a pregnancy test would still be advisable.

She is under 25, sexually active and has recently had an IUD fitted. The presence of an abnormal vaginal discharge and dyspareunia should alert you to an acute infection such as a sexually transmitted infection, endometritis or pelvic infection. She had an STI check prior to the IUD fitting, which was normal, and she has had no change in sexual partners, so an acute STI such as chlamydia seems unlikely.

If the history did not suggest other abdominal or urinary symptoms and the last bowel movement was recent with soft stools, constipation would be unlikely. A sexual history might reveal she had a history of treated chlamydia infection, but she has had the same partner for three years.

Annabelle is apyrexial, BP 110/80, pulse rate 70 regular. You note cervical excitation and left adnexal tenderness. Speculum examination revealed IUD threads of expected length with white cervical discharge.

What would you include in your immediate management for Annabelle?

There is no need to remove the IUD provided the PID is adequately treated and her symptoms improve [5]. An ultrasound scan may be useful if you suspect malposition or migration of IUD, but this is unlikely if the threads are of expected length.

A diagnosis of PID seems likely from her symptoms and examination findings. You should offer her antibiotics; the treatment regimen needs to eliminate risks of chlamydia, anaerobes and gonorrhoea, which are possible causes of PID. BASHH recommends the following:

- *ceftriaxone 500 mg IM stat + doxycycline 100 mg BD PO 14/7 + metronidazole 400 mg BD PO 14/7 OR*
- *ofloxacin 400 mg BD PO 14/7 and metronidazole 400 mg BD PO 14/7*

Partner notification (including STI check) and abstinence from sex during treatment would ensure the risk of reinfection is minimized. Follow-up is advised within a week and at the end of treatment to ensure symptoms have resolved and partner notification is complete.

Annabelle wants to know about the risk of infertility with PID. What would you tell her?

Chlamydia can be a cause of pelvic inflammatory disease as well as subfertility due to tubal scarring. However, you can reassure her that the risks are minimized by prompt treatment, effective partner notification and use of barrier contraception to reduce future episodes of STIs and PID.

Case History: Genital Sores

Liz is a married 27 year old. She presents to you with what she describes as 'painful lumps'" on the labia for a couple of days. What could she be describing?

It is often difficult to ascertain the diagnosis purely by a patient's description and in the early stages of infection. Genital warts and molluscum might be described as 'lumps' or even 'rash' by some patients, but they are not usually painful. The description might also include herpetic blisters (Figure 6.2) or hair follicle infection, which might be painful and swollen due to inflammation. Scabies infestation induces a hypersensitivity reaction so it is common to present with itchy red papules in the genital region. A sexual history and examination might help to narrow down the differential diagnoses.

Liz has been married for two years and she has had three long-term partners. She has had one normal STI test in the past and she believes she is at low risk of STIs. When you examine her you see a small crop of blisters on the left labia majora and a couple of small ulcers. You can also feel some swelling of the left inguinal nodes.

What is the most likely diagnosis? What test would you do to confirm the diagnosis? Herpes is best diagnosed by taking the fluid from the blister or ulcer for either viral culture or NAAT testing; some laboratories also offer an NAAT test for syphilitic ulcers. A generic skin swab for microscopy, culture and sensitivities (MC&S) will not detect syphilis or herpes. *Molluscum* usually presents with painless papules with clear fluid and central umbilification; it can only be diagnosed clinically, but in this case this is not a likely diagnosis.

Primary syphilis can be diagnosed using a swab from the ulcer either for NAAT testing or dark ground

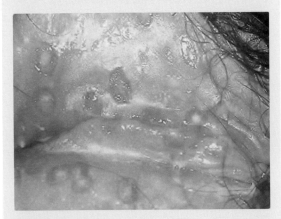

Figure 6.2 Herpes genitalis – female.

microscopy; the latter can only be done in GUM clinics. Treatment for syphilis requires intramuscular injection of antibiotics so should be referred to a GUM clinic if this is the suspected diagnosis.

There are two types of herpes viruses: HSV-1 and HSV-2. Not all cases of oro-labial herpes are caused by HSV-1 and not all cases of genital herpes are caused by HSV-2. Herpes virus is transmitted by close physical contact and can shed sporadically even between outbreaks of herpes blisters. Not everyone will have symptoms when they first acquire herpes and there is a long latency from exposure to clinical manifestation. Of people with positive serology for HSV antibodies, 80% are unaware that they have been infected. If symptoms occur, the first episode tends to be more severe and becomes milder with subsequent outbreaks. Serology for HSV is type-specific and needs careful interpretation. Antibody detection is not a reliable indicator of recent infection as it might be from a past asymptomatic infection. Oral antivirals should be given at early stages of symptoms or if new blisters are still forming. BASHH guidelines recommend any of the following regimes:

- Aciclovir 200 mg five times a day PO for five days (most cost-effective option)
- Aciclovir 400 mg TDS PO for five days
- Valaciclovir 500 mg BD PO for five days
- Famciclovir 250 mg TDS PO for five days.

Condoms might stop transmission especially between sero-discordant partners. Asymptomatic shedding is more likely in the first 12 months after infection and is more common with HSV-2 than HSV-1. The Herpes Virus Association (www.herpes .org.uk) produces useful information on how to explain and reassure people what this means for future sexual relations and in the case of women, pregnancy.

Case History: Fever, Tiredness and Rash

Mary is a 28-year-old woman who has returned from Tanzania four weeks ago and she presents to you with low-grade fever, rash, jaundice and tiredness. She had malaria prophylaxis before her four-week trip to see her family. She already had hepatitis A and typhoid injections five years ago.

What differential diagnoses might you consider?

Mary might be at risk of malaria and hepatitis A, despite travel vaccinations and malaria prophylaxis. Glandular fever, caused by Epstein–Barr virus, can be a cause of flu-like illness and abnormal liver function tests. She may be at risk of hepatitis B and HIV – both of these have similar routes of infection.

Why would you raise the issue of HIV testing on this occasion?

Acute hepatitis could cause fever, jaundice and tiredness, whereas acute HIV infection might present with fever, flu-like illness and sometimes a rash. Some people might not present with any of these at all. HIV is prevalent in the adult population in sub-Saharan countries such as Tanzania; however, you might need to check if she had been at risk of exposure, such as through sexual contact or otherwise. HIV and hepatitis B can both be transmitted sexually and through blood products. If she has a regular partner, they may be at risk too. If you have a patient who was born and grew up in a country where HIV is prevalent, it is entirely reasonable to offer them an HIV test if the risk assessment suggests they might be at risk, as NICE guidelines suggest [6].

You might feel her symptoms suggest malaria and send her urgently to your local hospital. However, many cases of acute HIV infection have been missed despite presenting to both primary and secondary care settings with symptoms suggestive of HIV [7]. There is no guarantee your secondary care colleagues would consider HIV testing. You might offer the only opportunity for a timely diagnosis for HIV.

What might be the barriers to raising the issue of HIV testing on this occasion?

Asking about HIV risk and recommending testing might need to be done sensitively. It is not uncommon for patients to feel surprised or even offended by your questioning. You might pre-empt such reactions by explaining why you are going to ask about sexual history and risk for HIV. She might not have been at risk at all, in which case an HIV test might not affect the outcome of the management.

The following suggestions are taken from *HIV in Primary Care* published by Medfash [8]:

- *You might be describing a common illness caused by viruses such as glandular fever or influenza. Some rare but important viruses may also be a cause and this includes HIV. I am not sure if you might be at risk of HIV?*
- *I am not sure if you might be at risk of HIV, but this is one infection that can affect your immune system and give you these symptoms. May I ask you some questions to check if you could be at risk?*

- *You have travelled to/come from/grew up in a county where HIV is quite common. Do you know anyone who has been affected by HIV?*

You should be able to assure confidentiality just like in a hospital or GUM clinic setting. You should also adhere to GMC guidance on confidentiality and when this can be breached, especially with respect to serious communicable diseases such as HIV, hepatitis and tuberculosis.

The Association of British Insurers (ABI) issued a statement in the 1990s stating that GPs are required to inform insurers *only if* an applicant is HIV positive, is awaiting an HIV test result or has any sexually transmitted infections with long-term health implications. GPs are *not required* to notify insurers of negative HIV tests or any single episode of minor sexually transmitted infections [9]. There are now travel and life assurance policies available for people with HIV who are stable on medications.

The UK National Guidelines for HIV Testing states the only purpose of the pretest discussion is to establish informed consent and a lengthy discussion is not necessary [10]. The issues covered might include:

- Benefits of HIV testing
- What 'positive' or 'negative' test results mean
- If test is negative, how they can continue to take steps to avoid HIV.

For somebody who might be at risk of HIV, or if you see someone who has a new diagnosis, you might wish to include in your discussion:

- HIV treatment is effective and will stop them from getting ill.
- They can take steps to prevent onward transmission.
- People with HIV can have healthy children if their HIV status is known early on in pregnancy.
- They will have more control over disclosing their status than if they find out while very ill with HIV infection.
- For people whose first language is not English, try saying 'your test result has come back and is HIV-positive, this means you have HIV', rather than saying your test is 'positive' which might be interpreted as 'good news'.

It is clearly devastating for someone to receive a positive HIV test result. They might have questions they wish to ask you. These might not be very different from anyone diagnosed with a life-threatening condition. However there might be an extra dimension because of the infectious nature. Questions might include:

- What is going to happen to me?
- Do I need treatment?
- Can this be cured?
- What should I tell my current/future partners?
- My partner does not have HIV – will they catch it from me one day? How can I stop this from happening? Can they sue me if they catch HIV from me?
- Can I have a baby?
- Do I have to tell anyone else such as my employers? Will they sack me?

A number of charities offer advice, information, counselling and support for those who are newly diagnosed and want more information. These charities and HIV clinics encourage people with HIV to register with a GP. All these questions can be answered by having a look at any of these websites:

- *Family planning association (FPA) www.fpa.org.uk*
- *Terrence Higgins Trust www.tht.org.uk*
- *National AIDS Trust www.nat.org.uk*
- *Positively UK www.positivelyuk.org*
- *National AIDS Manual NAM www.aidsmap.com.*

Many people diagnosed with HIV now will lead healthy normal lives with normal life expectancies because of highly effective anti-retroviral therapies. We will also see more people with HIV who are well and who may develop long-term conditions and have other primary care health needs. As GPs, we are often best placed to offer much of the primary care needs such as:

- Social welfare support
- Psychological support
- Contraception and preconceptual advice
- Health promotion such as lifestyle advice
- Screening such as *yearly* cervical cytology
- Health protection such as influenza, pneumococcal vaccinations.

Together with professional bodies such as BASHH, BHIVA (British HIV Association) and RCGP, we are all working together to help people with HIV get the best care from the right health care professionals. The BHIVA Standards of Care for People Living with HIV 2013 specifically mention the contribution of general practice in the care of people living with HIV [11].

Conclusions

STIs are common and many can be easily diagnosed and treated in UK primary care. Symptoms of some STIs can overlap with other conditions, so it is important to assess if someone is at risk by considering factors such as age, lifestyle and sexual behaviour through sensitive questioning and sexual history-taking.

Although many STIs are easily treated, some have long-term implications for a person's current and future relationships, as well as other aspects of their lives. Through better awareness, we can equip ourselves with the skills and knowledge to support our patients, so that dealing with sexual health issues feels less like 'opening a can of worms'.

References

1. Public Health England. Sexually transmitted infections and chlamydia screening in England 2013. 2014 20/6/2014. Report No.: Contract No.: 24.
2. Johnson AM, Mercer CH, Erens B, *et al*. Sexual behaviour in Britain: partnerships, practices, and HIV risk behaviours. *Lancet* 2001;358(9296):1835–1842.
3. Mercer CH, Fenton KA, Copas AJ, *et al*. Increasing prevalence of male homosexual partnerships and practices in Britain 1990–2000: evidence from national probability surveys. *AIDS* 2004;18(10): 1453–1458.
4. Mercer CH, Copas AJ, Sonnenberg P, *et al*. Who has sex with whom? Characteristics of heterosexual partnerships reported in a national probability survey and implications for STI risk. *Int J Epidemiol* 2009; 38(1):206–214.
5. Faculty of Sexual and Reproductive Healthcare. *Intrauterine Contraception*. London: Faculty of Sexual and Reproductive Healthcare, 2007.
6. National institute for Health and Care Excellence. *Increasing the Uptake of HIV Testing Among Black Africans in England*. London: NICE, 2011.
7. Ellis S, Curtis H, Ong EL, HIV diagnoses and missed opportunities. Results of the British HIV Association (BHIVA) National Audit 2010. *Clin Med* 2012; 12(5):430–434.
8. Madge S, Matthews P, Singh S, Theobald N, *HIV in Primary Care*. Lowbury R, editor. 3rd edition Medfash 2016.
9. Association of British Insurers. *HIV and Life Insurance: A Consumer Guide for Gay Men*. 2008.
10. British HIV Association, British Association for Sexual Health and HIV, British Infection Society. *UK National Guideline for HIV Testing 2008*. London: British HIV Association, 2008.
11. British HIV Association. *Standards of Care for People Living with HIV 2013*. London: British HIV Association, 2013.

Further Reading

Lazaro N, *Sexually Transmitted Infections in Primary Care*, 3rd edition Medfash. Available at: www.bashh.org/guidelines/.

Madge S, Matthews P, Singh S, Theobald N, *HIV in Primary Care, 2nd edition*. Medfash2011. Available at: www.medfash.org.uk/publications.

BHIVA. *UK National Guidelines for HIV Testing 2008*. Available at: www.bhiva.org/HIVTesting2008.aspx

BASHH Guidelines on www.bashh.org.

Cervical Pathology in Primary Care

Christine Corrin

Key Points

- Human papilloma virus infection is common, affecting the majority of men and women in the UK when they become sexually active. It is the persistence of infection which causes cervical problems.
- The high-risk strains of HPV, most commonly 16 and 18, cause cervical cancer, and immunization against these should be encouraged prior to the commencement of sexual activity.
- Cervical screening is important, including in those younger women who have been immunized against HPV infection.
- An asymptomatic cervical ectropion does not require treatment.
- Women presenting with postcoital bleeding require cervical examination and consideration of testing for sexually transmitted infections, especially chlamydia infection.
- Smears will not be examined by the cytology laboratory for women outwith the screening programme, if sent from primary care.
- Abnormal appearing cervices require referral to colposcopy as a fast-track referral. If cervical cancer is suspected, a cervical smear should not delay the referral.
- Women with cervical stenosis or atrophic vaginitis can be treated with a course of topical oestrogens to make the smear-taking easier and to reduce inadequate results.
- The role of HPV screening is changing. It is important to keep up to date with the latest developments.
- Cytology results reporting glandular abnormalities (CGIN) require fast-track referrals.
- Women presenting with postmenopausal bleeding require cervical examination, as cervical cancer may be the cause of the bleed.

Introduction

The prevalence of cervical cancer has reduced since the roll out of the national screening programme in 1998 and further reductions should be expected with the recent addition of vaccination against human papilloma virus (HPV) infection to the immunization programme. However, cervical disease is difficult to assess without a colposcope and many women present to primary care with postcoital bleeding or concerns about cytology results. Decisions regarding referral or explanation of results are important to ensure women are managed appropriately, while reducing unnecessary anxiety.

The relevance of HPV infection and the understanding of the important role this plays in the natural history of cervical neoplasia is rapidly developing, and changes to the screening programme will be made as this understanding progresses.

This chapter provides an overview of how the cervical anatomy changes, the cervical screening programme and how the results influence referral and management, as well as the impact that HPV testing will have on the future of managing cervical pathology.

The Cervix

The cervix is a tubular structure lying in the vagina at the entrance to the uterus.

The ectocervix is covered in squamous epithelium with the characteristic layers maturing from the basement layer up, forming a robust outer coating. The endocervix is lined with mucus-secreting columnar epithelium, with its fragile surface, just one cell thick. The area where the two types of epithelium meet is termed the squamocolumnar junction (SCJ).

Women's Health in Primary Care, edited by Anne Connolly and Amanda Britton. Published by Cambridge University Press
© Cambridge University Press 2017

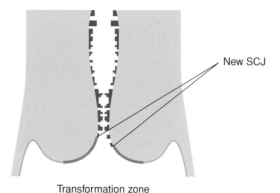

Transformation zone

Figure 7.1 The transformation zone.

Prepubertally the SCJ lies within the endocervical canal. Under the influence of oestrogen at puberty, the cervix everts, leaving the columnar epithelium exposed to the acid vaginal environment, which promotes transformation of the columnar epithelium to squamous epithelium. This results in a new SCJ. The area between the original SCJ and the new SCJ is termed the *transformation zone* (TZ) (Figure 7.1). It is in this region that most abnormalities develop and it is this area that should be sampled when taking a cervical smear.

Nabothian follicles are mucus-filled cysts often seen on the cervix (Figure 7.2). They result from mucus-producing glands trapped beneath squamous epithelium. They are a normal finding and always lie within the TZ. If a nabothian follicle is seen, that area should be included in the sampling area when taking a smear.

Occasionally clusters of nabothian follicles arise, which can appear alarming to the naked eye. It is appropriate, if there is any cause for concern, to refer for colposcopic examination, where the characteristic appearances with normal overlying vascular pattern can be visualized and appropriate reassurance given.

Case Scenario

Ella is a 19-year-old student who is embarrassed to explain her problem when she attends evening surgery. She has recently started a new relationship and she has noticed bleeding after each episode of sex.

An ectropion (Figure 7.3) describes the area when the columnar epithelium extends onto the ectocervix. It is a normal finding and requires no treatment if

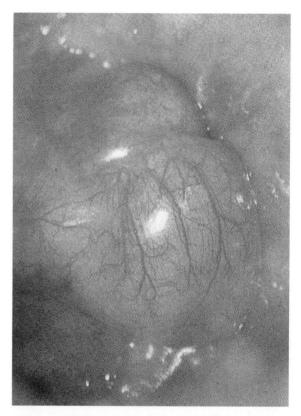

Figure 7.2 Colposcopic appearance of nabothian follicles with characteristic branching pattern of vessels overlying mucus-filled cysts. (For the colour version, please refer to the plate section.)

asymptomatic. Bleeding from an ectropion is common when taking a smear and is not an indication for referral [1]. Bleeding from the cervix at other times should be appropriately investigated, which includes swabs to

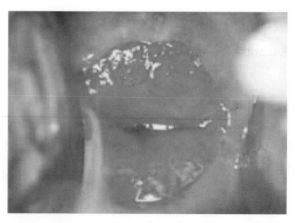

Figure 7.3 Ectropion. (For the colour version, please refer to the plate section.)

exclude a sexually transmitted infection causing a cervicitis of the exposed ectropion.

An ectropion can become more pronounced under the influence of oestrogen, commonly exacerbated by use of oestrogen-containing contraception.

Symptoms Associated with an Ectropion

The two most common symptoms associated with an ectropion are postcoital bleeding, resulting from trauma to the fragile endocervical tissue, and mucous discharge from the glands within the endocervical tissue.

Once confirmed that there is no abnormality, treatment can be hormonal, if appropriate, with a change from an oestrogen-containing contraceptive to a progesterone-only method, or by cautery. It is not always necessary to undertake formal electrocautery; the application of silver nitrate to small bleeding points may be sufficient.

If there is any concern about the appearance of the cervix a referral to colposcopy is required.

Postcoital Bleeding (PCB)

There are no current national guidelines for the management of PCB, which may arise from many causes. With a presentation of PCB, cervical examination is essential to determine whether colposcopy referral is indicated to exclude a malignancy before considering other investigation and treatment options.

Examination Findings

Indications for a Fast-Track Referral [1]

- Visible suspicious lesions.
- Post-menopausal PCB.
- Persistent PCB for more than four weeks in women over 35 years.

Cervical examination is essential as assessment of women presenting with any abnormal bleeding pattern, including PMB, IMB or PCB, to ensure the woman is appointed to the appropriate clinic to reduce any unnecessary diagnostic delay. Fast-track referral to colposcopy is indicated for those women with an abnormal appearance to the cervix.

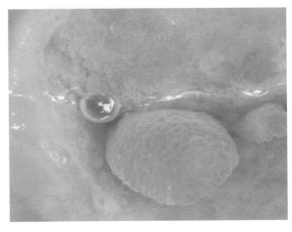

Figure 7.4 Cervical polyp. (For the colour version, please refer to the plate section.)

Indication for Early Referral (Four to Six weeks)

Persistent, unexplained PCB.

Prior to referral it is important to exclude infection being the cause, including sexually transmitted infections. The latest cytology report should be checked, but the smear should not be repeated if it is not due within the national screening programme (NHSCSP).

Non-Urgent Assessment

In a young woman with a short history of PCB (< four weeks) where the cervix and genital tract appear normal, it is reasonable to await results from swabs and a smear, if it is due, before proceeding to referral.

In the case of Ella, examination of the cervix is essential. Screening for infection demonstrated chlamydia infection and following treatment of her and her partner, her problem resolved.

Endocervical Polyps

Cervical polyps may arise from the ectocervix, endocervix or be endometrial in origin. Occasionally, a type-zero submucous fibroid may prolapse through the cervix and present as a polyp.

Small polyps may cause IMB, PCB or increased discharge, but the majority are asymptomatic and found during routine cervical screening.

Current recommendation is that cervical polyps should be removed and sent for histology by a practitioner with appropriate skills, although it is acknowledged that there is a very small risk of malignancy, 0.0–1.7% [2].

No further action is required if the polyp was small and asymptomatic, and histology is normal. If, however, symptoms persist after removal then further investigations, an ultrasound scan and/or hysteroscopy are warranted.

Congenital Anomalies

Embryologically, the cervix, along with the upper vagina, uterus and fallopian tubes, develop from bilateral paramesonephric ducts which fuse in the developmental process. Failure of fusion or incomplete fusion can lead to anomalies ranging from two distinct cervices to two ossei, with a common endocervical canal. Any such anomaly or failure to identify a cervix should trigger investigations as to the anatomy of the rest of the genital tract.

If there is more than one cervical os both must be sampled when taking cytology, put in separate containers and clearly marked.

The National Cervical Screening Programme [1]

There are approximately 3000 cases of cervical cancer registered annually in the UK, an incidence of approximately 10/100,000 women. It is the 12th commonest cancer in women in the UK and 4th commonest worldwide.

Following the introduction of the national screening programme in 1998, the incidence of cervical cancer in the UK halved and cervical screening is credited with saving 4500 lives a year in England.

Cervical screening has been demonstrated to be highly successful and so any alteration in the programme must improve outcome. The discovery that HPV is the major causative agent for cervical cancer has led to changes to the programme, which seem set to further decrease the incidence of cervical cancer in the UK.

In the UK all women are invited for screening every three years from age 25–50 and every five years from 50–65. Their first invitation arrives six months before their 25th birthday.

Tip: Remember this may be the first time a woman has ever had a speculum examination.

The only group of women eligible for more frequent screening are those who are HIV positive, who are invited annually. Other immunosuppressed women may be similarly at increased risk, but are not eligible under the NHSCSP for more frequent screening and require assessment or referral on an individualized basis.

There are no indications for early cervical screening in primary care or for additional routine smears, and the cytology laboratories will reject samples taken outside the screening programme. If there is clinical concern the woman should be referred for colposcopy.

Taking a Smear

When taking a smear it is important that the woman understands that the screening programme is to find women who may have 'precancer changes' which require further investigation. Under some circumstances a test for the presence of high-risk HPV (HR HPV) is included [3]. As HPV testing is relatively new, it is important that the reason for testing is discussed and an explanation of the findings given.

The participant needs to understand how she will receive her result and what will happen if the result is not normal. In England in 2013/14, 6.6% of smears showed some abnormality, with only 1.3% showing high-grade change [4]. Many women with an abnormal result are concerned that they have cancer and require appropriate reassurance.

When performing a smear, the entire cervix must be examined. Using a variety of sizes of Cusco speculum may help in difficult cases and if the cervix cannot be visualized, a bimanual examination will help identify its position. Failure to visualize the entire cervix is an indication for referral.

HPV testing is currently carried out on the same sample, if indicated.

Occasionally an additional endocervical sample is necessary in cervical stenosis in postmenopausal women or following a LLETZ procedure. If more than one sample is taken, both samples should be placed in the same pot. The only exception to this would be in the congenital presence of two cervices, when each cervix should be sampled separately and clearly labelled.

Cervical Cytology in Pregnancy [1]

- If cytology is up to date and negative this should be deferred until three months after delivery.
- Repeat screening as a follow-up after a low-grade abnormality should be delayed until three months after delivery.
- Repeat screening after a high-grade abnormality or any glandular abnormality cytology should be

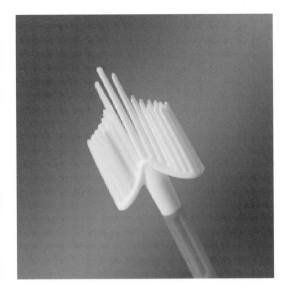

Figure 7.5 LBC cervical sampler.

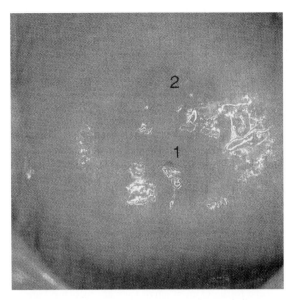

Figure 7.6 Stenosed cervix (1: cervical os; 2: transformation zone). (For the colour version, please refer to the plate section.)

performed during pregnancy to ensure treatment is not indicated.

Withdrawal from Routine Screening

There are occasions where it might be appropriate to consider withdrawal of a woman from the screening programme:

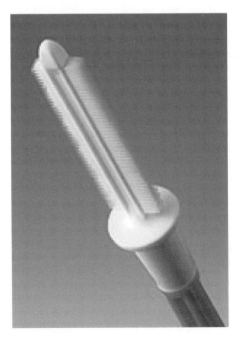

Figure 7.7 LBC endocervical sampler for use with stenosed cervix.

- Severe cervical stenosis where a smear that is representative of the TZ is impossible to obtain. Options include; cervical dilatation, hysterectomy or withdrawal from the screening programme. Dilatation or hysterectomy is recommended for those with previous high-grade CIN, CGIN or unexplained high-grade cytology. However, if these options are declined or not feasible, the woman may, with informed consent, withdraw from the screening programme.
- Women who lack capacity may find the procedure of taking a smear or performing a vaginal examination too distressing. Each woman needs to be considered according to her personal needs and withdrawal from screening may be appropriate. This decision should be reconsidered at regular intervals as risk factors and capacity may change.
- Some women choose to withdraw from the screening programme and must be provided with sufficient information to ensure this decision is fully informed. She may also be reinstated to the screening programme at any stage.

Ceasing Screening

Screening ceases age 65 unless the woman has not been screened since age 50 or she is due for follow-up after abnormal cytology.

Human Papilloma Virus (HPV)

HPV infection is associated with two common conditions encountered in gynaecological practice: abnormal cervical cytology and genital warts.

As the most important causative agent, evidence of HPV is found in more than 99% of cervical cancers.

There are more than 150 variants of HPV, which are divided into two groups, referred to as high risk and low risk. The high-risk group are those associated with a risk of developing cervical cancer. In the UK the two commonest HR types are 16 and 18, but other HR strains are more prevalent in other geographical locations.

The low-risk types, 6 and 11, are associated with the development of genital warts.

HPV testing has been introduced into the NHSCSP over the past few years and has added confusion and concern to the women when they are informed about their 'infection'. The importance of the current understanding of HPV is that testing in some instances improves the triage process for women requiring colposcopy appointments.

A few basics to aid understanding of the relevance of HPV infection include:

- HPV infection is common and transmitted via intimate sexual contact; 80% of the world's population contracts some type of the virus at least once in their lifetime, which can be a helpful statistic to reassure women who are feeling stigmatized by the finding.
- In the majority of women a normal immune system clears the virus with no requirement for treatment, but some women have persistent infection for many years. Previous smears were not tested for HPV, either because the sample did not warrant testing or predated the introduction of testing.
- Women do not have to assume that their current HPV infection has been acquired from a recent sexual encounter of themselves or their partner.
- The term high-risk requires clarification as this means they have a strain of HPV that requires colposcopic assessment and not that they are at 'high risk' of developing cervical cancer.

Smoking is associated with longer persistence of HPV compared with non-smokers [5].

HPV testing has been incorporated into the cervical screening programme in two situations (Table 7.1) [3]:

Table 7.1 HPV testing as part of screening

Smear result	HPV Test	
Negative	No	
Low-grade/BNC in squamous cells	Yes	HR HPV+ve – refer colposcopy HR HPV –ve – normal recall
High-grade	No	HR HPV assumed present
Invasion	No	HR HPV assumed present

1. Smears showing borderline nuclear change (BNC) in squamous cells or low-grade dyskaryosis.
2. As a test of cure after treatment.

A low-grade HR HPV negative smear result can cause anxiety and requires an explanation that there is virtually no risk of cervical cancer being present in the absence of HR HPV.

High-grade smears are not tested for HR HPV as it is assumed the virus is present and so anxieties about HPV may not arise until an HR HPV positive test of cure after treatment. Taking time to explain this is important.

HPV Vaccination

Since September 2008, HPV vaccination has been included in the NHS vaccination programme.

The current regime is to immunize girls aged 12–13 with two doses of the quadrivalent vaccine Gardisil (active against HPV Strains 6, 11, 16 and 18) at least six months apart in a 24-month period. This preparation protects against genital warts as well as cervical cancer. Girls who commence vaccination over the age of 15 are recommended to have three doses as the response is slightly reduced in this cohort.

Future vaccines will aim to prevent infection from additional HPV strains and a nonovalent vaccine has already been approved for administration.

The Australian programme also offers vaccination for boys which will additionally protect men against HPV-related cancers such as penile, anal, oropharyngeal and mouth cancers.

It is possible that HPV screening will replace cervical cytology as the primary screening tool in the future and trials are currently taking place. If the test is shown to be specific enough it could be used to identify the at risk population, reducing the need to perform smears on all women, but only on those who are found to be HPV positive.

Dyskaryosis and Cervical Intraepithelial Neoplasia (CIN)

Dyskaryosis refers to cytological abnormality and is used to describe the level of abnormality seen in a cervical smear sample. Dyskaryosis is classified as borderline, low-grade or high-grade.

The most obvious cytological characteristic is the higher the level of dyskaryosis, the more of the cell is occupied by the nucleus, referred to as a high nuclear-to-cytoplasmic ratio.

Cervical intraepithelial neoplasia (CIN) is a histological diagnosis. Results of biopsies and treatment specimens will refer to CIN. CIN is categorized as CIN1, 2 or 3. The term carcinoma *in situ* is still sometimes used to describe CIN3, which is misleading, as CIN3 is *not* cancer.

Squamous epithelium has several layers. CIN originates in the basal layers. CIN1 is present when the abnormality is confined to the lower third of the epithelium, CIN2, when the lower two-thirds are affected, and CIN3 refers to full thickness involvement.

Low-grade dyskaryosis equates to CIN1 and high-grade to CIN2 and 3.

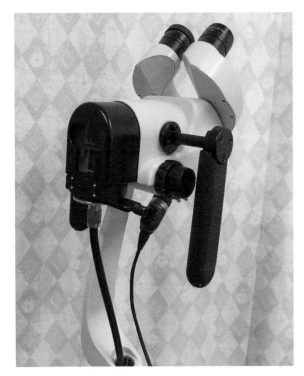

Figure 7.8 Colposcope.

Colposcopy

Colposcopy is the examination of the cervix using a magnification system. Colposcopic services in the UK are governed by the British Society for Colposcopy and Cervical Cytology (BSCCP). All colposcopists are required to retain BSCCP certification.

Indications for Colposcopy [1]

- Abnormal cytology
  - Borderline nuclear change (BNC) in squamous cells and HR HPV positive
  - Low-grade dyskaryosis and HR HPV positive
  - High-grade dyskaryosis
  - Suspicious for invasion
  - BNC in glandular cells
  - Possible glandular neoplasia

  Tip: It should be noted that borderline changes in squamous cells and low-grade dyskaryosis in the absence of HR HPV no longer warrants colposcopy referral.

- Clinically suspicious cervix. Refer on 2WW pathway

- Cervical abnormality including inability to identify cervix.
- Recurrent inadequate smears.
- Some women with PCB.

Colposcopic Examination

The woman is laid on a colposcopy couch with her legs supported and speculum examination is performed. The colposcope is a magnifying system that allows magnification from a distance and a clear visual assessment of the cervix. A screen may be available for the woman to also view the findings.

Solutions are applied to the cervix to aid diagnosis. *Acetic acid* alters the nuclear protein, rendering it opaque. When the light from the colposcope meets the cervix, it is reflected back from the opaque nucleus, appearing white to the colposcopist. The more dyskaryotic a cell, the larger the nucleus, the more light is reflected and the whiter the area appears.

Cytoplasm is glycogen-rich and stains dark brown with the application of *Schiller's iodine*. When little cytoplasm remains, as in a severely dyskaryotic cell, there will be little uptake of iodine.

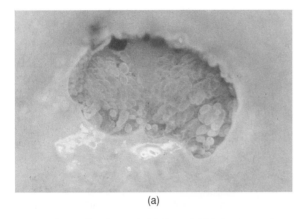

(a)

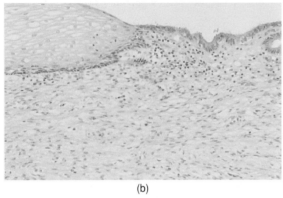

(b)

Figure 7.9 *Colposcopy.* (a) Colposcopic appearance of the external OS showing the SCJ. (b) Histology slide showing SCJ. (For the colour version, please refer to the plate section.)

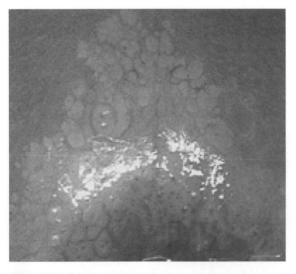

Figure 7.10 Colposcopic image showing mosaicism and punctation. (For the colour version, please refer to the plate section.)

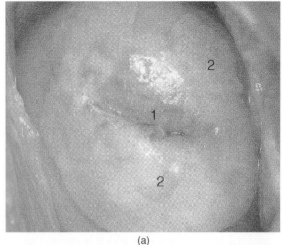

(a)

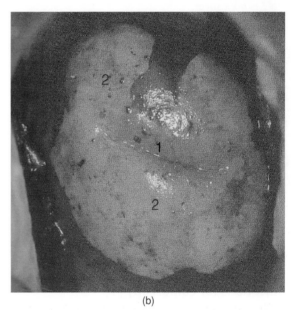

(b)

Figure 7.11 Effect of iodine on abnormal squamous tissue. (a) Before application of Shillers iodine (1: s–c junction; 2: aceto-white staining suggestive of CIN). (b) After application (1: s–c junction; 2: iodine – negative staining suggestive of CIN). (For the colour version, please refer to the plate section.)

Reports from colposcopy clinics often comment on the presence and density of acetowhite areas and the extent of the cervix staining iodine negative.

Other descriptive comments made in reports include the presence of mosaicism and punctation which refer to alterations in the vascular pattern. The more pronounced both features are, the more significant the abnormality.

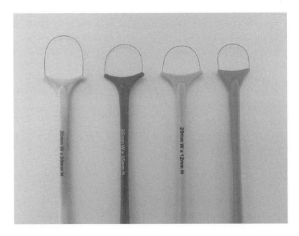

Figure 7.12 Loops used for LLETZ.

See and Treat

Many colposcopy clinics offer a see and treat policy for high-grade disease. If the referral smear is high-grade and colposcopic appearances show consistent findings, then treatment will generally be offered on the first visit. The concern associated with high-grade disease is that this is likely to progress to cervical cancer, whereas low-grade disease may not [6].

The commonest form of treatment offered is large loop excision of the transformation zone of the cervix (LLETZ) under local anaesthesia. Once the cervix is anaesthetized, a cone-shaped area of cervix will be removed using a heated loop of wire. Further diathermy will be applied after removal of the specimen to aid haemostasis and treat to a further depth.

Exceptions to See and Treat for High-Grade Disease

- There is evidence of a small increase in preterm delivery postLLETZ [7], so if there is a discrepancy between the smear result and the colposcopic appearance, a biopsy should be performed at first visit rather than proceeding to treatment.
- After LLETZ it is recommended that a woman abstain from intercourse, using tampons or swimming for four weeks, so if she is due to travel abroad within that time treatment may be delayed. There may also be difficulties with travel insurance if complications arise post-treatment. CIN is a slowly progressing condition and therefore deferring treatment until return from

holiday is unlikely to significantly increase risk, however colposcopic examination should be performed at first visit to exclude malignancy.
- Some colposcopists will treat with an IUD *in situ*, some prefer to remove and replace at the time of treatment and some will remove for treatment and recommend replacement at a later date. It is prudent to advise a woman referred to colposcopy with a high-grade smear that her IUD may have to be removed so she should refrain from intercourse or use an alternative reliable form of contraception for seven days prior to her colposcopy appointment to avoid either deferral of treatment or risk of pregnancy should the IUD be removed.
- Requirement for GA or treatment in another setting:
  - Very large lesions, especially those extending onto the vaginal walls.
  - Although most treatments are performed in the out-patient setting, the choice of opting for treatment under general anaesthetic should be offered to prevent women not attending their colposcopy appointment because of anxiety.
  - Some medical conditions, e.g. poorly controlled epilepsy.

Complications Post-LLETZ

Short Term

There is a risk of infection post-treatment or biopsy and a woman is informed that if she develops any signs of infection, e.g. offensive discharge, temperature, pelvic pain, she should seek advice from her GP. Antibiotics should be prescribed, including treatment for anaerobic infection.

Women must also be informed that if heavy bleeding occurs she should contact the unit who treated her. Contact numbers should be provided before leaving the colposcopy clinic.

Long Term [7]

There is some evidence that LLETZ can increase the risk of preterm delivery. The risk is only marginally increased over background risk after one treatment, but becomes more significant after multiple or larger treatments.

Cervical stenosis is rare, but can occasionally result in haematocolpos.

Other Treatment Methods

Destructive treatments using cold coagulation, cryotherapy or ball diathermy are not recommended for high-grade lesions, but are suitable for treating persistent low-grade disease or in the treatment of an ectropion.

Knife cone biopsy is sometimes used under general anaesthetic for large inaccessible lesions.

Laser treatment is occasionally used to take a cone or to vaporise low-grade lesions.

Hysterectomy is rarely required but may be recommended where there is persistent disease and little remaining cervix in women who have completed their families.

Management of Low-Grade Dyskaryosis HR HPV+ve [1]

Usually low-grade disease does not require excision, as approximately two-thirds of low-grade CIN (CIN1) will revert to normal spontaneously as the woman becomes immune to HPV.

Colposcopic examination with biopsies is, however, required in these women to make sure the diagnosis of low-grade disease is correct and add confirmation of this conservative approach.

Stopping smoking has been shown to increase the likelihood of clearing HPV and hence increase the chances of regression of CIN.

Otherwise follow-up is dependent on clinical appearances or biopsy results if taken and necessary.

Glandular Abnormalities [1]

Smear tests suggestive of abnormalities in glandular cells should all be referred for colposcopy urgently. These results are more difficult to interpret, the colposcopy is more challenging and there are few national guidelines for management.

The cytology lab will report on the site of origin of the abnormal glandular cells, either cervical or uterine, which aids referral to the correct clinic.

Generally where a result is suggestive of cervical glandular neoplasia, treatment will be recommended and carried out at first visit. Where the result is of BNC in glandular cells the management is more variable and each woman's situation is assessed individually. There

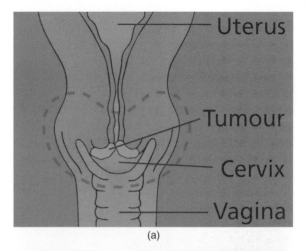

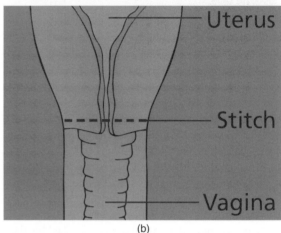

Figure 7.13 Trachelectomy. (a) Pre-op showing area removed. (b) Postprocedure. Images produced by Leeds Teaching Hospitals NHS Trust Medical Illustration Service.

is a much higher incidence of cancer with a BNC in glandular cells than where there is BNC in squamous cells and so it is appropriate that more treatments are performed, accepting that there will be some negative histology reports from treatment specimens. A multidisciplinary approach is essential with involvement of the patient in the decision-making process.

Follow-Up After LLETZ

HPV Test of Cure After CIN [1]

After LLETZ for CIN, most women will be discharged back to primary care, even if excision margins are not clear of CIN. It is likely that diathermy applied after LLETZ will have destroyed residual disease. A smear

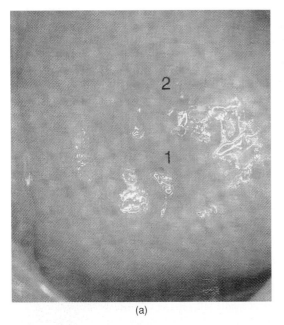
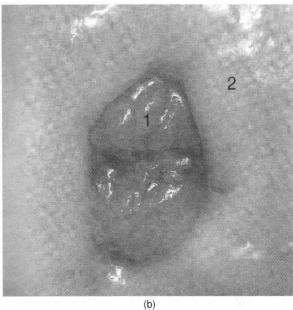

(a)   (b)

Figure 7.14 Common appearances post-LLETZ: (a) stenosis (1: cervical os; 2: transformation zone), (b) rosetting (1: columnar epithelium; 2: squamous epithelium). (For the colour version, please refer to the plate section.)

should be taken at six months which will be tested for the presence of dyskaryosis and for HR HPV.

The results of this smear could be:

- Negative for dyskaryosis and negative for HR HPV, in which case the woman is recalled at three years for a follow-up smear, regardless of age.
- Negative for dyskaryosis and positive for HR HPV and requires further colposcopy. Colposcopic findings and biopsy, if indicated, dictate follow-up requirements.
- Abnormal cytology requiring referral back to colposcopy.

If a woman is aged over 50 at treatment, her next smear should be at three years rather than five. If that smear is negative, she can revert to routine five-yearly recall.

HPV Tests of Cure After LLETZ for CGIN [1]

Following a LLETZ procedure for CGIN where histology indicates complete excision, an HPV test of cure is again indicated. If this is negative for dyskaryosis and HR HPV, a second test of cure is indicated a year later. If both tests are negative, normal recall can resume. A positive result will lead to continuing follow-up in the colposcopy service with women managed on an individual basis.

Incomplete excision of a glandular abnormality generally warrants further excisional treatment.

Cervical Cancer

Advice from the BSCCP states that it is difficult to comment on the rate of progression of untreated CIN3 to cervical cancer, as further studies are unethical. However, older literature reviews suggest that between 12 and 40% may progress [6].

The majority of cervical cancers arise from squamous cells, but about 15% are adenocarcinomas. There are other, rare cervical cancers, such as clear cell, small cell, lymphomas and sarcomas, and mixed squamous and glandular.

Cervical cancers are staged from 1–4, with subgroups, according to the FIGO classification.

Stage 1 cancers are confined to the cervix.

Stage 1A1 cancers, the earliest stage, where the tumour is less than 3 mm deep and less than 7 mm wide may be adequately treated with LLETZ or cone biopsy. Provided margins are clear, no further surgical intervention is required.

All cases of cancer will be discussed at an MDT meeting.

If a woman has a strong desire to retain fertility and the stage of cervical cancer is low (usually less than

1B1) and confined to the cervix, it may be possible, in a specialist centre, to offer radical trachelectomy where the cervix and lower third of the uterus is removed, along with pelvic node clearance.

There is a higher chance of miscarriage or premature delivery after trachelectomy. The baby must be delivered early, by LSCS [8].

More advanced cancers will be managed in specialist centres with radical surgery, radiotherapy and chemotherapy all playing a part, depending on staging and individual circumstances.

Tips

Topical oestrogen therapy is useful where there is difficulty in obtaining an adequate smear due to the SCJ lying high within the endocervical canal, i.e. postmenopausal women or those using long-term progesterone therapy.

The use of oestrogen treatment (or any other hormonal treatment) must be identified on the sample request form to ensure the cytologist understands the relevance of the histological changes.

Conclusion

Rates of cervical cancer have reduced in the UK since the introduction of the NHSCSP. Further reductions should be seen as the young women who are vaccinated against HPV infection reach screening age.

The role of HPV triage in the screening programme is changing and causing concern to women who do not understand the relevance of their results. It is important for all clinicians in primary care to be aware of changes to the programme so that they can support women appropriately if they have concerns.

References

1. Colposcopy and Programme Management. *Guidelines for the NHS Cervical Screening Programme, 2nd edn.* NHSCSP Publication No. 20, May 2010.

2. Mackenzie IZ, Naish C, Rees CMP, Manek S, Why remove all cervical polyps and examine them histologically? *BJOG* 2009;116(8):1127–1129.

3. HPV Triage and Test of Cure NHS Cancer Screening Programmes. Implementation Guide. NHSCSP good Practice Guide Number 3, July 2011.

4. HSIC Cervical Screening Programme England Stats for 2013/14, November 2014

5. Fonseca-Moutinho JA, Smoking and cervical cancer. *ISRN Obstet Gynecol* 2011:847684.

6. McCreadie MR, Sharples KJ, Paul C, *et al.* Natural history of cervical neoplasia and risk of invasive cancer in women with cervical intraepithelial neoplasia 3: a retrospective cohort study. *Lancet Oncol* 2008;9:425–434.

7. Castandon A, Brocklehurst P, Evans H, *et al.* Risk of preterm birth after treatment for cervical intraepithelial neoplasia among women attending colposcopy in England: retrospective-prospective cohort study. *BMJ* 2012;345:e5174.

8. Shepherd JH, Spencer C, Herod J, Ind TE, Radical vaginal trachelectomy as a fertility-sparing procedure in women with early-stage cancer-cumulative pregnancy rate in a series of 123 women. *BJOG* 2006;113(6):719–724.

Chapter

8

Management of Patients with Psychosexual Problems in Primary Care

Alison Vaughan and Leila Frodsham

Key Points

- When treating sexual problems, it is important to consider both psychological and physical factors.
- There is a degree of overlap between dyspareunia, vulvodynia and vaginismus.
- Consider advising women with dyspareunia to avoid penetrative sex in order to break the pain cycle.
- General behaviour mimics genital behaviour. Study one and you have insights into the other.
- IPM offers training that can be used to manage psychosexual problems in general practice.

The omnipresent process of sex, as it is woven into the whole texture of our bodies is the pattern of the whole process of our life.

Havelock Ellis

Sexual problems are common in the general population. The prevalence varies according to the type of questionnaires used and how the problem is defined.

Sexual Attitudes and Lifestyles in Britain: *Natsal 3*, 2013 [1], found that:

- 42% of men and 51% of women aged 16–74 interviewed who had had sex in the past year had experienced one or more sexual difficulties lasting a minimum of three months. This included lack of interest in having sex, feeling anxious during sex, pain during sex, vaginal dryness and problems getting or keeping an erection.
- One in six men and women feel that their health affects their sex life, but few seek help from health professionals.
- Only a quarter of men (24%) and under a fifth of women (18%) who say that ill-health affected

their sex life in the past year sought help from a health professional and when they did it was usually from a GP.

Nazareth *et al.* [2] looked at patients attending 13 GPs in London:

- Sexual difficulties were identified in 40% of women and 22% of men.
- Of these only 30% of women and 21% of men had sought sexual advice from their doctor.
- Only 22/773 (3%) women and 12/307 (4%) men had an entry in their family practice records relating to sexual difficulties in the previous two years.

Issues for Patients

- Not enough time; doctor was busy
- Too exposing; doctor uncomfortable
- Wanted a quick fix
- Wanted doctor to be expert
- Hoped doctor would pick it up
- Didn't know there was a problem.

Issues for Health Professionals

- 'How on earth can I do all that in a short consultation?'
- 'Might expose too much of myself?'
- Discomfort with not being able to fix a problem
- Lack of training
- 'Patient never told me there was a problem'
- 'I never see these cases' – consider, is this selective listening a defence against all of the above?

Women's Health in Primary Care, edited by Anne Connolly and Amanda Britton. Published by Cambridge University Press
© Cambridge University Press 2017

Presentation

This can be overt or covert. A small study carried out in general practice by Read *et al.* [3] confirmed a high prevalence of sexual problems. Specific complaints were:

- 45% painful sex
- 23% orgasmic difficulties
- Remainder mixed picture, e.g. painful sex accompanied by a loss of desire.

Some Examples of Covert Presentation

- Recurrent vaginal discharge with no diagnosis
- Inability to tolerate or avoids a vaginal examination
- Frequent failure to attend for cytology sampling
- Dissatisfaction with all methods of contraception
- Pelvic pain with no organic cause
- Medication or condition (e.g. diabetes) that causes sexual dysfunction, but the patient endures this until the doctor asks.

Sexual activity is dependent on physical and emotional factors. Physiological systems need to be intact, but also all kinds of emotions can enhance or subdue arousal and sexual activity. These emotional factors may not be experienced on a conscious level. Many doctors and patients see illness as either real or imagined; psychosexual medicine tries to take both sides into consideration. The term psychosexual medicine has been used since 1974 to describe a brief psychodynamic psychotherapeutic approach to managing sexual problems. Although used in specialist clinics, the technique was originally developed for brief consultations in general practice and contraception clinics.

The doctor who develops psychodynamic skills, but continues to treat the whole person, cannot forget physical doctoring and it is this combination of emotional and physical interest that provides the possibility of looking at the way in which the body and mind work together. The underlying causes of a problem may be physical or psychological in varying proportions, but rarely limited to one or the other. The attitudes, anxieties and fantasies revealed during the consultation and the physical examination are particularly relevant to the understanding of the sexual problem. Otherwise the doctor responds to the patient by being either overawed or not responding at all, so gives a

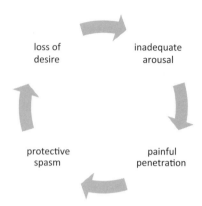

Figure 8.1 Cycle of vaginismus.

loss of desire → inadequate arousal → painful penetration → protective spasm

quick response without thinking or a generic response without hearing.

Sexual dysfunction is classified according to when in the sexual response cycle the problem occurs. Psychological issues can affect any part of this cycle.

Dyspareunia

This is defined as pain or discomfort that occurs in association with sexual intercourse. This is classified into superficial or deep, and has a number of physical causes. The patient might have feelings about this symptom or its physical cause, which should be acknowledged.

'This (lichen sclerosis) is eating away my love life.'

Vaginismus [4] has been defined as the persistent difficulty to allow vaginal entry of any object, despite the patient's conscious wish to do so.

'Foreplay is fun but when he tries to enter, he hits a wall. I hurt badly and he loses his erection.'

This recurrent involuntary spasm of the musculature of the outer third of the vagina is thought to be a defensive mechanism driven by fear. The fear can be physical, e.g. past history of deep dyspareunia from endometriosis, or emotional, e.g. wishes to avoid domination or rejection.

Vaginal dilators alone or vaginal surgery might attempt to address the sense of *physical size*, but not the sense of emotional size and associated feelings and fantasies.

'Am I a big enough woman for sex?'

According to anecdotal reports, patients with vaginismus can dress and appear younger than their years and may still have a strong bond with their mother.

Causes of Painful Intercourse

Superficial Pain

- Lack of sexual arousal – more common in diabetes, multiple sclerosis or spinal-cord injury, or inadequate stimulation by the partner, fatigue or fear of pain
- Vulvovaginitis caused by candidiasis, herpes, trichomonas
- Atrophic vaginitis
- Vulvar dermatatosis, e.g. lichen sclerosis
- Chemical irritation, perfumes, soaps
- Provoked vulvodynia
- Abnormalities of the hymen, vertical or horizontal vaginal septum
- Pelvic radiotherapy (resulting stenosis responds well to vaginal dilators)
- Trauma associated with genital surgery, e.g. episiotomy or prolapse repair
- Drugs that reduce lubrication, e.g. antihistamines, alcohol.

Deep Pain

- Endometriosis
- Pelvic inflammatory disease
- Irritable bowel disease.

Examination is required not just to detect pathology, but also to explore the fantasies that the patient has about her body. The act of undressing can undress the patient of their psychological defences and/or the barriers to seeing the problem.

> 'Chlamydia left me with a scar inside my vagina, no one can see this growth, but I think it's like a barrier which we can't get over.' Patient had been infected by her partner.

At this intimate examination the unconscious can emerge into the conscious, bringing with it fantasies of size, damage, feelings and appearance. These fantasies need respect, understanding not denial by reassurance. Though tempting to reassure patients that their anatomy is normal, it is more powerful to encourage them to see and feel it themselves. After surviving an examination, the patient can feel empowered to face their fears.

Case Scenario

Hera, age 20 years comes to see her GP complaining that 'something isn't right down below'. She wants a referral. The genitalia are normal, but the patient is not relieved.

'I wonder what you are really worried about?'

'Can't you see, they look like dragon's teeth?'

The doctor continues to reassure; 'Lots of women have asymmetrical labia.'

'My partner says, "Your dragon's teeth stop my willy working".'

Management must be tailored to the individual. Overcoming fear and building trust are essential, so a GP with a special interest and training in this area could manage this problem.

Some clinicians advocate the use of vagina dilators (trainers) and these may be useful for some women, e.g. those with vaginal stenosis after pelvic radiotherapy. However, case-control studies of women with and without vaginismus using electromyography have found no difference in their ability to contract and release pelvic floor muscles [4]. Therefore, the vagina needs relaxing not stretching. Encouraging the woman to put her own or her partner's finger into her vagina enables her to increase her confidence and familiarity with her body. If the woman is reluctant to engage with her own genitals, explore why, because this may lead to a disclosure of a physical fantasy. However, if the patient considers this to be homework it can rapidly become a chore. For women who fear vaginal specula and are unable to have a smear, consider lending them a device which they can get used to at home or suggest, during cervical sampling they assist you to insert the device. Avoiding penetrative sex when it is painful and using artificial lubricants (silicone-based ones are best) can prevent and break the vicious cycle. Other strategies include: progressive relaxation, sensate focus and hypnotherapy.

Refer those with underlying psychiatric problems, e.g. depression, to the mental health team.

Vulvodynia

This is defined as a burning pain occurring in the absence of relevant visible findings or a specific, clinically identifiable neurological disorder. Vulvodynia is categorized as generalized or localized, provoked, unprovoked or a mixture of the two [5,6].

Provoked vulvodynia is likely to be multifactorial in aetiology, though often a history of recurrent vulvo-vaginal candidiasis is reported. Pain is frequently felt at the introitus, during intercourse or on insertion of tampons. On examination, focal tenderness is elicited by gentle application of a cotton wool tip bud at the introitus, but there are no signs of inflammation. Normal vestibular erythema may be seen, but this is not a diagnostic sign.

Sexual problems are common:

- Superficial dyspareunia
- Reduced sexual arousal
- More negative sexual feelings
- Less interest in sex.

After exclusion of other treatable causes such as:

- Vulval candidiasis
- Herpes
- Dermatoses such as lichen planus and lichen sclerosis
- Neoplastic conditions such as vulval intraepithelial neoplasia and squamous cell carcinoma

no further investigations are required. The British Society for the Study of Vulval Disease recommends a multidisciplinary approach to patient care and that combining treatments can be helpful in dealing with different aspects of vulvodynia. Recommended regimes:

- Strict irritant avoidance. Use water or an emollient as soap substitute to wash. Oils (such as coconut) may act as a barrier to precipitating factors (allergens, chafing from clothing) and enable better lubrication for sexual function.
- Regular massage with a mild emollient may have a role in desensitizing the area.
- Topical local anaesthetic, e.g. 5% lidocaine ointment or 2% lidocaine gel. Use with caution because of possible irritation. Apply 15–20 minutes prior to penetrative sex. To reduce the risk of penile numbness, wash off the lidocaine just before sex, or use a condom.
- Women who experience vulvodynia may develop associated overactive pelvic floor muscles, which leads to a vicious cycle of worsening dyspareunia. A physiotherapist can identify high muscle tone,

spasm or poor relaxation within the pelvic floor muscles and treatment may result in symptom reduction, improvement of sexual functioning and quality of life.

- Amitriptyline gradually titrated up from 10 mg to 75 mg according to the response and side effects. Treatment should be maintained for three to six months before reducing gradually. Recent evidence does not indicate a benefit in most vulvodynia sufferers, but its use can be of benefit to those with anxiety and insomnia [7].
- Permission to stop penetrative sex, offer advice on lubricants and ways to improve intimacy through non-coital contact.
- Refer to psychosexual medicine clinic to explore the emotional and psychological aspects of vulval pain.

Loss of Desire

Case Scenario

35-year-old Juno strides confidently into her GP's office for an IUS insertion. Juno answers the doctor's questions with curt precision. The doctor is aware of feeling intimidated by this woman who makes the doctor feel inadequate. Juno has a young child, no current health problems and takes no medication apart from her contraceptive pill. She wants the IUS because her family is complete and she doesn't like the mood swings or loss of libido that the pill brings. The last comment is made in an undertone so could have been missed. The doctor echoes the patient's last words, though tempted to move on. Juno looks uncomfortable

'We rarely have sex.'

'Is that a problem for you?'

'No, but it is for my husband. It's ok once we start but I just can't initiate. Things will be different off the pill.'

'How unfortunate the pill affects you like this now; it never did all those years earlier.'

'I worry about getting pregnant again because I really don't want any more children.'

'I wonder what else was going on in your life when your libido changed?'

'Can't we get on? The difficulties in my sex life are all down to life issues which I need to sort. I suffered postnatal depression after my son was born. Look on the computer.'

'You're very angry.'

'Of course I'm bloody angry. You're not getting on with your job, childbirth has ruined my life, whereas my husband's life has stayed exactly the same. He's had it easy.'

'Must be difficult making love to someone you feel resentful toward.'

'Tell me about it…Yet, I should not complain because he's a good man – just a hopeless help.'

Silence. Juno cries.

'I wonder what those tears are about.'

'He's not really hopeless, I am. I just can't tell him how I feel. You see I really want another baby and am getting too old to wait. However, I couldn't work full time with two children, but we need my salary. Part of me doesn't want this device fitted, but he will think me stupid if I don't go ahead.'

'How do you know he will react like that? Can't be easy to be abandoned in bed if you're hiding your feelings and don't feel very confident about yourself.'

Silence.

'Right let's get on with it. By the way can I have this removed after a year? I am going to have that talk with my husband.'

Other Areas/Approaches that Could have been Made

- Possible reoccurrence of her depression.
- Medication.
- Change in role from wife to mother. For some people certain roles are more immediately powerful in terms of how the individual sees themselves. The mother role can eclipse the role of lover.
- Partner is no longer attractive.
- Female sexual response cycle is different to men's in that woman may engage in sex with a partner for a broad range of reasons other than actual sexual desire, i.e. sexual desire can emerge during sex even though it wasn't present at all before the sex started.

- If the presenting problem had been a lifelong loss of interest in sex, this may be connected with the individual not having developed as a sexual person.
- If there was a total loss of desire there may be a need to explore an organic disorder, for example, depression, chronic disease, pituitary, thyroid or adrenal disorders.

Anorgasmia

Orgasm is a normal reflex that requires adequate physical stimulation and an emotional ability to let go.

The majority of women climax clitorally. Some may feel under pressure from the partner to do so vaginally, otherwise he will consider himself a failure.

'If you really loved me you would come at the same time.'

Physical reasons are rare, but they include:

- Hypopituitarism
- Multiple sclerosis, diabetes; both disrupt neurological pathways
- Pelvic surgery. This can not only lead to neurological disruption, but also psychological issues over loss of sexual organs
- Dermatological conditions
- Drugs, e.g. antidepressants (especially SSRIs), some beta blockers.

Psychosocial/psychosexual reasons are more common.

In women the orgasmic reflex is easily disturbed by situational factors or relationship problems.

'I just can't seem to let go when I know my teenage son is in the next bedroom.'

The psychosexual reasons are varied. The Institute of Psychosexual Medicine in their research into adult survivors of childhood sexual abuse with sexual difficulties in adulthood [8] found that almost a quarter complained of an inability to achieve an orgasm.

Menopausal Issues

Sexual function alters with age and the menopause. Older women have concerns that include vaginal dryness, loss of libido, pain and body image issues.

A 52-year-old complaining to her GP about dyspareunia:

'*Any attempts at penetration leave me in searing agony. Foreplay irritates. I think my insides are shrivelling up just like my skin. Sex is a chore, but if I don't do it he'll go back to his mistress.*'

Her atrophic vaginitis was successfully treated with oestrogen cream and vaginal moisturisers (Hyalofemme®), plus lubricants. However, her GP also gave her time to express anger and hurt at her husband's affair and come to terms with her own changing body.

Testosterone therapy in conjunction with oestrogen therapy may be indicated in women with surgical menopause.

Gott *et al.* [9] found that despite recognizing on a theoretical level that sexuality remained important to older people, sexual health is not proactively discussed by GPs with older patients. The researcher found that the reasons for this were:

- Within primary care, sexual health tends to be equated with younger people.
- Sex is not seen as a legitimate topic for discussion with this age group.
- GPs had not received any training in this area.

The following model L.O.F.T.I. [10] can be used as an aid for consultation about sexual problems. Look back at the consultation with Juno and see how the model was used.

Listening

- What is and is *not* said and *when.*
- Listening to *silence* and note *when.*
- The *patient's story* and not the doctor's. Note the patient's tone and use of language.

Observing

- *Referral.* Why has the patient chosen to see that particular doctor? Have they been sent by another member of the practice team or by their partner? Patients may choose to discuss sexual problems with a GP they do not usually see – a locum or registrar.
- The *presentation.* 'When did the problem start?' (Lifelong or acquired.)
  'Did anything else happen at the time it started?' (Any trigger factors?)
  The patient may not spontaneously disclose something significant that happened at the time

the problem started because it seems too trivial or was too terrible to mention.
'Does it always happen or is it connected to a particular situation.' (Situational.)

- The *appearance* and *behaviour* of the patient. Perhaps they keep cancelling appointments or their outward demeanour is at odds with their story.

Feeling

- What's the *feeling* in the room and in the doctor? Patient's subconscious feelings are transferred to the doctor.
- Learn to tolerate confusion and ignorance.

Thinking about the doctor–patient relationship

- What is going on between the doctor and the patient? How did the patient behave in the doctor's presence?
- What sort of doctor did the patient turn you into? A teacher, a parent?
- How did it feel to be with this patient?
- Defences of the doctor, e.g. order investigations for no clear reason.
- The defences of patient, e.g. 'I really want this smear but my period has come yet again.'
  De-doctor, 'You are not getting on with your job.'
- Why present and why now? What is the patient's motivation?

Interpreting

Check out your findings with the Expert (the patient), e.g. 'Must be difficult making love to someone you feel resentful toward.'

The Genital Examination

Patients present to doctors expecting a physical and psychological examination of their complaints.

The genital area of the body is not called private parts for nothing. By removing the clothes and protective anatomy, the inner self is revealed. People in this exposed and vulnerable position can blurt out things that surprise not just the doctor, but also themselves. If the doctor finds themselves avoiding examination of a particular woman, consider why. Is this the patient's fear that they have something too terrible to be shown?

Case Scenario

Artemis, aged 24 years complained that sex was so painful she couldn't tolerate penetration. When her GP went to examine her she sat up on the couch, knees drawn up to chin, with a protective swaddling of NHS blue roll. The doctor felt uncomfortable about examining her.

'Are you sure you want me to examine you today?'

'I hate all this'

'This?'

'Examinations, doctors ... sex.'

'Sex?'

'I don't want to have sex because I'm afraid of the pain.'

'Tell me about this pain.'

'I can't, it's too deep ... its beyond everything.'

Tears.

Silence.

'It brings back the pain when a neighbour raped me and put his fist inside me when I was 15.'

Trauma, like sexual abuse or assault may be provoked to remerge by a new event and cause problems, or memories, more endurable in later life, can prompt the patient into seeking help for the first time.

How Can I Train?

The ability to recognize psychosexual difficulty is an essential part of everyday practice. Patients may wish to keep separate their physical complaints from their sexual problems, but some prefer to stay with their GP. For GPs who wish to acquire psychosexual therapy as a specialist skill, the following organizations can be approached:

Institute of Psychosexual Medicine (IPM): Psychosexual medicine is a type of brief therapy practised by doctors, based on psychoanalytical principles, but drawing on medical knowledge and skills. This approach allows the biological, socio-cultural and psychological needs of the patient to be addressed and is considered to be 'holistic'. Some of the basic skills taught by IPM are available to some allied health professionals. http://www.ipm.org.uk/23/information (accessed September 2016).

College of Sexual & Relationship Therapists (COSRT): The focus of therapy is to provide a safe space and regular time to talk about what is going on in the life of the client(s). The treatment may utilize a variety of techniques dependent on the individual's needs. If the client(s) decides, with the therapist, that there are any physical factors that need to be checked, then they will be referred to their doctor. http://www.cosrt.org.uk (accessed September 2016).

When to Refer

The GP needs to determine if the patient wishes or needs to be referred and then to whom. Services for sexual dysfunction vary across the UK, so a GP will need to know who the local experts are. IPM and COSRT keep lists of accredited practitioners on their websites.

GPs views on their management of sexual dysfunction (Humphery and Nazareth, 2001 [11]):

- 'It is an important topic that needs more research and investigation. I feel that there is a lot of misery waiting to be discovered and treated.'

- *But* 'this is not a priority area; there are no targets and so no reimbursement for extra work.'

Yeah, *BUT:*

- 'At the time when one is with a distressed patient, the priority seems high for the individual.'

References

1. NATSAL Sexual attitudes and lifestyles in Britain: Highlights from Natsal-3. 2013. http://www.natsal.ac.uk/media/2102/natsal-infographic.pdf

2. Nazareth I, Boynton P, King M, Problems with sexual function in people attending London general practitioners: cross sectional study. *BMJ* 2003;327:423.

3. Read S, King M, Watson J, Sexual dysfunction in primary medical care; prevalence, characteristics and detection by the general practitioner. *J Publ Health Med* 19(4):391–397.

4. Crowley T, Goldmeier D, Wadsworth J, Hiller J, Diagnosing and managing vaginismus. *BMJ* 2009 338:b2284.

5. Nunns D, Mandal D, Byrne M, Guidelines for the management of vulvodynia. *Br J Dermatol* 2010;162:1180–1185.

6. Edwards SK, Bates CM, Lewis F, Sethi G, Grover D, 2014 UK guideline on management of vulval conditions. *Int J STD AIDS* 2015 26(9): 611–624.

7. Leo RJ, Dewani S, A systematic review of the utility of antidepressant pharmacotherapy in the treatment of vulvodynia pain *J Sex Med* 2013;10: 2497–2505.

8. Vanhegan G, Treatment of psychosexual disorders in previously abused patients. *Br J Family Planning* 1996;22:191–193.

9. Gott M, Hinchliff S, Galena E, General practitioner attitudes to discussing sexual health issues with older people. *Social Sci Med* 2004;58(11):2093–2103.

10. Botell J, Training lectures in psychosexual medicine; skills of psychosexual medicine. *J Inst Psychosexual Med* 2001;26:24–28.

11. Humphrey S, Nazareth I, GP's views on their management of sexual dysfunction. *Family Pract* 2001;18:516–518.

Further Reading

Skrine R, Montford H (editors), *Psychosexual Medicine: An Introduction*. 2001 Arnold.

Skrine R, *Blocks and Freedoms in Sexual Life: A Handbook of Psychosexual Medicine*. 1997 Radcliffe Medical Press Ltd.

British Society of Sexual Medicine. www.bssm.org.uk (accessed September 2016).

Sexual Advice Association. www.sexualadviceassociation.co.uk (accessed September 2016) has useful information sheets for patients.

VulvalPain Society. www.vulvalpainsociety.org (accessed September 2016).

Self-Help Books

Valins L, *When a Women's Body Says No to Sex*. Penguin 1988.

Chapter 9

Infertility Management in Primary Care

Clare Searle

Key Points

- Fertility problems are common and affect up to one in seven couples.
- Fertility consultations are often emotional and require time and sensitivity to fully explore the relevant factors and concerns.
- Likely barriers to success should be addressed early to optimize outcomes, including lifestyle issues for both partners.
- Fertility concerns require 'couple-centred' care, so both partners should be involved at all stages and be able to support each other.
- Basic investigations are necessary from both partners prior to referral.
- Understanding of local referral pathways and criteria is important.
- Women with a past gynaecological history of note or aged over 35 should be referred into a specialist fertility clinic after six months of trying to conceive naturally.

Introduction

Reproductive medicine has developed rapidly over recent years and now a very complex array of possibilities and alternative options for parenting exists. In today's world, having a family is by and large possible, though in many cases this often includes options whereby parents accept that to achieve this, their babies may not be entirely their own biological material.

On the whole, fertility is much more complicated than it ever has been, and this is particularly true in primary care, where the process of investigations for fertility really begins. These consultations require a truly holistic approach, patience, support and guidance.

Therefore, in this chapter, we aim to give an overview of recent advances, current trends and present guidance to equip primary care clinicians to be best placed to support couples in their decision-making.

Principles of Care

Infertility is broadly defined as a failure to conceive after one year of regular unprotected penetrative sexual intercourse. Couples in whom there are reasons for subfertility, or who are over the age of 35 years, should be identified as high risk and referred on at six months. Ideally, regular intercourse should occur two to three times per week, throughout the month, and not just around the time of ovulation [1].

The Broader Issue

Due to changing social habits and cultural diversity, NICE estimates that on average, one in seven couples will have difficulty conceiving. Though the statistics are not all bleak, 84 out of 100 couples will become pregnant within one year of trying and this will rise a further 8% by the second year [2].

It is important to consider the variety of relationships in this process. In the majority we are discussing heterosexual couples struggling to conceive, but as mentioned before, variety exists and similar considerations must be given to same sex couples and those wishing to conceive without a current life partner.

In addition to this, the cause of infertility can be due to female and male factor causes or indeed a combination. It is important that all involved keep an open mind and bear no judgement [3].

Women's Health in Primary Care, edited by Anne Connolly and Amanda Britton. Published by Cambridge University Press © Cambridge University Press 2017

Female Infertility

The causes of female infertility may be broadly divided into three groups: failed ovarian function, anatomical abnormalities and environmental factors.

Failed Ovarian Function

Failure to ovulate is thought to account for around 25% of presentations, and is usually related to abnormal hormone function.

Hormonal Dysfunction

This is the most common cause for anovulation. The process of ovulation depends upon a complex balance of hormones and their interactions to be successful. Any disruption in this process can hinder ovulation. There are three main causes of this problem:

- *Hypogonadotrophic hypogonadism.* The hypothalamus is the portion of the brain responsible for sending signals to the pituitary gland, which, in turn, sends hormonal stimuli to the ovaries in the form of follicle-stimulating hormone (FSH) and luteinizing hormone (LH) to initiate egg maturation. If the hypothalamus fails to trigger and control this process, immature eggs will result. This is the cause of ovarian failure in 20% of cases. The most common presentation of this is in women with a low BMI and/or high exercise regimens.
- *Pituitary gland problems.* The pituitary is responsible for producing and secreting FSH and LH. The ovaries will be unable to ovulate properly if either too much or too little of these hormones are produced. Common causes include physical injury, tumours and chemical imbalances, e.g. Sheehan's syndrome.
- *Ovarian problems.* In approximately 50% of cases, the ovaries do not produce normal follicles in which the eggs can mature. Ovulation is rare if the eggs are immature and the chance of fertilization becomes almost non-existent. Polycystic ovary syndrome is the most common disorder responsible for this problem. Symptoms include amenorrhoea, hirsutism, anovulation and infertility. The syndrome is characterized by a reduced production of FSH, and normal or increased levels of LH, oestrogen and testosterone. This abnormal ratio of gonadotrophins causes partial development of ovarian follicles, follicular cysts therefore develop which are detectable on ultrasound. Please refer to Chapter 14 on Polycystic Ovary Syndrome.

Scarred Ovaries

Physical damage to the ovaries may result in failed ovulation. For example, extensive, invasive or multiple surgeries for repeated ovarian cysts may cause the capsule of the ovary to become damaged or scarred, such that follicles cannot mature properly and ovulation does not occur. Infection may also have this impact.

Premature Ovarian Insufficiency and 'Age-Related Infertility'

More and more women are finding their natural supply of eggs is running out. The explanation is usually age. Human biology dictates that a woman's store of eggs is fixed from birth. From puberty onward that store begins to deplete each month, programmed to be exhausted at menopause, when reproductive life comes to an end. Most studies show this decline occurs around age 35 with the menopause transition phase beginning around age 45 and menopause at age 51. In premature ovarian insufficiency this process of decline happens much faster, and loss of ovarian function, similar to the menopause occurring at age 40.

There has been increasing media interest in this area, given the pattern of many older women becoming first time mothers. The technique of vitrification, with rapid freezing of cells preventing the formation of ice crystals known to damage the genetic structure of the egg, was initially used to preserve fertility ahead of cancer treatments [4], but, privately, it is increasingly being used to buy a little time as the biological clock continues to tick. There is little published evidence about the reliability of egg freezing and the chance of then going on to a healthy term pregnancy with a thawed egg. This is a very complex dilemma: on the one hand it encourages forward thinking and empowerment of women, whilst on the other it is widely criticized for the implication that young women should soldier on at work through their child-bearing years.

Figures from the Office of National Statistics (ONS) show women are giving birth later year on year. In 2010 the average age of women giving birth to their first child was 27.8 years in comparison to 26.5 years in 2000 (Figure 9.1).

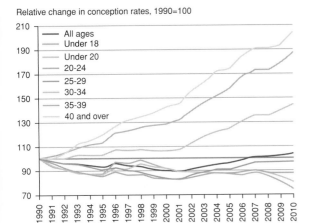

Relative change in conception rates, 1990=100

Figure 9.1 Average age of women giving birth to their first child, 1990–2010.
Source: Office for National Statistics. Conceptions in England and Wales, 2010. (For the colour version, please refer to the plate section.)

Consequentially, even if a woman achieves a pregnancy at an older age, the risk of miscarriage is higher due to poorer quality eggs.

Anatomical Issues

- *Uterine leiomyomas.* Fibroids are very common, typically affecting women aged 30–45 and often cause no symptoms unless they grow large enough to press on other organs. Depending on their position within the uterus, they can interfere with embryo implantation, whilst large fibroids may distort the shape of the abdomen or narrow the uterine cavity, leading to increased risk of miscarriage or preterm delivery.
- *Poorly functioning fallopian tubes.* Tubal disease affects approximately 25% of infertile couples and varies from mild adhesions to complete tubal blockage. Treatment for tubal disease can be surgical and, owing to the advances in microsurgery and lasers, success rates (defined as the number of women who become pregnant within one year of surgery) are as high as 30% overall; however, in many cases recognizing this as 'absolute infertility' and moving to *in vitro* fertilization (IVF) early is recommended. The main causes of tubal damage include:
  - *Infection.* This is caused by both bacteria and viruses, usually transmitted sexually. These infections commonly cause inflammation

resulting in tubal scarring and damage. Sometimes a hydrosalpinx, a condition in which the fallopian tube is occluded at both ends and fluid collects in the tube, can be seen on ultrasound scans.
  - *Abdominal diseases.* The most common of these are appendicitis and colitis, causing peritoneal inflammation which can affect the fallopian tubes and lead to scarring and blockage.
  - *Previous surgery.* Pelvic or abdominal surgery can result in adhesions that alter the tubes in such a way that eggs cannot travel through them.
  - *Ectopic pregnancy.* Pregnancies that occur within the tube rather than uterus often cause irreversible tubal damage.
  - *Congenital defects.* In rare cases, women may be born with genetic defects leading to tubal or uterine abnormalities, e.g. septate uterus.

Endometriosis

Endometriosis has long been implicated in affecting the fertility potential in various ways [5]. The fecundity of normal couples is approximately 15–20% per month and is directly affected by maternal age, whereas the fecundity of women suffering from endometriosis drops to 2–10% per month [1]

Endometriotic spots occur not only in the uterus (adenomyosis), but elsewhere in the abdomen, commonly affecting the fallopian tubes, ovaries, pouch of Douglas and the pelvic peritoneum. A positive diagnosis can only be made by diagnostic laparoscopy.

Male Infertility

Sperm Disorders

Problems with the production and maturation of sperm are the most common causes of male infertility [6]. Sperm may be immature, abnormally shaped, or unable to move properly. Or normal sperm may be produced in abnormally low numbers (oligospermia) or seemingly not at all (azoospermia). This problem may be caused by many different conditions, including the following:

- *Infection or inflammation*, e.g. STIs, prostatitis or mumps virus.
- *Endocrine or hormonal disorders*, e.g. Kallmann syndrome (an absence of or decrease in the function of the male testes).

- *Immunological disorders*; some men produce antibodies to their own sperm.
- *Environmental and lifestyle factors.*
- *Genetic diseases*, most of which are either directly or indirectly associated with sperm abnormalities.
- *Anatomical abnormalities.* Obstructions of the genital tract can cause infertility by partially or totally blocking the flow of seminal fluid. This is commonly due to infection and inflammation, previous surgery or the presence of varicose veins in the scrotum (scrotal varicoceles).
- *Immotile cilia syndrome.* Here, the sperm count is normal but the spermatozoa are non-motile, e.g. Kartagener's syndrome.
- *Mitochondrial deletions.* Mitochondria are structures in the cell responsible for energy production. There are actually a set of genes in the mitochondria separate from the normal chromosome set contained in the nucleus. Recently, it has been discovered that these genes, when altered or deleted, can affect a person's health and/or fertility.
- *Liver disease, renal disease, or treatment for seizure disorders.*
- *Other factors.* Other factors may arise from the defective delivery of sperm into the female genital tract. This could be caused by impotence or premature ejaculation.

Environmental Factors

Changing Family Demographics

Increasing numbers of people are in same sex relationships, and solo mothers (or fathers) are now raising children from birth without a partner. According to figures from the Human Fertilisation and Embryo Authority (HFEA) the numbers of such women are rising and in 2012, 963 had fertility treatment with donor sperm at a UK licensed clinic [7]. Though this is not NHS funded, it is important to recognize that women should be fully counselled about their options.

Initial Assessment

The first consultation is important, as time is paramount for a successful outcome. Determining the woman's goals is key to preventing unhelpful investigations and wasting time.

Women may present with straightforward 'failure to conceive', but commonly they have stopped the combined pill and been tracking their cycle more carefully and have read to some extent around the problem.

Women often present alone for the first consultation and this allows exploration of any guilt or stigma attached to her failure to conceive, and sensitivity when teasing out histories of previous pregnancies, pelvic infection and sexual abuse. This can evoke significant negative emotions for women and can be part of a past not shared with their current partner. Going forward, this gives the opportunity to encourage future transparency with their partner, as they are usually the major support system for the woman. Psychological support and counselling may also be helpful. However, the primary aim should not be lost or overshadowed by the psychological element, as this will often be resolved by achieving an ongoing pregnancy in itself. Following this first consultation, both partners should be encouraged to attend and share appointments.

Infertility History: General

For both parties identify basic history:

- Age
- Smoking status
- Alcohol consumption
- BMI
- History of STIs
- Frequency of unprotected vaginal sexual intercourse
- History of surgery to abdomen or genital organs
- Previous history of major medical or surgical illness.

Infertility History: Female

- Nature of relationship; heterosexual, same sex, single parent
- Length of time trying to conceive
- Parity
- Smear results
- Menstrual history; age started, duration, regularity of cycle, contraception
- Sexual history; pain during intercourse
- Intermenstrual or postcoital bleeding
- Consanguinity
- Genetic abnormalities
- Psychosexual difficulties.

Infertility History: Male

- Any previous fathered pregnancies
- Problems with erection and/or ejaculation
- Previous history of trauma, torsion or operation to testes
- Use of steroids, e.g. for muscle building.

A questionnaire may be useful which includes all the relevant sections to avoid omissions and save time.

Examination

Examination is done to exclude any major findings and identify any higher-risk patients for early onward referral. This would include patients with a fibroid mass, evidence of hirsutism and clinical signs of polycystic ovaries and patients where the pelvis feels fixed or there is nodularity suggestive of endometriosis.

In cases of abnormal semen analysis, examining the male might reveal small or undescended testis, hernia or hydrocele.

Advice

All patients at first consultation should be informed that:

- Lifestyle factors such as weight, smoking and alcohol intake play a major role in fertility, and should be optimized to have the best chance of becoming pregnant. A BMI of >19 but <30 is ideal for both men and women. Smoking cessation is essential.
- Vaginal sexual intercourse two to three days every week is advisable.
- Female fertility and (to a lesser extent) male fertility declines with age.
- Stress can reduce libido and frequency of intercourse, which can contribute to the fertility problems.
- Contacting a fertility support group or having counselling may be helpful.

Local guidelines differ, but ideally patients must have stopped smoking for at least 6 months and have a BMI of <30 to qualify for NHS treatment. If couples are made aware of the guidelines early on, it gives them an opportunity to achieve target BMI even before investigation or treatment starts. It will also help with spontaneous conception.

Advice for specific risk factors

- *Tight underwear.* There is an association between elevated scrotal temperature and reduced semen quality, but it is uncertain whether wearing loose-fitting underwear improves fertility.
- *Occupation.* An enquiry about occupation should be made as some occupations involve exposure to hazards that can reduce male/female fertility; appropriate advice should be offered.
- *Drug use.* Advice should be provided regarding prescription, over-the-counter or recreational drugs which may interfere with male and female fertility.
- *Folic acid.* Women should take folic acid (recommended dose: 0.4 mg/day) before conception and up to 12 weeks' gestation to reduce the risk of having a baby with neural tube defects. Women with a child with a neural tube defect, or who are taking anti-epileptic or diabetic medication, should be recommended a higher dose of 5 mg/day.
- *Complementary therapy.* The effectiveness of complementary therapies for fertility problems has not been properly evaluated; further research is needed before such interventions can be recommended.

Investigations

There is evidence that being treated by a specialist team is likely to improve the effectiveness and efficiency of treatment and is known to improve people's satisfaction with treatment, so while these initial investigations should be done in primary care, further investigation and management requires referral.

Primary Care Investigations

- Female tests
  - FSH and LH – must be done between days 2 and 4 of the cycle
  - Day 21 progesterone (if irregular cycle, can be repeated a week later)
  - FBC, TFTs, oestradiol, prolactin and testosterone
  - Rubella and chlamydia screening
- Male tests
  - Semen analysis – if first results are abnormal, repeat test no sooner than three months later.

If azoospermia or severe oligozoospermia is detected, repeat test as soon as possible.

- If repeat semen analysis is abnormal, then FSH, LH, prolactin, testosterone, TSH tests and genetics tests such as karyotyping, CFTR mutation and Y-chromosome microdeletion should be performed. These may be performed by the specialist fertility team.

Baseline tests are imperative as further more intrusive investigations should only be proceeded with if the couple are both actively engaged.

Investigations Usually Conducted Within an Infertility Service

- *Ovarian reserve testing.* In primary care the use of a day 2–4 FSH is crucial in decision-making for the patient. The current threshold for FSH is above 8.9 IU/L for a low response, and below 4 IU/L for a high response.

  These become of huge significance to women on their journey through delay in fertility.

  Additionally, two other tests of ovarian reserve are supported through NICE:

  - total antral follicle count, ≤4 for a low response and >16 for a high response
  - anti-müllerian hormone (AMH), ≤5.4 pmol/L for a low response and ≥25.0 pmol/L for a high response [8]

  These will usually be offered in a specialist clinic setting to support the decision-making for NHS IVF referral. The woman's age and other parameters are commonly no more than markers of the ageing ovary.

- *HSG.* The simplest test to check a woman's tubal patency is with an x-ray and dye test called a hystero-salpinogram. The radio-opaque dye is inserted through the cervical os, so is similar to having a smear test allowing an outline of the uterus and tubes. HSG can identify areas of adhesions (scarring), polyps and fibroids, as well as congenital abnormalities. The dye may show up blockages anywhere along the tube.

- *HyCoSy.* Hystero-salpingo-contrast sonography uses an ultrasound scan and contrast medium to get a more detailed image of the uterus, ovaries and tubes. This test is used to check for polycystic ovaries, fibroids, polyps and other problems in the pelvis, as well as tubal patency.

- *Laparoscopy.* This is a more invasive investigation, but it is often considered the 'gold standard'. It is usually performed if a woman has a history of pelvic surgery (such as an appendectomy), pelvic pain or other symptoms, or if an HSG highlights a possible problem. Laparoscopy has the advantage of being able to examine the outside of the tubes and uterus to check for adhesions and endometriosis. A dye is usually passed through the inside of the tubes to check they are patent. An exploratory laparoscopy allows treatment of conditions such as endometriosis or adhesions at the same time. A hysteroscopy may be performed at the same time as laparoscopy to assess the uterine cavity.

NICE CG 156 recommends women with no known co-morbidities (such as pelvic inflammatory disease, previous ectopic pregnancy or endometriosis) should be offered HSG or, where appropriate expertise is available, HyCoSy, to screen for tubal occlusion. This is a reliable test for ruling out tubal occlusion and is less invasive. It makes more efficient use of resources than laparoscopy. A systemic review and meta-analysis showed a 92% sensitivity for diagnosing tubal occlusion and 95% specificity [9] in HSG and similar results for HyCoSy.

Management Strategies

The most cost-effective management strategies are provided by attempting to minimize the group of 'unexplained' infertility.

- *Ovulation disorders: polycystic ovaries.* Ovarian stimulation treatments include clomifene citrate, metformin or a combination of these drugs. If there is resistance to clomifene one of the following second-line treatments should be considered: laparoscopic ovarian drilling, combined treatments of clomifene and metformin or gonadotropins.

- *Tubal and uterine disorders.* For women with mild tubal disease, tubal surgery may be more effective than no treatment. Women with hydrosalpinx should be offered salpingectomy, preferably by laparoscopy, before IVF.

  Women with amenorrhoea and intrauterine adhesions should be offered hysteroscopic adhesiolysis to restore menstruation and improve their chance of pregnancy.

- *Managing endometriosis.* There has not been shown to be an association between the extent of the disease and the severity of the symptoms. Women with mild, moderate or severe disease should be offered laparoscopic surgical ablation or resection of endometriosis plus adhesiolysis to improve fertility. Women with ovarian endometriomas should also be offered laparoscopic cystectomy.

Male Factor Infertility

Dependent on the cause and severity the following may be considered:

- Assisted reproductive technologies:
  - *Artificial insemination.* This procedure places large numbers of healthy sperm either at the entrance of the cervix or into the partner's uterus, to have direct access to the fallopian tubes.
  - *IVF, GIFT and other techniques. In vitro* fertilization and gamete intrafallopian transfers have been used to treat male infertility. As is the case with artificial insemination, IVF and similar techniques offer the opportunity to prepare sperm *in vitro*, so that oocytes are exposed to an optimal concentration of high quality, motile sperm.
  - *Microsurgical fertilization* (microinjection techniques, such as intracytoplasmic sperm injection). This treatment is used to facilitate sperm penetration by injection of a single sperm into the oocyte.
- *Drug therapy.* A small percentage of infertile men have a hormonal disorder that can be treated with hormone therapy.
- *Surgery.* This is designed to overcome anatomical barriers that impede sperm production and maturation or ejaculation. Procedures to remove varicose veins in the scrotum (varicocele) can occasionally serve to improve the quality of sperm.

Unexplained Infertility

A great deal of research has gone into the medical management of unexplained infertility and it is clear there is much overtreatment. Firstly, in a recent meta-analysis from Holland, the authors point out that treatment often seemed to delay the much wanted successful outcome [10]. Secondly, some mild causes of infertility – for example, low sperm count – condemn already anxious couples to more psychological distress. Thirdly, it is very clear that where no cause is found, there is an excellent chance of having a pregnancy naturally without expensive treatment.

Perhaps the message should be – 'Just think of the number of women who became pregnant spontaneously after several treatment cycles have failed'. NICE 2013 states that women with unexplained fertility should not be treated with ovarian stimulation drugs, but should be encouraged to have regular unprotected sex for a total of two years (this includes up to one year before investigations) before IVF will be considered.

Prediction of IVF Success

Clearly the key to cost-effective management is the identification of those most likely to achieve a live birth through IVF, which has led to the introduction of access criteria.

Currently NICE guidelines suggest women under the age of 42 should be offered at least one full cycle of IVF treatment if they have evidence of a good ovarian reserve.

Other criteria, such as excluding those with a live child have been added; however, due to current financial pressures there is widespread variation on the adoption of the NICE guideline which is leading to a concern about a 'postcode lottery' in provision and care.

Post-treatment Outcomes

Fertility care doesn't end with a positive pregnancy test. Many of the couples who have been through fertility care will have increased risks relating either to their fertility problem or maternal age alone. In addition to this, despite the HFEA aim to reduce twin pregnancy rates down to 10% for IVF patients, the rates can still be considerably higher between centres. Twin pregnancies are by definition a high-risk pregnancy and NICE supports single embryo transfer in those with higher chances of successful treatment.

It is important to stress that NICE CG 156 recommends informing people considering IVF that the absolute risks of long-term adverse outcomes in children born as a result of IVF are low.

Conclusion

It is essential to introduce discussions of family planning to women in their 20s and 30s early on in general practice. Contraception consultations present a golden opportunity for this, as well as educating patients to be thoughtful about their general and sexual health. Moreover, it is never too early to address fertility-related lifestyle factors with patients, and raise awareness of declining fertility and increased risks of pregnancy, including miscarriage, with age.

Investigations in primary care should be undertaken promptly to prevent delay in initiating treatment and referral; recognizing 'at risk groups' early on allows referral without delay.

The first consultation is essential to managing expectations. The patient should have a clear idea of the process ahead and the time scales involved. As a GP it is critical to know the local criteria for NHS-funded treatment to best inform the patient, allowing them a head start on stopping smoking and reducing their weight where possible. Empathy and transparency of the clinician as well as local support groups and fertility forums may be invaluable in supporting patients along their journey.

References

1. National Institute for Health and Clinical Excellence (NICE). Fertility: assessment and treatment for people with fertility problems (update). (Clinical guideline 156.) 2013. www.nice.org.uk/CG156 (accessed September 2016).

2. Human Fertilisation and Embryology Authority (HFEA). Facts and figures. 2006. www.hfea.gov.uk (accessed September 2016).

3. Brkovich A, Fisher W, Psychological distress and infertility: forty years of research. *J Psychosom Obstet Gynaecol* 1998;19:218–228.

4. Roberts J, Ronn R, Tallon N, Holzer H, Fertility preservation in reproductive-age women facing gonadotoxic treatments. *Curr Oncol* 2015;22(4): e294–304.

5. Bulletti C, Coccia ME, Battistoni S, Borini A, Endometriosis and infertility. *J Assist Reprod Genet* 2010;27(8):441–447.

6. Jungwirth A, Diemer T, Dohle G, Giwercman A, Guidelines on male infertility. European Association of Urology 2015. http://uroweb.org/wp-content/uploads/17-Male-Infertility_LR.pdf (accessed September 2016).

7. Human Fertilisation and Embryology Authority (HFEA). Fertility treatment in 2010: Trends and figures. 2011. www.hfea.gov.uk (accessed September 2016).

8. La Marca A, Sighinolfi G, Radi D, *et al*. Anti-Müllerian hormone (AMH) as a predictive marker in assisted reproductive technology (ART). *Hum Reprod Update* 2010;16(2):113–130.

9. Maheux-Lacroix S, Boutin A, Moore L, *et al*. Hysterosalpingosonography for diagnosing tubal occlusion in subfertile women: a systematic review with meta-analysis. *Syst Rev* 2013;2:50.

10. Kersten F, Hermens RP, Braat DD, *et al*. Overtreatment in couples with unexplained infertility. *Hum Reprod* 2015;30(1):71–80.

Chapter 10

Ectopic Pregnancy from a Primary Care Perspective

Jacqui Tuckey and Chantal Simonis

Key Points

- Always include ectopic pregnancy in your differential diagnosis for women of reproductive age with abdominal pain.
- Pain and bleeding in early pregnancy is an ectopic pregnancy until proven otherwise.
- Not all women with ectopic pregnancy have typical symptoms.
- Most women with ectopic pregnancy do not have any known risk factors.
- Women with a history of ectopic pregnancy should be offered access to early ultrasound scanning in any subsequent pregnancy to determine location.
- No method of contraception is contraindicated in a woman solely because she has had an ectopic pregnancy.
- The psychological sequelae of ectopic pregnancy are often overlooked.

Case Scenario: Laura

Laura is a 37-year-old patient presenting to a tertiary fertility clinic with a four-year history of secondary subfertility. She had a right salpingectomy for ectopic pregnancy in a previous relationship. Diagnostic laparoscopy in 2014 had shown an absent right fallopian tube, a normal, patent left tube and the presence of minimal endometriosis. Her partner had a normal semen analysis and two conceptions with a previous partner (resulting in a termination of pregnancy and an ectopic).

The couple underwent an IVF cycle resulting in the transfer of two embryos. Two weeks later a urinary pregnancy test was positive. Laura attended at seven weeks' gestation for an early pregnancy scan. On questioning, she commented that she had noticed a small amount of brown vaginal loss the week before. This had settled and she had not had any pain.

Transvaginal pelvic ultrasound scan showed an empty uterus with a thickened endometrium. A left adnexal mass could be seen and there was a small amount of blood in the pouch of Douglas. Laura was transferred straight to the gynaecology ward and underwent emergency laparoscopy. This confirmed the diagnosis of left ampullary ectopic pregnancy and she underwent laparoscopic salpingectomy.

Introduction

An ectopic pregnancy is one which implants outside of the endometrial cavity. Without timely diagnosis and treatment it may be a life-threatening situation [1]. Most ectopic pregnancies are tubal (98%), with the remainder occurring in the abdomen, ovary or cervix [2]. Of tubal pregnancies, 80% occur in the ampulla.

Prevalence

There are approximately 11,800 ectopic pregnancies in the UK each year, a prevalence of 11:1000 pregnancies [3]. The incidence is increasing worldwide, mainly due to the increased incidence of pelvic inflammatory disease caused by *Chlamydia trachomatis*. Ectopic pregnancy is more common following IVF, with an incidence of 4% [4]. This is because of the proportion of women undergoing assisted conception who have underlying tubal pathology. For individual women with known tubal damage, however, their risk of ectopic pregnancy is lower after IVF than if spontaneous pregnancy occurs.

Heterotopic pregnancy, with the presence of a simultaneous intra- and extra-uterine pregnancy, occurs in 1:4000 pregnancies. It is more common after

Women's Health in Primary Care, edited by Anne Connolly and Amanda Britton. Published by Cambridge University Press © Cambridge University Press 2017

IVF because of the increase in multiple pregnancies. It is of vital importance, therefore, that a health care professional carrying out pelvic ultrasound scan for pregnancy is informed if the patient has had IVF and how many embryos have been replaced. Any practitioner must be adequately trained and must fully assess the pelvis, even if an intrauterine pregnancy is seen, or this rare type of pregnancy will potentially be missed.

Risk Factors

The main risk factor for ectopic pregnancy is tubal damage from previous ectopic pregnancy, pelvic inflammatory disease, endometriosis or tubal surgery. Faulty implantation of developing embryos occurs because of a defect in the anatomy or function of the damaged fallopian tube. The incidence of tubal damage increases with successive episodes of PID (13% after a single episode, 35% after two and 75% after three episodes) [5]. Overall, a patient with a history of ectopic pregnancy has a 10–25% chance of a further ectopic pregnancy and a 50–80% chance of an intrauterine pregnancy.

There has been much written about the risk of ectopic pregnancy with IUD use for contraception. A meta-analysis [6] of case-control studies published in the 1990s reported no increased risk of ectopic pregnancy associated with current copper IUD use. NICE guidance [7] on long-acting reversible contraception (LARC) states that the risk of ectopic pregnancy associated with the use of copper IUDs is lower than using no contraception. The UK Medical Eligibility Criteria (UKMEC) for contraceptive use [8] considers past ectopic pregnancy to be a condition for which there is no restriction for the use of IUDs. The absolute risk of ectopic pregnancy is not increased by the use of intrauterine contraception, because the method is highly effective. However, if a woman becomes pregnant using an IUD, it is likely to be ectopic and so this must be excluded. The bottom line is that IUDs are better at preventing pregnancies in the uterus than the tube. Faculty of Sexual and Reproductive Healthcare guidance on intrauterine contraception [9] says that women should be advised that the overall risk of ectopic pregnancy is very low, approximately 1 in 1000 at five years of use and no particular device has a lower rate. Women choosing intrauterine methods of contraception should be informed about symptoms of ectopic pregnancy.

Complications

Ectopic pregnancy presents a major health problem for women of reproductive age. Failure to make a prompt diagnosis can result in tubal rupture, which in turn can lead to haemorrhage, shock, DIC and ultimately death. The Confidential Enquiry into Maternal Death, last reported in 2011 [10], for the triennium 2006–8 showed a reduction in case fatality rate to 16.9/100,000 ectopic pregnancies. This suggested that previous messages concerning the prompt diagnosis of this potentially fatal condition may have been acted upon – but there is still room for improvement. There were 11 early pregnancy deaths in this period; six were ectopic and care was considered to be substandard in half of them. The Confidential Enquiry has now been replaced by MBRRACE UK (Mothers and Babies: Reducing Risks Through Audits and Confidential Enquiries). The format and focus has changed and it will report yearly. In December 2014 figures were published for 2009–12, during which time there were 357 maternal deaths (10:100,000 births). Twelve of these were early pregnancy deaths, but the number of ectopic pregnancies was not specified.

A significant consequence of ectopic pregnancy is tubal subfertility. Approximately 40% of women with a history of ectopic pregnancy will not be able to conceive an intrauterine pregnancy spontaneously [2]; 25% of couples having assisted conception treatment will have a diagnosis of tubal subfertility.

When to Suspect an Ectopic Pregnancy

One of the concerns of the Confidential Enquiry into Maternal Deaths, was the difficulty in diagnosing the condition. In our case study, Laura was a fertility patient with a history of previous ectopic pregnancy. She had minimal symptoms, yet the pregnancy was easily detected on ultrasound scan – this is not a common scenario. About one-third of women will have no known risk factors and atypical presentation is common [11].

Ectopic pregnancy should be suspected in women who are pregnant, or have missed a period, with vaginal bleeding or abdominal pain. Review of studies reported in the NICE guidelines [11] report that 93% of women present with abdominal or pelvic pain, 73% with amenorrhoea and 64% with vaginal bleeding. Many women have poor recall for their menstrual history and it is crucial to remember that what is described as a period may not be. Less common symptoms include gastrointestinal symptoms, dizziness, fainting and shoulder tip pain.

The report of the Confidential Enquiry states that GPs should ask all women of reproductive age who have abdominal pain with diarrhoea and vomiting about the risk of pregnancy. A third of women with ectopic pregnancy do not present with vaginal bleeding. If there is any doubt, a urinary pregnancy test (UPT) should be carried out in the surgery. NICE recommend that all health care professionals caring for women of reproductive age should have access to pregnancy tests. The Confidential Enquiry report goes further in suggesting that GPs should consider carrying a pregnancy test in their emergency bag. Fainting and dizziness is uncommon with gastroenteritis, but may occur with a bleeding ectopic pregnancy.

How to Manage a Suspected Ectopic Pregnancy

Management depends primarily on how stable the patient is. Women with bleeding or other symptoms of an early pregnancy complication should have their pulse and blood pressure assessed. Those women who are not haemodynamically stable should be transferred to hospital by ambulance, without undertaking a pelvic examination and with intravenous fluids, if available. Women who are haemodynamically stable should have a UPT to confirm pregnancy and then an abdominal examination should be carried out. If abdominal tenderness is elicited, an ectopic pregnancy should be strongly suspected and immediate admission arranged to an early pregnancy assessment unit (EPAU) or out-of-hours gynaecology service. If abdominal pain and tenderness is absent, a pelvic examination should be carried out to check for pelvic or cervical motion tenderness, and if present urgent admission arranged as above. It is recommended by the NICE Guideline Development Group (GDG) that palpating for adnexal masses when performing pelvic examination for women with pain should be avoided because of the risk of tubal rupture.

Laura was asymptomatic and haemodynamically stable. She did, however, have clear ultrasound findings consistent with an ectopic pregnancy. Had she presented to her GP with this scenario, a same-day referral to an early pregnancy assessment unit would have been the appropriate course of action; a high index of suspicion would have been required.

Early Pregnancy Assessment Unit

Assessment and ultrasound scanning facilities should ideally be available seven days a week for the management of women with complications of early pregnancy; they should offer a dedicated service provided by health care professionals competent to diagnose and care for women with pain and bleeding in early pregnancy. These units should have the facility to accept self-referrals from women with previous ectopic pregnancy and recurrent miscarriage. In the primary care setting, expectant management may be used for women less than six weeks' gestation with bleeding, but no pain. Women need to be given clear advice on symptoms to be aware of and how to get help in an emergency. It is vital that GPs know their own local facilities and referral pathways.

The recommendations for women less than six weeks' gestation are based on evidence reviewed by NICE [11] that demonstrates that ultrasound scanning does not always confirm a diagnosis at less than six weeks and many women have spotting in early pregnancy that resolves without needing investigation. Additionally, the expert reviewers were of the opinion that a negative UPT virtually rules out an ectopic. Remember, there are always exceptions and it is crucial to be guided by the patient's signs and symptoms. It is not always possible to be certain of gestation and women are often poor historians when it comes to their menstrual history.

Support and Information Giving

Early pregnancy complications can cause significant distress to women and their partners, even when the pregnancy is unplanned. Past history will contribute to how the patient copes with the situation in which she finds herself. Women will react differently to early pregnancy complications and need to be provided with information and support in a sensitive way. If you make a referral, it is important to explain why and what she can expect to happen next.

Diagnosis in Secondary Care

Women who are haemodynamically unstable will be admitted for urgent surgical management. For stable women in whom an ectopic pregnancy is suspected, a transvaginal ultrasound will be carried out to determine if the pregnancy is intrauterine, definite or probable ectopic, a molar pregnancy or a pregnancy of unknown location. If the diagnosis is uncertain, serial human chorionic gonadotrophin (hCG) levels, repeat transvaginal scans or laparoscopy may be used. It is important that the woman understands that it can sometimes require repeated investigations to make a diagnosis – this clearly may add to her distress.

Treatment Options

The treatment options for a haemodynamically stable woman are surgical, medical or, rarely, expectant. A small proportion of women with a pregnancy of unknown location who have minimal or no symptoms and remain well can simply be watched. Intervention may take place if symptoms develop or worsen, or if hCG levels are not steadily falling.

Laparoscopic surgery may involve removal of the tube (salpingectomy) or tubal incision and removal of the pregnancy (salpingotomy). Following salpingotomy, serial hCG levels will be required to ensure that no persistent trophoblast remains. Salpingectomy is the treatment of choice if the tube is very diseased or damaged as there is a high risk of recurrence. Salpingotomy should be offered, as an alternative, to women with contralateral tubal damage, but up to 1:5 will require further treatment, either medical or surgical. Women who are rhesus negative and undergo surgical management should be offered anti-D prophylaxis.

Medical management with methotrexate may be offered to women as a first-line treatment, provided they can return for follow-up. They must have no significant pain, an unruptured ectopic pregnancy with an adnexal mass less than 35 mm and no visible heartbeat, hCG level <1500 IU/L and no intrauterine pregnancy on scan. Provided women are appropriately selected, success rates are comparable to laparoscopic salpingotomy.

Methotrexate is a folic acid antagonist which can be given intramuscularly (IM) or injected into the ectopic pregnancy. Direct injection into the ectopic requires laparoscopy and success rates are lower than with systemic methotrexate. The currently used regimen is IM methotrexate 50 mg/m^2 (the body surface area of a patient is calculated from a formula using weight and height measurements). Serum hCG levels are checked on days four and seven and the dosage repeated if they have not fallen by at least 15% [12]. Serum hCG levels are continued weekly until a negative result is obtained. Approximately 14% of women will require a repeat dose and less than 10% will require subsequent

surgical intervention; 75% of women will experience pain and a proportion of women will require hospital admission for observation. Some will report conjunctivitis, stomatitis and gastrointestinal upset.

A number of systematic reviews have examined reproductive outcomes following surgical treatment, but there are no RCTs. There is a suggestion that intrauterine pregnancy rates may be higher following salpingotomy, but the benefit is likely to be small [12]

In view of her previous history of ectopic pregnancy, it was appropriate that Laura was advised to have a salpingectomy. She had four years of secondary subfertility following her first ectopic and therefore medical management or conservative surgery would not have been a prudent choice for a clearly damaged tube.

Fertility After Ectopic Pregnancy

A woman who has an ectopic pregnancy will want to know what her chances are of having a baby in the future. Studies suggest that about 60% of women who have an ectopic pregnancy will go on to have a spontaneous, viable intrauterine pregnancy [13]. After one ectopic pregnancy the risk of recurrence is 5–20%; this rises to 32% after more than one ectopic.

Controversy exists about the role of surgical treatment in optimizing future fertility. An observational population-based study of 1064 women with ectopic pregnancy 1992–2008 in France gives good information about these issues [14]. The two-year cumulative rate of intrauterine pregnancy (IUP) was 67% after salpingectomy, 76% after salpingotomy and 76% after medical treatment. It must not be forgotten that other factors have an impact on pregnancy rates, with a significantly lower rate for women >35 years. The two-year cumulative risk of recurrence was 18.5% after surgical treatment and 25.5% after methotrexate.

A more recent retrospective cohort study of 618 patients compared outcomes according to the type of surgical treatment [15]. Two-year IUP rates were 55.5% after salpingectomy, 50.9% after salpingotomy and 40.3% after tubal reanastomosis. The recurrence rates at two years were 8.1%, 6.3% and 16.7%, respectively.

Laura's only option for fertility was further assisted conception; fortunately she had some frozen embryos in storage and the plan for her was to use these next. Despite the absence of both fallopian tubes, she will still have a very small risk of cornual ectopic pregnancy. Surgical removal of the tubes will always be as complete as possible, but a cornual stump will remain. Laura will need to have an early ultrasound scan at approximately six weeks' gestation in any future pregnancy to confirm location.

Follow-Up

The psychological cost of ectopic pregnancy is frequently overlooked, as it is often not viewed in the same way as other pregnancy loss [4]. It is thought that women have the same grief reaction as women who experience miscarriage, but they may also have the additional stress of concern about future fertility.

Follow-up is an important part of the process. Sadly this is not always offered in the hospital setting and may fall to the GP, thus it is important to be well informed. It is vital to ensure that any arrangements that have already been made for antenatal care are cancelled and this requires vigilance. There is nothing more distressing to a woman who has experienced an early pregnancy loss than receiving, for example, an appointment for a nuchal scan, and such appointments are not automatically cancelled. Laura had not yet arranged antenatal care with her GP, although he was, of course, advised of her ectopic pregnancy. Laura and her partner were offered counselling within the subfertility clinic setting. It is a requirement of the Human Fertilisation and Embryology Authority (HFEA) that clinics offering assisted conception offer access to specialist counselling if required.

The woman needs to be given the opportunity to discuss any questions she may have about her treatment, future fertility and risk of recurrence. Subsequent pregnancies should be reported promptly so that early location scanning can be arranged. Psychological wellbeing needs to be assessed; grief, anxiety and depression are common after early pregnancy loss and may be as intense as that following any other form of bereavement. Distress is commonly at its worst after four to six weeks and may last for many months. Referral for counselling, preferably with a counsellor experienced in dealing with women after pregnancy loss, if available, may be appropriate. The Ectopic Pregnancy Trust (www.ectopic.org.uk) is a charity supporting those who have experienced ectopic pregnancy and health care professionals looking after them. The Miscarriage Association (www.miscarriageassociation.org.uk) offers similar support.

Don't forget that, like any other conception, an ectopic pregnancy may have been unplanned and unwanted; contraceptive advice may be required. The issues around IUD use have been discussed above, but the recommendations from the Faculty of Sexual and Reproductive Healthcare (FSRH) are that no form of contraception is contraindicated after ectopic pregnancy. Women need reliable, effective contraception; a method with a low failure rate will have a low risk of ectopic. Even women who wish a further pregnancy may require short-term reliable contraception until they have recovered both emotionally and physically, and are ready to try again. Women who are treated with methotrexate should be advised to avoid pregnancy for three months as there is a possible teratogenic risk – this needs to be clearly stated when they choose this treatment method. As she no longer had either fallopian tube, Laura could not conceive spontaneously and therefore did not require contraceptive advice.

Conclusion

Ectopic pregnancy is a common complication of early pregnancy, and the incidence has risen worldwide due to the increase in pelvic infection, mainly as a result of chlamydia infection. It can result in significant morbidity, affecting both physical and mental health. Future fertility is affected and there is a risk of recurrence, which varies depending on method of treatment undertaken. Tubal infertility accounts for the diagnosis in about a quarter of couples attending an infertility service.

Ectopic pregnancy can be difficult to diagnose and this was one concern raised by the Confidential Enquiry into Maternal Deaths. Deaths from early pregnancy complications are low, but there are a consistent small number of deaths from ectopic pregnancy, many of which are avoidable. Any maternal death is a tragedy; we will only avoid deaths from ectopic pregnancy by vigilance. The adage that a woman of reproductive age at risk of pregnancy with abdominal pain has an ectopic pregnancy until proven otherwise is one that is well worth remembering.

References

1. Farquhar CM, Ectopic pregnancy. *Lancet* 2005; 366(9485):583–591.

2. Barnhart KT, Clinical practice: Ectopic pregnancy. *NEJM* 2009;361(4):379–387.

3. Draycott T, Lewis G, Stephens I, Executive summary: Eighth Report of the Confidential Enquiries into Maternal Deaths in the UK. *BJOG* 2011;118(Suppl. 1): e12–e21.

4. Tay JL, Moore J, Walker JJ, Ectopic pregnancy. *BMJ* 2000;320(7239):916–919.

5. Sepilian VP, Ectopic pregnancy. 2014 (updated). *Medscape*: 2041923.

6. Xiong X, Buekens P, Wollast E, IUD use and the risk of ectopic pregnancy: A meta-analysis of case-control studies. *Contraception* 1995;52:23–34.

7. National Institute for Health and Clinical Excellence (NICE). Long-acting reversible contraception: the effective and appropriate use of long-acting reversible contraception. 2005.

8. Faculty of Sexual and Reproductive Health Care. UK medical eligibility criteria for contraceptive use (UKMEC 2009). 2009.

9. Faculty of Sexual and Reproductive Health Care. Intrauterine Contraception. Clinical Effectiveness Unit. June 2015.

10. CMACE. Saving mothers' lives. Reviewing maternal deaths to make motherhood safer: 2006–2008. *BJOG* 2011;118 (S1): 1–203. Chapter 6: Deaths in early pregnancy.

11. National Collaborating Centre for Women's and Children's Health Ectopic pregnancy and miscarriage. Diagnosis and initial management in early pregnancy of ectopic pregnancy and miscarriage. (full NICE guideline) Clinical guideline 154. 2012 www.nice.org .uk (accessed September 2016).

12. RCOG Green top Guideline No. 21, Tubal pregnancy, management. 2014 www.rcog.org.uk (accessed September 2016).

13. Sivalingham V, Duncan W, Kirk E, Shepherd L, Horne A, Diagnosis and management of ectopic pregnancy. *J Fam Plann Reprod Healthcare* 2011;37(4): 231–240.

14. De Bennetot M, Rabischong B, Aublet-Cuvelier B, *et al.* Fertility after tubal ectopic pregnancy: results of a population-based study. *Fertil Steril* 2012;98(5):1271–1276.

15. Li J, Jiang K, Zhao F, Fertility outcome analysis after surgical management of tubal ectopic pregnancy: a retrospective cohort study. *BMJ Open* 2015;5(9): e007339.

Management of Miscarriage in Primary Care

Sally Kidsley and Najia Aziz

Key Points

- Miscarriage is defined as the spontaneous loss of a pregnancy before 24 weeks' gestation.
- Miscarriage occurs in up to 25% of pregnancies and 50% of cases of miscarriage are due to chromosomal abnormalities.
- Recurrent miscarriage is three or more consecutive miscarriages.
- Most common signs associated with threatened miscarriage are pain and bleeding, it is extremely important to exclude ectopic pregnancies in women who have bleeding and pain in early pregnancy. Therefore it is essential that primary care practitioners are able to perform a quick and sensitive pregnancy test.
- An ectopic pregnancy may also present with pain and no bleeding. Primary care clinicians must have a low threshold for performing a pregnancy test in sexually active women presenting with pelvic pain.
- Miscarriage can have a long-lasting, psychological effect on the woman and her partner, and ongoing emotional support may be needed during the loss and in future pregnancies.
- The management of missed miscarriage includes the following choices: expectant, medical and surgical. It is important that the woman (and her partner, if appropriate) is involved in making the choice.

Definition

A miscarriage is defined as the spontaneous loss of a pregnancy before 24 weeks' gestation [1]. About 15–25% of recognized pregnancies end in miscarriage, 85% of which will occur before 10 weeks of gestation [2,3].

Miscarriage can have a massive psychological impact on the woman and her partner, and this impact may persist for many months after the miscarriage itself [4]. However, it is important to reassure women that a miscarriage will usually not affect her ability to become pregnant again and carry a future pregnancy to full term [5].

Types (Classification)

Miscarriage is usually defined as below, and the management will be different for each type [3,6]:

- *Threatened miscarriage*: usually mild symptoms of bleeding with little or no pain. The cervical os is closed.
- *Inevitable miscarriage*: usually presents with heavy bleeding with clots and pain. The cervical os is open. The pregnancy will not continue and will proceed to incomplete or complete miscarriage.
- *Incomplete miscarriage*: this occurs when the products of conception are partially expelled. Many incomplete miscarriages can be unrecognized missed miscarriages.
- *Missed miscarriage*: the foetus is dead, but retained. The uterus is small for dates. A pregnancy test can remain positive for several days after the foetus has died. It usually presents with a history of threatened miscarriage and persistent, brown discharge. Early pregnancy symptoms may have decreased or gone.
- *Recurrent miscarriage*: when a woman suffers three or more consecutive miscarriages.

Causes

In the majority of miscarriages no cause will be found, although it is thought that chromosomal

---

Women's Health in Primary Care, edited by Anne Connolly and Amanda Britton. Published by Cambridge University Press
© Cambridge University Press 2017

abnormalities can account for about 50% of cases [3]. This lack of understanding often adds to the concerns and upset of the parents as they look for a reason or something to change in order to prevent the problem recurring.

Other causes may include:

- Abnormal foetal development
- Genetically balanced parental translocation
- Uterine abnormality
- Incompetent cervix (second trimester miscarriage)
- Placental failure
- Multiple pregnancies
- Immunological issues
- Infections
- Endocrine, e.g. luteal phase deficiency, polycystic ovarian syndrome.

Risk Factors

In most cases there are no obvious factors that could have predicted a miscarriage, but there are some risk factors where miscarriage is more likely to occur [1]:

- High BMI (>30 kg/m^2) is associated with reduced fertility and increased risk of miscarriage
- Low BMI (<18 kg/m^2)
- Age over 35 years [4]
- The longer the length of time it takes the woman to conceive, the higher the chance of miscarriage
- A new partner
- Paternal age over 45 years
- Sustained stress, particularly at work
- Multiple pregnancies.

Differential Diagnosis [6]

Bleeding in early pregnancy is common and occurs in approximately one-third of pregnancies [3]. It is important to determine the cause of her bleeding, as there are several issues which may be totally unrelated to the pregnancy and some causes are more serious than others. She will obviously be anxious about the pregnancy and will want to understand if this is normal viable pregnancy bleeding, which requires reassurance, or whether she is experiencing a miscarriage.

The main causes of bleeding in early pregnancy can be:

- Normal viable pregnancy
- Ectopic pregnancy

- Molar pregnancy
- Cervical polyps
- Cervical ectropion
- Gynaecology cancers.

Abdominal pain is also relatively frequent in early pregnancy and is more concerning. This must be investigated to exclude the following:

- Ectopic pregnancy
- Torsion or rupture of ovarian cysts
- Fibroid torsion
- Urinary tract infection
- Appendicitis.

Case Scenario

Gemma is a 32-year-old primary school teacher who attends evening surgery in tears. She and Adam, her partner, have been trying to conceive for 18 months and she is now seven weeks' pregnant. She started bleeding when at school earlier today and has requested an emergency appointment.

She tells you that her bleeding has been light and painless.

It was important that Gemma was seen as an emergency appointment because of the anxiety she has about her pregnancy. It is important that she is carefully questioned about any pain she is experiencing and about the amount of bleeding she has had, which will give some indication about the urgency of her management.

Any woman who presents in early pregnancy with bleeding needs to be told that this is a threatened miscarriage. Threatened miscarriage is the most common complication of early pregnancy, occurring in approximately 20% of pregnant women before 20 weeks of gestation. Although many women who have threatened miscarriage go on to have a successful pregnancy, there is an increase in risk of miscarriage in the same pregnancy of 2.6 times and 17% of women with threatened miscarriage go on to have further complications in the same pregnancy. In the UK, it is estimated that around a quarter of a million women each year suffer a miscarriage. This loss is associated with a significant amount of physical and psychological morbidity and they require sensitivity and support.

A woman who presents with bleeding and associated pain, or pain alone, in early pregnancy, needs to have an ectopic pregnancy excluded as a matter of urgency. Ectopic pregnancies affect about 11 in every 1000 pregnancies, but these women have increased problems with morbidity and a maternal mortality rate of 0.2% linked to the ectopic pregnancy.

There are also many women who have no symptoms or signs at all during their early pregnancy but will be diagnosed with a missed miscarriage at their first antenatal scan.

It is important for all working in primary care to understand the referral route into the local early pregnancy assessment unit or emergency gynaecological unit to avoid delay in managing cases of early pregnancy bleeding. Most painless bleeds can wait for an appointment within a day or two, as long as the blood loss is not too much. It is also important to have access to in-house pregnancy testing for women who present with pelvic pain ± vaginal bleeding, as a low threshold for urgent referral should be made in women with a positive pregnancy test and any concerns that the presentation may be due to an ectopic pregnancy; about a third of women with an ectopic pregnancy will have no known risk factors. A woman with a positive pregnancy test and pain needs urgent assessment. A transvaginal, rather than an abdominal, ultrasound scan is the gold standard route of examination in early pregnancy, and the woman should be advised of this before attending, to minimize the distress it could engender [1,3]. Women should also be reassured that the scan will have no detrimental effect on the pregnancy itself.

Case Scenario

Gemma is referred into the local EPAU and an appointment is made for the following morning. She is given advice about how to manage if she develops heavier bleeding or significant pain overnight. She is told to attend the unit at 9am, having only had a drink of water.

The following are the recommendations set out by NICE in the guideline on ectopic pregnancy and miscarriage regarding the diagnosis and management of early pregnancy complications [6]:

- Refer women who are haemodynamically unstable, or in whom there is significant concern about the degree of pain or bleeding, directly to A&E.
- Be aware that atypical presentation for ectopic pregnancy is common.

Box 11.1

Symptoms and signs of ectopic pregnancy include:
- Common symptoms:
  · Abdominal or pelvic pain
  · Amenorrhoea or missed period
  · Vaginal bleeding with or without clots
- Other reported symptoms:
  · Breast tenderness
  · Gastrointestinal symptoms
  · Dizziness, fainting or syncope
  · Shoulder tip pain
  · Urinary symptoms
  · Passage of tissue
  · Rectal pressure or pain on defecation
- Most common signs:
  · Pelvic tenderness
  · Adnexal tenderness
  · Abdominal tenderness

- Be aware that ectopic pregnancy can present with a variety of symptoms (Box 11.1).

Refer to an EPAU women with bleeding or other symptoms and signs of early pregnancy complications who have:

- A pregnancy of six weeks' gestation or more or
- A pregnancy of uncertain gestation.

The urgency of this referral depends on the clinical situation.

As pregnancy tests become cheaper to buy and more sensitive, women are presenting very early in a pregnancy with vaginal bleeding. These women are equally as anxious and expect referral for urgent assessment and scan. NICE have advised expectant management for women with a pregnancy of less than six weeks' gestation who are bleeding, but not in pain, as an ultrasound scan in these women can be unreliable and may not be sensitive enough to be able to confirm a viable pregnancy. These women require supportive and reassuring management, including:

- Repeating a urine pregnancy test after 7–10 days and return if it is positive
- A negative pregnancy test means that the pregnancy has miscarried
- To return if their symptoms continue or worsen.

Women who return with worsening symptoms and signs that could suggest ectopic pregnancy should be referred to an EPAU for further assessment. The decision about whether she should be seen immediately or within 24 hours will depend on the clinical situation as above.

Emotional Support and Information Giving

Women who present with bleeding in early pregnancy, and their partners, require information and support. Their reaction to complications or the loss of a pregnancy will be variable and as expected in primary care, all health care professionals managing such cases need to be trained in sensitive communication [7].

Women and their partners should be kept fully informed about the possible causes, anticipated course of the problem and investigations they will receive and when. The evidence-based information should be provided in a variety of formats including:

- When and how to seek help if existing symptoms worsen or new symptoms develop, including a 24-hour contact telephone number.
- What to expect during the time she is waiting for an ultrasound scan.
- What to expect during the course of care (including expectant management), such as the potential length and extent of pain and/or bleeding, and the possible side effects. This information should be tailored to the care she receives.
- Information about postoperative care (for women undergoing surgery).
- What to expect during the recovery period – for example, when it is possible to resume sexual activity and/or try to conceive again, and what to do if she becomes pregnant again. This information should also be tailored to the care she receives.
- Information about the likely impact of her treatment on future fertility.
- Where to access support and counselling services, including leaflets, web addresses and helpline numbers for support organizations.

These consultations require sufficient time to discuss issues during the course of their care with additional appointments if required and a follow-up appointment should be offered to all women following pregnancy loss.

Management of Miscarriage [3,6,8]

The management options for miscarriage are:

- Expectant
- Medical
- Surgical (local and general anaesthetic).

> **Case Scenario**
>
> Gemma is seen in the EPAU on the following day and has a transvaginal ultrasound scan. The scan confirms a non-viable pregnancy. She is given the option of expectant, medical or surgical treatments and she opts for expectant management.

Expectant Management

A woman with a confirmed diagnosis of miscarriage can be offered expectant management for 7–14 days (as the first-line management strategy), assuming there is no other concern, such as infection or increased bleeding risk, e.g. history of coagulopathies.

She should be informed about the risk of infection (1 in 100) and the risk of haemorrhage warranting blood transfusion (2 in 100). In some women, bleeding and pain will not occur at all during expectant management, which will indicate that the process of miscarriage has not started. In some women, bleeding will persist or increase, which will suggest incomplete miscarriage. In both of these scenarios, a repeat scan is offered and all treatment options (continued expectant, medical or surgical management) are discussed, allowing her to make an informed choice. If she opts for continued expectant management a further review is arranged at 14 days after the first follow-up appointment.

Women undergoing expectant management of miscarriage are offered oral and written information about what to expect throughout the process, advice on pain relief and where and when to get help in an emergency. Once expectant management is completed, a woman is advised to undertake a urine pregnancy test after three weeks and to contact the health care professional if it is positive.

Medical Management

According to the NICE guidelines [6], vaginal misoprostol can be offered for the medical treatment of a missed or incomplete miscarriage. A woman can choose to have her treatment administered orally if this is her preference. The following treatment options are suggested:

- *Missed miscarriage*: a single dose of 800 micrograms of misoprostol
- *Incomplete miscarriage*: a single dose of either 600 or 800 micrograms of misoprostol.

All women receiving medical management of miscarriage are offered pain relief and anti-emetics as needed. She is informed about what to expect throughout the process, including the length and extent of bleeding and the potential side effects of treatment, including pain, diarrhoea and vomiting. She should also be advised to undertake a urine pregnancy test after three weeks following her medical management and to contact a health care professional if it is positive. The risk of infection and haemorrhage is the same as for expectant management.

Surgical Management

The options for surgical management include:

- Manual vacuum aspiration
- Surgical management under general anaesthesia.

Manual vacuum aspiration (MVA)

Manual vacuum aspiration is undertaken under local anaesthetic in an outpatient or clinic setting. A local anaesthetic is injected into the cervix and the cervix is then dilated (if needed) gradually. A narrow suction tube is inserted into the uterus to remove the pregnancy tissue by aspiration. The procedure normally takes about 10 minutes in total.

Surgical management

Surgical management is carried out in theatre under general anaesthetic. All women undergoing surgical management of miscarriage are provided with oral and written information about the treatment and what to expect during and after the procedure. The risks associated with surgical management are:

- Infection (2–3 in 100)
- Perforation of uterus (1 in 200), plus possible damage to other organs and blood vessels
- Haemorrhage (less than 1 in 200)
- Repeat procedure for evacuation of retained products

- General anaesthetic reaction (1 in 10,000) and death (1 in 100,000) or local anaesthetic reaction (in case of MVA)
- Hysterectomy (1 in 30,000), if there is uncontrolled bleeding or severe damage to uterus.

Case Scenario

Gemma miscarries at home and after a few days her bleeding settles. She returns to the surgery to ask for a sick note as she feels unable to return to her busy job working with young children just yet. She is tearful and anxious about the same problem happening if she was to become pregnant again.

She has been advised to look at the Miscarriage Association website and offered a further appointment after a week for further support. Adam has been very supportive, but he has had to return to work as he is self-employed as a joiner.

Postmiscarriage Care [3,6]

Women should be informed about how to access support and counselling services, including leaflets, web addresses and helpline numbers for support organizations. The Royal College of Obstetricians and Gynaecologists and the Miscarriage Association has useful patient information leaflets that can be accessed through their website [9].

Women who do not wish to become pregnant should be advised to commence contraception immediately after the miscarriage. Further information on the use of contraception can be obtained from the Faculty of Sexual and Reproductive Healthcare or Family Planning Association websites [3,7].

Anti-D rhesus prophylaxis should be given at a dose of 250 IU (50 micrograms) to all rhesus-negative women who have a surgical procedure to manage an ectopic pregnancy or a miscarriage.

Anti-D rhesus prophylaxis is not given to women in the following cases:

- Medical management for an ectopic pregnancy or miscarriage
- Threatened miscarriage or complete miscarriage
- Pregnancy of unknown location.

Recurrent Miscarriage [10]

Recurrent miscarriage is defined as:

- Three or more consecutive miscarriages before 10 weeks' gestation.

- One or more morphologically normal foetal loss occurring after 10 weeks' gestation.

The risk of recurrent miscarriage is higher if:

- A women is overweight
- A woman is over the age of 35 and her partner is over the age of 40.

The known causes of recurrent miscarriage are:

- Anti-phospholipid syndrome (APLS)
- Blood clotting disorders (factor V Leiden, factor II (prothrombin), gene mutation and protein S deficiency)
- Chromosomal abnormalities
- Cervical incompetency
- Other causes that may play a part but there is not enough evidence: uterine anomalies (bicornuate or septate uterus), polycystic ovarian syndrome (PCOS), infections (toxoplasmosis, rubella) and immune problems (raised levels of uterine NK cells).

All women who have had recurrent miscarriage should be offered a referral to the gynaecology department for an appointment for investigations. The recommended tests include:

- Assessment for antiphospholipid antibodies (lupus anticoagulant and anticardiolipin). Two tests are done 6–12 weeks apart. If antiphospholipid antibodies are found, treatment with aspirin and heparin is considered in future pregnancies.
- Pelvic ultrasound to detect uterine abnormalities. If the ultrasound shows any abnormality, then hysteroscopy or laparoscopy is offered to confirm the diagnosis.
- Investigations for genetic abnormalities in both partners.
- Investigations for foetal genetic abnormalities (if foetal tissue is available).
- Thrombophilia screen (if history of late miscarriages).

A woman should be advised that it may not be possible to determine the cause of her recurrent miscarriage, but women in whom no cause is found may be reassured that the prognosis for a future successful pregnancy is 75%.

The Miscarriage Association has produced the following patient information leaflets:

- Investigations following recurrent miscarriage
- Antiphospholipid syndrome and pregnancy loss.

Psychological Effects

It is clear from research that health care professionals can make a huge difference to a woman's experience of early pregnancy complications and loss. The health care professional is unable to do much in terms of changing the outcome of the pregnancy, but actually, just by being sympathetic, taking some time, listening to the woman, and really understanding that this may be a very significant loss in her life and that of her partner, it can really make a big difference to her [1].

The language used when describing miscarriage can have both a negative and a positive effect on the woman and her partner. The RCOG recommends that a more patient-focussed terminology should be adopted.

It is very common for women and their partners to blame themselves after a pregnancy loss, and the first thing a health care professional needs to do is to reassure the woman and her partner (if appropriate) that this is not the case [5]. This is often worse if the couple have been trying to conceive for a long time, so being aware of the history of the woman and her partner is vitally important.

In terms of alcohol, caffeine, stress and allergy to her partner's sperm, there's certainly no evidence that any of these make any difference to the outcome of the miscarriage [1].

Sometimes, women and their partners feel they must just get on with their lives, regardless, and haven't been given the opportunity to talk about the pregnancy loss. It is important, as a health care professional, to realise that women and their partners often experience common bereavement reactions, including sadness, anger and guilt that is expected with any other bereavement.

The bereavement process with miscarriage is often made more difficult because there is no foetus to bury and mourn, and sometimes it is difficult for the woman and partner to find the right amount of time and support to deal with their loss[4].

Within the first six months following miscarriage, 30–50% of women will have symptoms of depression, and the woman needs to be reassured that this is common and likely to improve with time, but that it should be addressed and managed as appropriate [1].

There can be lots of stresses on a relationship anyway and often the partner who is trying to support the woman feels like he is unable to grieve himself and, as with other problems around perinatal mental health, his needs are often ignored. So as a health care professional it is important to also consider the partner in cases of miscarriage.

Open and empathetic listening and sign-posting to relevant information and support groups can really support the couple at this distressing time. Some women appear to cope well initially after the miscarriage and require support later, so the initial contact should make sure she is aware that she can return later if she feels this would be helpful.

> **Case Scenario**
>
> Gemma returned to clinic after a week to request a renewal of her sick note for a further week. She had found the on-line information supportive and had spoken to a couple of her friends, who she had found out had already had a miscarriage. She found this support helpful and was planning to return to work on the following Monday.

Conclusion

Miscarriage is a common complication, but not an insignificant part, of early pregnancy and needs to be recognized as an important part of the life of a woman, and her partner. It is important that one is aware of the causes of bleeding in early pregnancy, and who requires referral urgently and who can be managed by referral to the local EPAU.

Support of the woman and her partner is essential because of the concerns and guilt this issue can cause, and the impact on their psychological wellbeing. Counselling should be offered as a choice to women after a miscarriage [8]. Better mental health outcomes have been associated with having a choice in the treatment option [4]. The woman should also be reassured that the treatments for miscarriage are safe and that they will not affect future pregnancies [5].

Most women will have no recurrence of the problem, but those who have recurrent miscarriages need referrals and investigations.

Further information is available from The Miscarriage Association www.miscarriageassociation.org.uk (accessed September 2016).

References

1. Miscarriage: Management in Primary Care. BMJ Learning. 2013. http://learning.bmj.com/learning/module-intro/.html?moduleId=10042839 (accessed September 2016).

2. Darney BG, Weaver MR, Stevens N, Kimball J, Prager SW, The Family Medicine Residency Training Initiative in Miscarriage Management: Impact on practice in Washington state. *Family Med* 2013;45(2): 102–107.

3. Prine LW MacNaughten H, Office management of early pregnancy loss. *Am Fam Physician* 2011;84(1): 75–82.

4. Smith LF, Frost J, Levitas R, Bradley H, Garcia J, Women's experience of three early miscarriage management options; a qualitative study. *Br J Gen Pract* 2006;56(524):198–205.

5. Smith LF, Ewings PD, Quinlan C, Incidence of pregnancy after expectant, medical or surgical management of spontaneous first trimester miscarriage: long term follow-up of miscarriage treatment [MIST] randomised controlled trial. *BMJ* 2009;339:b3827.

6. NICE. Ectopic pregnancy and miscarriage: Diagnosis and initial management in early pregnancy of ectopic pregnancy and miscarriage. NICE guidelines [CG154]. December 2012.

7. Cameron MJ, Penney GC, Terminology in early pregnancy loss: what women hear and what clinicians write. *J Fam Plann Reprod Health Care* 2005;31 (4):313–314.

8. Levine K, Cameron ST, Women's preferences for method of abortion and management of miscarriage. *J Fam Plann Reprod Health Care* 2009;35(4): 233–235.

9. Jansson C, Adolfsson A A Swedish study of midwives' and nurses' experiences when women are diagnosed with a missed miscarriage during a routine ultrasound scan. *Sex Reprod Healthcare* 2010;1(2):67–72.

10. RCOG. Recurrent Miscarriage, Investigation and Treatment of Couples (Green-top 17, May 2011 (available online at http://www.rcog.org.uk; accessed September 2016).

Chapter 12

Pregnancy-Related Issues Relevant for Primary Care

Jenny Blackman

Key Points

- Preconceptual counselling is essential for women with complex medical needs.
- Optimize medical conditions before pregnancy and provide appropriate contraception until this is achieved.
- Check medication for women of reproductive age and wherever possible use agents with a known low-risk profile for pregnancy.
- It is important to be able to explain common pregnancy symptoms from a physiological point of view.
- Liaise between specialties and refer women with pre-existing conditions to joint medical/obstetric clinics.
- Use the RCOG (Royal College of Obstetricians and Gynaecologists) Green Top Guidelines for pregnancy-related queries such as chickenpox exposure, genital herpes and obstetric cholestasis.
- Reading the triennial Confidential Enquiry Into Maternal Mortality summary will provide the latest recommendations.
- The recommended vaccination schedules in pregnancy should be known.
- Use the postnatal follow-up visit to give specific lifestyle advice and advice regarding future pregnancies, such as for women with gestational diabetes or hypertension in pregnancy.

Introduction

This chapter focuses on common pregnancy-related symptoms and key issues relevant to primary care in the preconceptual, antepartum and postnatal periods. Intrapartum events and obstetric emergencies are not covered here.

Using cases to illustrate clinical scenarios related to the pregnant patient, this chapter aims to give stepwise and logical approaches to common problems with discussion around the subject after each one.

Type 1 Diabetes

Case Scenario 1

A 22-year-old patient comes to see you. She has had type 1 diabetes since the age of 15. Last month she had a first trimester miscarriage. She thinks she might have thrush again and is requesting treatment.

She has been taking long- and short-acting insulin, but struggles with her blood sugar control at times because of a stressful job and shift work.

She has a BMI of 29.

There is no other relevant past history and she does not smoke.

She is in a stable long-term relationship with a supportive partner.

Her presenting complaint should be investigated with a vaginal swab for *Candida* and treatment as necessary. The consultation should also be used to explore whether her recent pregnancy was planned or unplanned.

If she is hoping to conceive again, her diabetic control should be reviewed and the opportunity taken to address aspects from a preconceptual point of view.

Discussion regarding a suitable contraceptive may be appropriate if she is not planning another pregnancy or until her diabetic control is optimal.

She should be aiming for the same capillary plasma target ranges as all people with type 1 diabetes: fasting glucose 5–7 mmol/L on waking and 4–7 mmol/L before meals. The Diabetes in Pregnancy Pathway published by NICE in 2015 [1] emphasizes the importance of preconceptual care for women with pre-existing type 1 diabetes, aiming for a pre-pregnancy HbA1c of 48 mmol/mol and strongly advising against pregnancy if the HbA1c is greater than 86 mmol/mol.

Women with diabetes who have a BMI greater than 27 should be given advice on weight management in line with NICE guidance on obesity.

Careful counselling about the risks of pregnancy with diabetes includes consideration of effects of the pregnancy on disease and effects of the diabetes on the pregnancy for both the mother and fetus. This counselling is particularly important as the risks are reduced with tighter diabetic control. Maternal diabetes is associated with an increased risk of miscarriage, congenital abnormalities, pre-eclampsia, infections, sudden intrauterine fetal demise, macrosomia and intrauterine growth restriction. There is an increased chance of caesarean delivery and intrapartum problems such as shoulder dystocia.

Folic acid at the higher dose of 5 mg daily is recommended from three months prior to conception in all diabetic women.

Women with type 1 diabetes who are planning to become pregnant should be offered ketone testing strips and a meter and advised to test for ketonaemia if they become hypoglycaemic or unwell. They should also be advised that nausea and vomiting, often associated with early pregnancy, may affect blood glucose control.

Diabetic women should be informed of the increased risk of hypoglycaemia and impaired awareness of these episodes in pregnancy.

There is an increased progression of nephropathy and retinopathy for diabetic women in pregnancy. Retinal screening and renal function should be performed preconceptually if not done within the past three months.

Early referral to a joint obstetric and endocrine clinic is advised, preferably preconceptually.

With improved diagnosis, management and organ transplantation, many people with conditions that historically had a high childhood morbidity and mortality such as renal disease and cardiac conditions are now in a position to contemplate pregnancy. For these women, pregnancy is usually still a huge undertaking and a challenge for obstetric and medical teams.

The effects of pregnancy on the disease, the effects of the condition on the mother and the fetus during pregnancy and the implications of any medications in pregnancy are important considerations for any woman with a pre-existing medical condition.

Some conditions carry implications of passing on a genetic disorder and should be offered genetic counselling. This enables full discussion regarding partner testing, options for pre-implantation genetic diagnosis and prenatal testing if appropriate.

In order to allow time for input from other specialties, investigations to assess the predicted risks for pregnancy, and optimizing medications and for the woman to make an informed choice, reliable contraception should be discussed.

Long-term prognosis should be considered as many women with complex medical conditions may survive pregnancy, but not see their children grow up.

Nausea and Vomiting in Early Pregnancy

Case Scenario 2

A 22-year-old Asian lady presents with persistent vomiting. She has been unable to tolerate food and can only sip water. She has an appointment to see the midwife for a booking visit next week and thinks she is seven weeks pregnant. You saw this lady frequently in the first trimester of her previous pregnancy with severe nausea and vomiting requiring admission on two occasions.

Nausea and vomiting in the first trimester of pregnancy is extremely common, but hyperemesis gravidarum occurs in less than 2% of pregnancies. Hyperemesis is intractable vomiting commencing in the first trimester with signs of dehydration requiring admission. It is a diagnosis of exclusion.

As there is not one confirmatory test, it is essential to exclude other causes of nausea and vomiting by means of history, examination and urine testing. The most common of these is a urinary tract infection. Rarer causes include Addison's disease, peptic ulcer disease, pancreatitis and thyrotoxicosis. Physical examination will establish the degree of dehydration. Postural hypotension and tachycardia are important signs. Urine will show ketones. A previous history of hyperemesis makes the diagnosis more likely.

Any lady who is ketotic and unable to maintain adequate hydration should be admitted to hospital for early and aggressive treatment. Complications of hyperemesis include Mallory–Weiss tears, Wernicke's encephalopathy due to thiamine deficiency, hyponatraemia, thrombosis, depression and psychological effects. Less severe vomiting can be managed by liaising with the early pregnancy unit clinic. An ultrasound should be performed to date the pregnancy and exclude multiple pregnancy and molar pregnancy [2].

Common recommendations include taking small and frequent meals, avoiding spicy or fatty foods and avoiding noxious sensory stimuli. However, there are few studies evaluating this advice [3].

Acupressure and electrical stimulation wrist bands as interventions have mixed evidence. Acupuncture may have some benefit.

Several randomized trials have shown the benefit of ginger without adverse outcomes.

Vitamin B6 used on its own is associated with reduced nausea. There is good evidence for the safety and effectiveness of an H1 receptor antagonist antihistamine (such as cyclizine or promethazine) with pyridoxine for nausea and vomiting in pregnancy. Patients should be informed that all anti-emetics, including antihistamines, are unlicensed for the treatment of nausea and vomiting in pregnancy in the UK [4].

Dopamine antagonists such as metoclopramide stimulate gut motility and have been shown to be effective in decreasing vomiting, and are considered safe with regards to teratogenicity [5].

Centrally acting serotonin antagonists such as ondansetron have limited data regarding efficacy and safety, but one large study in Denmark which found no association between ondansetron and adverse fetal outcome has led to its increased use [6].

Epilepsy

Case Scenario 3

A 19-year-old woman with epilepsy comes for review. She has not had fits for the past 8 months. She has been taking lamotrigine for several years. She is unsure of the date of her last menstrual period, but thinks it was more than five weeks ago and had a positive pregnancy test. She is unsure how she feels about pregnancy as she often rows with her partner and he is unemployed at present.

Epilepsy is a high-risk condition in pregnancy. However, the majority of pregnancies proceed without difficulties. Women who have been free from seizures for many years are unlikely to experience seizures in pregnancy providing their medication is continued. The greatest risk of seizures is at the time of labour and delivery. Sudden unexplained death in epilepsy (SUDEP) remains the predominant cause of death in epilepsy in pregnancy.

The risks of uncontrolled convulsive seizures outweigh the potential teratogenic risk of medication and women with epilepsy are advised to continue their medication during pregnancy. Most studies show a two- to threefold increase in major fetal malformations (neural tube defects, orofacial clefts and heart defects) for women on anti-epileptic medication, compared with the general population. Phenytoin, primidone, phenobarbitone, carbamazepine and sodium valproate all cross the placenta and are teratogenic. The risk of fetal malformation increases with use of multiple agents [2].

Abrupt withdrawal or changes in medications are not recommended, even in women presenting with an unplanned pregnancy taking high-risk medication. Changes should be in consultation with a specialist team and allow the woman to make informed choice about the balance of risks.

Most women with epilepsy of child-bearing age are currently prescribed lamotrigine. The dose may need to be increased two- to threefold during pregnancy.

Preconceptual counselling and discussion in early pregnancy for women with epilepsy is often overlooked, but should be robustly delivered in all care settings and on an opportunistic basis. Early referral for joint care with the obstetrician and neurologist is indicated. All women should be prescribed 5 mg folic acid daily, if possible for three months prior to conception.

Repeatedly, national confidential enquiries into maternal mortality and morbidity such as the MBRRACE report [7] have highlighted poor communication and lack of joined-up thinking between primary care, obstetrics and other hospital specialties as key factors. There were 14 epilepsy-related maternal deaths between 2009 and 2012. Two of these were from drowning and entirely preventable by strong advice against bathing/washing over a bath of water to all women with epilepsy who are of child-bearing age.

Group B Streptococcus

Case Scenario 4

You are looking at some results on behalf of a colleague. A pregnant woman was recently seen with vulval irritation and vaginal discharge in the second trimester of pregnancy. A vaginal swab showed *Candida* and Group B streptococcus.

This lady only needs treatment for *Candida*. The community midwife needs to be aware of the result showing Group B streptococcus, as this patient should be offered intravenous antibiotics in labour.

Group B streptococcus does not usually cause severe infections in well adult women (unlike Group A streptococcus, which can cause a rapid and severe sepsis in pregnancy and the pueperium). However, Group B streptococcus is recognized as the most frequent cause of significant infection in the neonate in the first week of life.

There is often confusion about the significance of Group B streptococcus found during pregnancy. The UK National Screening Committee does *not* recommend routine screening for Group B streptococcus as there is insufficient evidence that the benefits outweigh the risks and it has not been shown to be cost effective [8].

Therefore, vaginal swabs should not be taken during pregnancy without clear clinical indication.

If, however, a swab is indicated by vaginal discharge or prelabour spontaneous rupture of the membranes and Group B streptococcus is identified, *intrapartum* intravenous antibiotics are offered to women.

If a woman has a urine infection with Group B streptococcus, a course of antenatal antibiotics is given and antibiotics are recommended during labour.

Intrapartum antibiotics are offered to women who have had a previous newborn with Group B streptococcal infection.

Chickenpox Exposure

Case Scenario 5

You have been asked to phone a lady back who phoned the receptionist in a panic this morning. She is 27 weeks pregnant and this is her first pregnancy. She is booked with the midwife, is low-risk, has no relevant past history and has been well in her pregnancy.

The day before yesterday she went to her nephew's birthday party and her sister phoned to say that he is covered in what appears to be chickenpox.

You need to establish the risk for this exposure by asking if she has had chickenpox before or has scars from past chickenpox. If this is the case she can be reassured.

Next you need to establish if significant exposure has occurred. This is defined as face to face contact or being in the same room for more than 15 minutes [9].

More than 90% of women born in the UK are immune to varicella zoster. However, if there is no definite history of infection, maternal blood can be tested to see if she is seropositive. If this is the case, she can be reassured.

Contracting varicella zoster is not known to increase the risk of miscarriage, but carries a small risk of fetal varicella syndrome under 28 weeks' gestation. In the last four weeks of pregnancy there is significant risk of varicella infection in the newborn.

Varicella immunoglobulin (VZIG) can be given up to 10 days after exposure to non-immune women. This is not only for fetal effects of varicella zoster infection, but because chickenpox during pregnancy has greater risks to the pregnant women than in the non-pregnant state.

If chickenpox develops, then treatment is with aciclovir.

Seronegative women could be offered immunization outside of pregnancy.

Vaccinations in Pregnancy, Normal Pregnancy Physiology and Management of Anaemia

Case Scenario 6

You see a 34-year-old lady who is currently 29 weeks into her fifth pregnancy. She asks you whether or not she should have the flu vaccine. She saw on the news that it is not a very effective injection this season, but her midwife has suggested she has it. She also mentions how tired she is and says she feels short of breath climbing the stairs at home.

Influenza vaccination (inactivated vaccine) is recommended for all pregnant women. There are several benefits to receiving the vaccine, including protection for both mothers and their babies and avoiding the complications that arise from the flu. In a recent MBR-RACE report (2009–2012), 1 in 11 of the women who died had flu. This was during the flu pandemic, but half of the flu-related deaths were considered preventable, as they had not received vaccination [10]. The flu vaccination also protects newborn babies up to six months of age.

Pertussis vaccine is also recommended in pregnancy. The vaccine is safe for both mother and baby in the third trimester. Vaccination is offered between 28 and 32 weeks, but can be given up to 38 weeks' gestation. This vaccination programme was initiated in 2012 in response to a pertussis outbreak and there has been a decrease in the number of whooping cough cases in babies below six months of age.

The following vaccinations are contraindicated in pregnancy: BCG, measles, mumps, rubella, varicella, vaccinia and HPV [11]. Women who are found in pregnancy to be non-immune to rubella should be offered rubella immunization (MMR vaccine) after delivery, which is considered safe if breast-feeding.

Physiological changes in normal pregnancy mean that most women are aware of feeling more short of breath. This is partly due to the effects of progesterone on ventilation.

A full blood count to screen for antenatal anaemia is routinely taken at booking and the 28-week midwife visit. Physiological changes lead to a normal dilutional anaemia. However, pregnancy also causes a significant increase in iron and folate requirements. The definition of normal haemoglobin levels in pregnancy are >110g/dL in the first trimester and >105 g/dL in the second and third trimesters.

Dietary advice and a trial of oral iron is the first-line management of anaemia in pregnancy, providing haemoglobinopathy has been excluded. Serum ferritin is the most useful parameter for assessing iron deficiency and levels below 15μ/L are diagnostic of iron deficiency and below 30μ/L should prompt treatment. An increase in haemoglobin must be demonstrated after two weeks, otherwise further tests are required [12].

Referral and consideration of parenteral iron should be initiated from the second trimester onwards for all women with confirmed iron deficiency who fail to respond or are intolerant of oral iron.

Iron deficiency is associated with preterm delivery, low birth weight and possibly abruption and increased peripartum blood loss.

Itching in Pregnancy

Case Scenario 7

A lady comes to see you at 34 weeks' gestation in her second pregnancy. She is very distressed by severe itching.

Itching in pregnancy is a common symptom, causing significant distress and loss of sleep for some women.

Obstetric cholestasis is a diagnosis to consider. It can cause widespread itching, but often affects the palms and soles. If this lady had obstetric cholestasis previously then this makes the diagnosis more likely as it has a high recurrence rate. A rash is not a feature of obstetric cholestasis. Liver function is abnormal and both liver function and the itching resolve after birth. (Alkaline phosphatase is increased in normal pregnancy as it is made by the placenta so this does not indicate disease).

Other causes of itching and liver dysfunction such as drugs, hepatitis, autoimmune conditions and gall stones need to be excluded.

Other pregnancy specific conditions to be considered in any woman with abnormal liver function are pre-eclampsia and acute fatty liver of pregnancy.

Women with obstetric cholestasis should be referred to an obstetric team and will have weekly liver function tests and consideration of timing of delivery. Over the years, obstetric cholestasis has caused anxiety and iatrogenic prematurity because of the association with stillbirth. The current additional risk of stillbirth above that of the general pregnant population has not been determined, but is likely to be small.

Once the woman has delivered, symptoms and liver function should return to normal. Checking liver function tests can be deferred until the postnatal check. She can be reassured about the lack of long-term sequelae for herself and her baby [13].

Women who have had obstetric cholestasis should avoid the combined oral contraceptive pill.

Postnatal Hypertension

Case Scenario 8

You are asked to see a 33-year-old lady 10 days postnatally. Unfortunately there is very little information on the discharge summary about her antenatal care, but she tells you that she had to be induced at 37 weeks' gestation because her blood pressure was very high, she had a headache and her blood tests were abnormal. She laboured quickly and had a normal birth. She has recovered well and feels well now.

Her midwife has now handed over care to the health visitor but asks if her labetolol can be 'weaned off'.

Ideally this lady should have been discharged with a clear plan regarding the postnatal period, but often this is not the case. The dangers of hypertension during the postnatal period are of eclampsia and stroke.

All women should be aware of symptoms such as headache, nausea, vomiting, visual disturbance and epigastric pain. The blood pressure should be checked by the community midwife on alternate days for two weeks after discharge for women with hypertension during pregnancy and/or labour. Any woman with a diastolic blood pressure greater than 90 with symptoms or sustained over four hours or a systolic blood pressure greater than 150 should be reviewed and have blood taken for FBC, renal and liver function.

Most women with antenatal hypertension will need antihypertensives for two weeks following delivery. Blood pressure medication can be reduced when the BP is consistently 130–140/80–90 mmHg [14].

If medication is still required at six weeks postdelivery then investigation for other causes is warranted as 13% of women thought to have gestational hypertension or pre-eclampsia have underlying disease. Urine should be checked at the six-week postnatal check and if proteinuria still exists then renal function should be reviewed and further investigated.

Severe early onset (requiring delivery before 34 weeks) pre-eclampsia has a recurrence rate of 40% in future pregnancies, although this usually occurs two to three weeks later and is less severe. Mild pre-eclampsia at term has a recurrence risk of 10% [15].

Screening for pre-eclampsia would happen automatically in a future pregnancy as blood pressure, symptoms and urine testing are addressed routinely at each point of contact with the community midwife for every woman.

In her next pregnancy she should take low dose aspirin 75 mg daily from 12 weeks of gestation. In addition to women with previous pregnancy-related hypertension, other women who should receive low-dose aspirin include women with pre-existing hypertension, diabetes, chronic kidney disease and those with a history of autoimmune disorders such as SLE or antiphospholipid syndrome and women with more than one of the following risk factors – primigravida, maternal age above 40 years, pregnancy interval of greater than 10 years, BMI above 35, family history of pre-eclampsia and multiple pregnancy. Evidence shows a 17% reduction in the risk of developing pre-eclampsia if low-dose aspirin is taken by these women [16].

Gestational Diabetes

Case Scenario 9

A 36-year-old lady had her second baby six weeks ago. She had a glucose tolerance test at 28 weeks because her BMI is 44. She was diagnosed with gestational diabetes (GDM) and was taught how to monitor her blood sugars. Her GDM was managed with diet and she had extra growth scans. She was induced at 38 weeks and had an emergency caesarean delivery for fetal distress. She was not given any further advice apart from that she did not need to monitor her blood sugars after delivery.

A fasting glucose test should be offered 6–13 weeks postnatally to exclude diabetes. If this is below 6.0 mmol/L she will need an annual HbA1c test to check her blood glucose level is normal and she should be told she has a moderate risk of developing type 2 diabetes in the future, with appropriate advice and guidance (NICE – Preventing type 2 diabetes).

She has a significant risk of developing gestational diabetes in future pregnancies. She should be given lifestyle advice and encouragement to normalise her BMI.

Women with a fasting glucose of 6.0–6.9 mmol/L should be told that they have a high risk of developing type 2 diabetes. Women with a fasting level greater than 7.0 mmol/L are highly likely to have type 2 diabetes and therefore need confirmatory tests [1].

All women who have had a previous caesarean delivery are considered high risk for future pregnancies and are usually seen at 20 weeks' gestation for discussion about mode of delivery. There is a 72–75% chance of a successful vaginal birth in the woman's next pregnancy and the scar rupture rate is approximately 0.5%. All women who have had a previous caesarean are advised to labour with fetal monitoring and intravenous access in a hospital delivery suite [17].

References

1. NICE. *Diabetes in pregnancy: management from preconception to the postnatal period*. Clinical Guideline NG3. National Institute for Health and Care Excellence, Feb 2015.

2. Nelson-Piercy C, *Handbook of Obstetric Medicine, 5th edn*. CRC Press; 2015.

3. Boelig RC, Berghella V, Kelly AJ, Barton SJ, Edwards SJ, Interventions for treating hyperemesis gravidarum. *Cochrane Database Syst Rev* 2013;(6):CD010607.

4. Gadsby R, Barnie-Adshead T, Severe nausea and vomiting of pregnancy: should it be treated with appropriate pharmacotherapy? *Obstetr Gynaecol* 2011;13(2):107–111.

5. Mella MT, *Nausea/vomiting of pregnancy and hyperemesis gravidarum*. Maternal-fetal evidence Based Guideline 2. Inform Healthcare, 2011:72–80.

6. Pasternak B, Svanström H, Hviid A, Ondansetron in pregnancy and risk of adverse fetal outcomes. *N Engl J Med* 2013;368(9):814–823.

7. MBRRACE (Mothers and Babies: Reducing the risk through audits and confidential enquiries across the UK) Saving Lives, Improving Mothers' Care. Lessons learned to inform future maternity care from the UK and Ireland Confidential Enquiries into Maternal Deaths and Morbidity 2009–2012. 2014.

8. Royal College of Obstetricians and Gynaecologists. Group B Streptococcal Disease, Early onset. Green-top Guideline no. 36. RCOG. 2012.

9. Royal College of Obstetricians and Gynaecologists. Chickenpox in Pregnancy. Green-top Guideline no. 13. RCOG. 2015.

10. Knight M, Key messages from the UK and Ireland confidential enquiries into maternal death and morbidity. *Obstetr Gynaecol* 2015;1:72–73.

11. Arunakumari PS, Kalburgi S, Sahare A, Vaccination in pregnancy. *Obstetr Gynaecol* 2015;17(4):257–263.

12. British Society for Haemoatology. UK guidelines on the management of iron deficiency in pregnancy. British Committee for Standards in Haematology. 2011.

13. Royal College of Obstetricians and Gynaecologists. Obstetric Cholestasis. Green-top Guideline no. 43. RCOG. 2011.

14. NICE. Hypertension in pregnancy: diagnosis and management. Clinical Guideline CG107 National Institute for Health and Care Excellence. 2010.

15. Smith M, Waugh J, Nelson-Piercy C. Management of postpartum hypertension. *Obstetr Gynaecol* 2013;15(1):45–50.

16. Mone F, McAuliffe F M. Low-dose aspirin and calcium supplementation for the prevention of pre-eclampsia. *Obstetr Gynaecol* 2014;16(4):245–250.

17. Royal College of Obstetricians and Gynaecologists. Birth after previous caesarean birth. Green-top Guideline no. 45. RCOG. 2015.

Chapter 13

Postnatal Care in Primary Care

Judy Shakespeare

Key Points

- If women are not breastfeeding they need adequate contraception from three weeks postnatal.
- If a woman consults a GP saying she thinks she has a perinatal mental health problem, she is almost certainly right. Do not dismiss her or normalize her symptoms.
- Venous thromboembolism can occur even if a woman has been adequately anticoagulated.
- Infection can be serious in the postnatal period: there are red flags for admission.
- Prescribing in pregnancy and breastfeeding needs careful consideration of risks and benefits. If necessary, take advice before stopping old or starting new medication.

At the postnatal examination:

- Use a template.
- Ask about mental health first before physical health.
- Pregnancy is a 'stress test' for life in women. The postnatal discharge letter should offer advice about future health screening requirements; i.e. annual HbA1C following GDM.
- Preconception care should start at the postnatal check.
- Offer advice about lifestyle issues, such as weight, exercise, smoking and alcohol.

This chapter aims to cover the normal and abnormal postnatal period relevant to general practitioners. It considers the time after discharge from hospital and does not consider care for the baby. Both mental and physical health are considered.

Definition: the postnatal period is the period beginning immediately after the birth of a child and extending for about six weeks. This is roughly the time it takes for a woman's body to return to the non-pregnant state. For postnatal mental illness (PMI) the period extends to 12 months after childbirth.

Normal Physiological Changes in the Postnatal Period

The Uterus

The pregnant term uterus weighs about 1000 g, but by six weeks after birth it weighs 50–100 g. The endometrial lining rapidly regenerates and by the 16th day, it is restored throughout the uterus, except at the placental site. The size of the placental bed decreases by half immediately after birth because of uterine contractions. Vaginal discharge (lochia) comes from the placental bed. After initial uterine contraction, the volume of lochia rapidly decreases. Lochia lasts an average of five weeks, but this is variable (15% of women still have lochia six or more weeks postnatal).

Vagina

The vagina shrinks rapidly in size, but never to its prepregnant size. By three weeks, the rugae start to reappear in women who are not breastfeeding. In breastfeeding mothers, who have persistently decreased oestrogen levels, the vaginal epithelium remains atrophic for a variable period and women may experience dyspareunia.

Perineum

The swollen and engorged vulva rapidly resolves within one to two weeks. Most of the muscle tone is

Women's Health in Primary Care, edited by Anne Connolly and Amanda Britton. Published by Cambridge University Press
© Cambridge University Press 2017

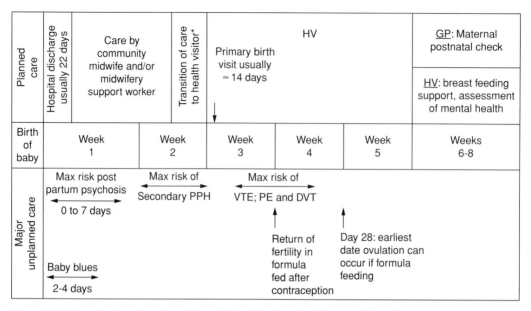

Figure 13.1 Planned and major unplanned postnatal care by primary health care professionals.

regained by six weeks, but it may not return to normal, depending on the extent of injury during birth.

Abdominal Wall

The abdominal wall remains soft and poorly toned for many weeks.

Ovaries

The resumption of normal ovarian function is variable, with a mean time to first menses of seven to nine weeks in formula-feeding mothers. However, ovulation can occur as early as 28 days after birth. Hence contraception is needed from 21 days.

In breastfeeding women, the resumption of menses is variable and depends on how much and how often the baby is fed and supplementary formula feeding. Anovulation in lactating women is caused by elevated prolactin levels. If women are less than six months postnatal, amenorrhoeic and fully breastfeeding, the lactational amenorrhoeic method (LAM) is over 98% effective in preventing pregnancy [1]. The risk of pregnancy for women using LAM is increased if breastfeeding decreases (particularly stopping night feeds), when menstruation recurs, or more than six months postnatal.

Breasts

After a miscarriage or termination, lactation can be experienced from 16 weeks' gestation. If not breastfeeding, the prolactin level returns to normal within two to three weeks. The colostrum is already present in the breasts at birth and suckling by the newborn triggers its release during the first two to four days. For most women having their first baby the milk will 'come in' at three to four days, but this may be sooner after subsequent births.

Transition to Motherhood

Becoming a mother is a major life transition and women usually spend time considering and imagining the kind of mother they will be when their baby is born; but the reality may be different. If a woman is more able to adjust her expectations of herself and the relationship with her baby, she may cope better.

Routine Postnatal Care

This is covered by NICE postnatal care guidelines and quality standards [2,3]. The care that women can expect to receive is illustrated in Figure 13.1.

Timeline of Routine Postnatal Care Pathway and Key Complications

Routine postnatal care is not the responsibility of GPs. Although many women appear to recover well after pregnancy, incontinence, perineal pain, anxiety and depression are common and can persist for months or years. About a quarter of women now have a caesarean section and maternal factors such as obesity, older age and conditions such as diabetes or hypertensive disorders increase the risk of intervention and hence complexity of postnatal care.

The Maternal Postnatal Examination (PNE)

The PNE, usually at six to eight weeks, is the only part of routine postnatal care for which a GP is responsible; 90% of women report having received it four to eight weeks after birth, but an online survey of 4000 self-selected women found a third reported that their six-week routine GP appointment did not meet their emotional needs and almost half that it was not thorough enough [4]. The evidence base for the purpose and content is poor. NICE postnatal care guideline [2] says vaguely:

'At the end of the postnatal period, the coordinating healthcare professional should ensure that the woman's physical, emotional and social wellbeing is reviewed. Screening and medical history should also be taken into account.'

There is a need to redefine the purpose and content of the PNE. Here is a framework that could be used:

Organization of the Practice

- Decide who will do it; the usual GP, the woman's choice or a practice doctor with a special interest?
- Will women be invited for the check and if so, by whom and how will they do this?
- Will it happen with the baby check?
- How much time is needed?
- Develop a practice template for consistency.

The tasks for the PNE:

'Women need to be clear about what the appointment will cover and that a separate time will be available for the baby's check. The check should include assessing:

- how a woman has made the transition to motherhood, including her mental health;

- her recovery from the birth, using direct questions about common morbidities;
- longer term health risks for any morbidity identified;
- any further help she might need whether connected with the birth or not; and what advice she might need about future family planning.
- Provide follow-up care for diabetes, hypertension, anaemia, sepsis, mental health or conditions which may have complicated pregnancy, may impact on another pregnancy and future life' [5].

Case Scenario: A Complex Pregnancy with Multimorbidity

Jane is aged 38 years, had her first child six weeks ago and attends for her postnatal check. She is obese (BMI 35) and developed gestational diabetes (GDM) and pre-eclampsia during pregnancy. Her pregnancy was managed by the joint obstetric–diabetic clinic and she had a normal birth at 39 weeks. There were no other problems during pregnancy. She was managed by diet alone and her blood sugar and blood pressure were normal on discharge from hospital, with no proteinuria.

- Her *discharge letter* should contain information and recommendations for her care.
- She has made the *transition to motherhood* well and has no mental health problems.
- She has *recovered* well with no persistent morbidities.
- She has *risk factors* for her next pregnancy and her future health
- She has multi-morbidities: *obesity, GDM* and *pre-eclampsia*. Consider each condition separately.
- *Contraception* needs to be considered for each condition and a decision made that balances her choice against risks identified, using UKMEC [6].

Obesity

Jane's eating habits and physical activity levels could influence the health of the wider family, including her children. Supporting her in the postnatal period to change her eating habits and physical activity levels may improve the health and risk for the whole family. It may also improve the outcomes of future pregnancies.

At her PNE she should be weighed and her BMI calculated. She should be offered a referral for advice on healthy eating and exercise [3].

Table 13.1 Postnatal tests and follow-up after gestational diabetes [7]

Fasting plasma glucose mmol/l at 6–13 weeks	< 6.0	6.0–6.9	≥7
HbA1c mmol/mol (%) at 13 weeks or later	<39 (5.7%)	39–47 (5.7–6.4%)	≥48 (6.5%)
Current risk of diabetes	Low	High	Confirms current diabetes
Future risk of diabetes	Moderate	High	N/A
Advice	Weight control, diet and exercise (lifestyle advice)	In addition to lifestyle advice see NICE preventing type 2 diabetes guideline	Refer for care for type 2 diabetes
Contraception	If her BP is normal she should choose a form of contraception based on her own preferences [6].		
Advice for next pregnancy	Consult early in pregnancy 75 g two-hour OGTT as soon as possible after booking		Preconception care to optimize diabetes control, renal and retinal screening
Follow-up	Annual FBG or HbA1c	Annual weight/BMI Annual FBG or HbA1c	As for type 2 diabetes

Gestational Diabetes Mellitus

Women diagnosed with GDM have a sevenfold increased risk of type 2 diabetes. Jane is likely to develop GDM in subsequent pregnancies, but could reduce her risk if she lost weight [7].

In addition to addressing her obesity with lifestyle advice, Jane should have either a fasting plasma glucose at 6–13 weeks postnatally or an HbA1c after 13 weeks (unreliable before then). Table 13.1 shows how to interpret results from postnatal testing after GDM and follow-up.

If her BP is normal she could choose any form of contraception [6].

She needs annual review of her BP, fasting blood glucose or HbA1c and cardiovascular risk, with ongoing lifestyle advice

Pre-Eclampsia

Jane has a risk of recurrence of subsequent pregnancy hypertensive disorders and pre-eclampsia (Figure 13.2) [8].

She also has an increased lifetime risk of hypertension and cardiovascular disease. Unfortunately, pregnancy hypertension is not included as a risk factor in the QRisk2 tool so it is difficult to accurately predict her risk.

Figure 13.2 Risks for future pregnancies of hypertension in pregnancy.

Women who have had **gestational hypertension** should be told that their risk of developing:

- gestational hypertension in a future pregnancy ranges from about 1 in 6 (16%) pregnancies to about 1 in 2 (47%) pregnancies

- pre-eclampsia in a future pregnancy ranges from 1 in 50 (2%) to about 1 in 14 (7%) pregnancies.

Women who have had **pre-eclampsia** should be told that their risk of developing:

- gestational hypertension in a future pregnancy ranges from about 1 in 8 (13%) pregnancies to about 1 in 2 (53%) pregnancies

- pre-eclampsia in a future pregnancy is up to about 1 in 6 (16%) pregnancies

- pre-eclampsia in a future pregnancy is about 1 in 4 (25%) pregnancies if their pre-eclampsia was complicated by severe pre-eclampsia, HELLP syndrome or eclampsia and led to birth before 34 weeks, and about 1 in 2 (55%) pregnancies if it led to birth before 28 weeks.

NICE clinical guideline 107 Hypertension in pregnancy

Postnatal Mental Health Problems

These conditions are common and affect about 20% of postnatal women. Treatment is clear, evidence based and effective [9,10]. A tool for GPs to understand the management of PMIs, as recommended by NICE, has been produced by the RCGP [11]. Not all postnatal mental illness (PMI) is depression and Table 13.2 shows the rates of different disorders. PMI ranges from the 90% of mild-moderate illness that can be managed in primary care to severe illness that needs to be managed by specialist perinatal psychiatrists.

Baby Blues is not PMI; it affects most women within a few days of birth. This can include feeling upset, with mood swings, and wanting to cry for no particular reason. These feelings disappear after a few days and never last longer than two weeks.

Mild-moderate PMIs are important because of the devastating effects and distress they can have on women who are not identified early and treated adequately. They can compromise the healthy emotional, cognitive and physical development of the child, with long-term consequences [12]. Although effects on the children are marked, for example maternal anxiety doubles the risk of mental health problems in the child from 5% to 10%, the effect is not inevitable and in the absence of social adversity and if they are of short duration, the risks to the child are generally low [13]. PMIs can have lasting effects on partner and family relationships. There is emerging evidence that 10% of fathers may suffer perinatal depression, or a range of anxiety symptoms [14].

Women who have experienced postnatal depression are at risk of suffering further episodes of illness, both following subsequent deliveries and also unrelated to childbirth. After one postnatal episode the risk of recurrence is 25%.

Table 13.2 Rates of perinatal psychiatric disorder per thousand maternities

Postnatal psychosis	2/1000
Chronic serious mental illness	2/1000
Severe depressive illness	30/1000
Mild-moderate depressive illness and anxiety states	100–150/1000
Post-traumatic stress disorder	30/1000
Adjustment disorders and distress	150–300/1000

JCC-MH: Guidance for commissioners of perinatal mental health services. RCPsych 2012

There are barriers to the identification of PMI; only half of mothers meeting diagnostic thresholds for perinatal depression and anxiety are currently identified [15] despite frequent routine contact with a range of primary care services at this time. NICE recommends that women should be asked at each postnatal contact about their emotional health and encouraged to discuss how they are feeling (Figure 3.2).

A recent report [16] has shown that the greatest barrier to providing better support to women is the low level of identification of need. Barriers to identification were identified, including the following.

Barriers to Identification for Women

- Poor awareness of perinatal mental illness among women, their partners and families
- Stigma and fear among women that their baby might be taken away
- Feeling dismissed or overly reassured when discussing their problems with GPs.

Barriers to Identification for GPs

- Time pressures on GP consultations
- Insufficient training and confidence among GPs in managing PMI
- A lack of contact between GPs and women during pregnancy and inconsistent team-working between GP practices and midwives and health visitors
- A lack of focus on mother and baby wellbeing after initial six- to eight-week check
- A lack of specialist resources to refer to.

Red flag for GPs

- If a woman consults a GP saying she thinks she has a perinatal mental health problem, she is almost certainly right. Do not dismiss her or normalize her symptoms

  There is more information available in the RCGP perinatal mental health toolkit (www.rcgp.org.uk/clinical-and-research/toolkits/perinatal-mental-health-toolkit.aspx; accessed September 2016).

Managing Common Maternal Morbidities After Birth

'After Pains'

After pains are common and caused by involutionary uterine contractions. They last for two–three days after

At a woman's first contact with services in pregnancy and the postnatal period, ask about:

- any past or present severe mental illness

- past or present treatment by a specialist mental health service, including inpatient care for any severe perinatal mental illness in a first-degree relative (mother, sister or daughter).

- refer to a secondary mental health service (preferably a specialist perinatal mental health service) for assessment and treatment, all women who:

  - have or are suspected to have severe mental illness

  - have any history of severe mental illness (during pregnancy or the postnatal period or at any other time).

At a woman's first contact with primary care or her booking visit, and during the early postnatal period, consider asking the following **depression** identification questions as part of a general discussion about a woman's mental health and wellbeing:

- During the past month, have you often been bothered by feeling down, depressed or hopeless?

- During the past month, have you often been bothered by having little interest or pleasure in doing things?

Also consider asking about **anxiety** using the 2-item Generalized Anxiety Disorder scale (GAD-2):

- Over the last 2 weeks, how often have you been bothered by feeling nervous, anxious or on edge?

- Over the last 2 weeks, how often have you been bothered by not being able to stop or control worrying?

NICE antenatal and postnatal mental health CG 192. 2014

Figure 13.3 NICE guidance for assessing mental health

birth and are worse in multips. Breastfeeding stimulates the uterus to contract and increases the severity of the pains. Non-steroidal anti-inflammatory drugs are better than placebo at relieving pain, but paracetamol is no better than placebo.

Perineal Pain

Perineal pain may be caused by trauma, stitches, infection, constipation, haemorrhoids or an anal fissure.

Perineal lacerations occur in 85% of vaginal deliveries. Obstetric anal sphincter injury causes more perineal pain than other perineal trauma. Spontaneous second-degree tears are less painful than episiotomies. Although perineal pain affects most mothers, it usually resolves within two months of birth, but about 20% still report perineal pain and dyspareunia at six months.

Prevention may be possible; *antenatal* digital perineal massage reduces the likelihood of perineal trauma (mainly episiotomies), ongoing perineal pain and is generally well accepted. The impact is more obvious for women having their first birth. Reliable information on the benefits of massage and how to do it can be found on the internet.

Constipation

Postnatal constipation is estimated to affect 24% at three months postnatal. Haemorrhoids, episiotomy pain, damage to the anal sphincter or pelvic floor muscles during childbirth and iron supplementation all increase the risk. A high-fibre diet and increased fluid intake can prevent constipation, but there is a lack of good evidence about treating women, although a bulk-forming laxative would be first choice if diet and fluids are ineffective.

Haemorrhoids and fissures should be treated as in the general population.

Back Pain

Backache is reported by about half of women during pregnancy. An additional 14% report new onset after birth, with varying findings about the relationship to epidural anaesthesia; most of these women have recovered within six months. Factors correlated with persistent postnatal back pain are pain before pregnancy, pain during pregnancy, physically heavy work and multiple pregnancy. NICE advises that back pain after birth should be treated as at any other time [2].

Incontinence

About a third of women leak urine after birth and many still report it 12 years later. Faecal incontinence of varying severity occurs in about 10% of women, and over a third of these women still report it 12 years later. Most women with incontinence after birth do not seek any advice or treatment.

Pelvic floor muscle training (PFMT) is an effective treatment for women with persistent postnatal urinary incontinence and can also help women with faecal incontinence. Antenatal PFMT may help higher-risk women, such as primips and women with a large baby. The more intensive the programme the greater the treatment effect.

Divarication of the Recti Abdominal Muscles (DRAM)

DRAM results from stretching of the linea alba during pregnancy and is a common problem after pregnancy. It usually corrects itself by eight weeks, but may persist. Although most women are asymptomatic, except cosmetically, it can lead to back pain and occasionally hernias. A systematic review of various exercise regimes was inconclusive about the benefit, but for most women, referral to a physiotherapist for pilates or other core-strengthening exercises are recommended. Surgery, a 'tummy tuck', is a last ditch cosmetic treatment.

Breastfeeding Problems

In general, this is the field of expertise of midwives, health visitors and breastfeeding counsellors and not GPs. However, you should know how to access the breastfeeding resources available in your locality.

Painful Nipples

Painful nipples are common and there are no effective specific treatments that are better than applying expressed breast milk or nothing. For most women, nipple pain reduces by seven to ten days after birth.

Mastitis

Of lactating women, 10–33% get mastitis; breast abscesses are less common. The usual organism is *Staphyloccocus aureus*.

Infection tends to localize to a segment (blocked milk duct) but it can spread to an entire breast quadrant. Women complain of pain, difficulty breastfeeding, engorgement, redness and cracked nipples; but they may also present with fever, fatigue or rigors (sepsis), without breast localization.

Management

- Assess for systemic inflammatory response syndrome (SIRS) and red flag sepsis and act accordingly (see Figure 13.4)
- Continue breastfeeding as milk stasis causes mastitis. If feeding is too painful a woman should hand express or use a breast pump to encourage milk flow from the engorged segment. The antibiotic of choice is flucloxacillin 500 mg QDS for 10 days or erythromycin 500 mg QDS if penicillin-allergic. Co-amoxiclav or clarithromycin are alternatives in more severe infection or intolerance.
- Analgesia (paracetamol) and ice packs/warm compresses/a warm bath or shower may help.
- Refer to breastfeeding expert to check attachment and feeding technique.
- Refer to hospital if symptoms are not settling after one course of antibiotics or if an abscess forms. Immediate referral to hospital is indicated if the woman with mastitis is clinically unwell, if there is no response to oral antibiotics within 48 hours, if mastitis recurs or if there are very severe or unusual symptoms [17].

'Red flag' signs and symptoms should prompt urgent referral for hospital assessment and, if the woman appears seriously unwell, by emergency ambulance:

- pyrexia more than 38°C
- sustained tachycardia more than 90 beats/minute
- breathlessness (respiratory rate more than 20 breaths/minute; a serious symptom)
- abdominal or chest pain
- diarrhoea and/or vomiting
- uterine or renal angle pain and tenderness
- woman is generally unwell or seems unduly anxious or distressed.

RCOG Green Top guidelines 64b 2012

Figure 13.4 Indications for hospital referral in sepsis.

Tiredness

Every mother is tired after birth, but most do not consult with it. Other possibilities are anaemia, depression or hypothyroidism, and NICE recommends taking it seriously [2].

Anaemia

Postnatal anaemia is defined as Hb <10 g/dL and results from postpartum haemorrhage or a low Hb during pregnancy. Women should be offered iron 100–200 mg daily for at least three months before having a repeat FBC and ferritin to ensure Hb and iron stores are replete. There is no indication to do a routine Hb unless there are symptoms or risk factors

Thyroid Problems

Postnatal thyroiditis, an auto-immune disease, affects about 5% of women and is the commonest cause of postnatal thyroid dysfunction. It presents with painless swelling of the thyroid gland; one-third of patients will only have a thyrotoxic phase; one-third only a hypothyroid phase and one-third will have both phases. Clinical symptoms can mimic typical fatigue following birth, as well as postnatal depression and Graves' disease. It is associated with abnormalities of thyroid hormones and positive autoantibodies. Differentiation of the hyperthyroid phase of postnatal thyroiditis from Graves' disease is important because Graves' disease requires antithyroid therapy (which

does not work in postnatal thyroiditis). A low uptake on a radioisotope uptake scan confirms the diagnosis.

Mild cases need no treatment. If the hyperthyroid symptoms are troublesome, a peripherally acting beta blocker drug is indicated. Symptomatic postnatal hypothyroidism should be treated with levothyroxine. By 12–18 months most women recover, but 20% need long-term replacement.

Significant Postnatal Physical Illnesses

Secondary Postpartum Haemorrhage (PPH)

Secondary PPH is defined as abnormal or excessive bleeding between 24 hours and 12 weeks postnatally. It is usually caused by endometritis, with or without retained products of conception. It affects 1–3% of women. Risk factors are complicated deliveries, including caesarean section and anaemia. Most cases are caused by Group A streptococcus.

Genital tract sepsis is a major cause of maternal death and should be treated aggressively with intravenous antibiotics (see Figure 13.4) [17,18]. Recommended antibiotics are clindamycin plus gentamicin, meaning that if the diagnosis is suspected the woman should be admitted (Figure 13.4). Surgical treatment is needed if there is excessive or continuing bleeding, irrespective of ultrasound findings.

Epilepsy

The immediate postpartum period is high risk for increased seizure frequency or for the first onset of seizures due to increased stress, sleep deprivation, missed medication, changes in the bio-availability of medication and anxiety. Women are also at risk of sudden unexpected death in epilepsy (SUDEP). They need advice about medication and breastfeeding and about reducing risk from seizures by not bathing or sleeping alone. An epilepsy specialist nurse or midwife could be helpful for GP and patient [17].

Venous Thromboembolism

Thrombosis and thromboembolism are the leading cause of direct maternal death [17]. A systematic review of risk of postnatal VTE found that the risk varied from 21- to 84-fold from the non-pregnant state. The absolute risk peaks in the first three weeks postnatal (421 per 100,000 person-years). A PE is still possible, even when a patient has had adequate thromboprophylaxis. Brief faintness and shortness of breath are common premonitory signs and buttock pain can suggest a pelvis vein thrombosis. Routine observations: (temperature, pulse, BP, respiratory rate, O_2 sats, peak flow) and a chest examination are important, and tachycardia and reduced O_2 sats are suggestive of the diagnosis, even if the woman appears well. D-dimer and Wells scores are not validated for use in pregnant and postnatal women, so urgent diagnostic imaging is needed to exclude a PE [19].

Bereavement

One in 200 births ends in stillbirth and one in three stillbirths occurs at term. About 1 in 450 pregnancies lead to neonatal death (death in the first four weeks after pregnancy). An independent study giving a national picture of the NHS care experienced by parents of babies who died before or during birth or as newborns was published in 2014 [20]. There are several important messages for GPs. Firstly, the high rate of anxiety and depression in the mothers *and fathers*. Secondly, the value mothers *and fathers* attach to support from GPs; around 10% of parents were visited at home after the bereavement and this was especially appreciated. Thirdly, only just over 50% of women who had a bereavement had a PNE, usually because they were not invited. This is an important time to check for mental health problems, to offer support, signpost to other resources and to discuss issues for another pregnancy.

Significant Psychiatric Illness

Severe PMI, caused by severe depressive disorder or postnatal psychosis, is a leading cause of maternal death throughout the first postnatal year and the majority of women who kill themselves have a previous history of severe mental illness [21]. Hopefully, GPs, with their knowledge of past medical history from the chronological medical record, will have passed this information on to midwifery services at the time of booking. These women should have been referred to a perinatal psychiatrist after booking, so a care plan is be in place before delivery for prevention, early detection and treatment [9].

The acute onset of postnatal psychosis (PP), one of the most severe forms of illness seen in psychiatry, is rare and a GP is likely to see a case only about once every 10 years; 50% of women who develop PP have a strong risk factor (previous psychosis, bi-polar disorder).

Most PP starts within two weeks of birth, with more than 50% starting on days 1–3. Of women who develop psychosis, 50% will have no significant psychiatric history and therefore have no plan in place. Sudden onset and rapid deterioration are typical and the clinical picture often changes rapidly, with wide fluctuations in the intensity of symptoms and severe swings of mood. They can have mania and depression at the same time, resulting in agitation, trouble sleeping and significant change in appetite, psychosis and suicidal thoughts. Suspected PP is 'red flag'.

> **Red Flag**
>
> Postpartum psychosis is a psychiatric emergency and requires specialist assessment and treatment within four hours [9].

Prescribing in Breastfeeding Women

Prescribing in breastfeeding needs careful consideration of risks and benefits. The BNF identifies drugs under their specific headings:

- use with caution or contraindicated in breastfeeding, e.g. lithium
- can be given to the breastfeeding mother because present in milk in amounts unharmful to the infant
- might be present in milk in significant amount but not harmful.

With newer drugs a GP can get advice from the Specialist Pharmacy Service (SPS; www.sps.nhs.uk/home/medicines/; accessed September 2016) or a US site, LactMed (toxnet.nlm.nih.gov/newtoxnet/lactmed.htm; accessed September 2016).

References

1. Clinical Effectiveness Unit, Faculty of Sexual Health and Reproductive Healthcare. *Postnatal Sexual and Reproductive Health*. FRSH. 1989.

2. National Institute of Health and Care Excellence. Routine postnatal care of women and their babies. Clinical Guideline 37. 2014.

3. National Institute for Health and Care Excellence. Quality Standard for Postnatal Care. NICE quality standard QS 37. 2013

4. NCT and Netmums Six Week Check survey. Briefing document. http://www.nct.org.uk/press-release/nct-netmums-research-finds-six-week-postnatal-check-unsatisfactory (accessed September 2016).

5. NHS Better Births. Improving outcomes of maternity services in England: A Five Year Forward View for maternity care. 2016. https://www.england.nhs.uk/wp-content/uploads/2016/02/national-maternity-review-report.pdf (accessed September 2016).

6. Faculty of Sexual Health and Reproductive Health Care. Summary sheets for UK medical eligibility criteria. 2010

7. National Institute for Health and Care Excellence. Diabetes in pregnancy: management of diabetes and its complications from preconception to the postnatal period. NICE NG3. 2015.

8. National Institute for Health and Care Excellence. Hypertension in pregnancy: the management of hypertensive disorders during pregnancy. NICE CG 107. 2010.

9. National Institute for Health and Care Excellence. Antenatal and postnatal mental health: clinical management and service guidance. NICE CG192. 2014.

10. Scottish Intercollegiate Guideline Network/Health Improvement Scotland. Management of perinatal mood disorders. Guideline No 127. 2012.

11. Shakespeare J, Practical implications for primary care of the NICE guideline CG192 Antenatal and postnatal mental health. RCGP. 2015. http://www.rcgp.org.uk/clinical-and-research/toolkits/~/media/92F73D8AA0014DEAB37B55CDF7F2CE2B.ashx (accessed September 2016).

12. Bauer A, Parsonage M, Knapp M, Iemmi V, Bayo A, *The Costs of Perinatal Mental Health Problems*. Centre for Mental Health and London School of Economics. 2014.

13. Stein A, Pearson RM, Goodman SH, *et al.* Effects of perinatal mental disorders on the fetus and child. *Lancet* 2014;384(9956):1800–1891.

14. Paulson JF, Bazemore SD, Prenatal and postpartum depression in fathers and its association with maternal depression: A meta-analysis. *JAMA* 2010;303(19):1961–1969.

15. Ramsay, R, Postnatal depression. *Lancet* 1993;341: 1358.

16. Khan L, *Falling through the Gaps: Perinatal Mental Health and General Practice*. Centre for Mental Health. 2015.

17. Knight M, Kenyon S, Brocklehurst P, *et al.* (eds.) on behalf of MBRRACE-UK. *Saving Lives, Improving Mothers' Care: Lessons Learned to Inform Future Maternity Care from the UK and Ireland Confidential Enquiries into Maternal Deaths and Morbidity 2009–12*. National Perinatal Epidemiology Unit, University of Oxford. 2014.

18. RCOG. Bacterial sepsis following pregnancy. Green Top Guideline No. 64b. 2012.

19. Greer I, Thomson A, The acute management of thrombosis and embolism during pregnancy and the puerperium. RCOG Green-top guideline no. 37b. RCOG. 2010.

20. Redshaw M, Rowe R, Henderson J, *Listening to Parents after Stillbirth or the Death of their Baby after Birth*. National Perinatal Epidemiology Unit. 2014.

21. Knight M, Tuffnell D, Kenyon S, *et al.* (editors) on behalf of MBRRACE-UK. *Saving Lives, Improving Mothers' Care: Surveillance of Maternal Deaths in the UK 2011-13 and Lessons Learned To Inform Maternity Care from the UK and Ireland Confidential Enquiries into Maternal Deaths and Morbidity 2009-13*. National Perinatal Epidemiology Unit, University of Oxford. 2015.

Polycystic Ovary Syndrome
Management of a Long-Term Condition in Primary Care

Anne Connolly and Virginia A. Beckett

Key Points

- Polycystic ovary syndrome is a common endocrine disorder with short- and long-term health consequences, the majority of which can and should be managed in primary care.
- The condition can be diagnosed from history and examination using the Rotterdam criteria.
- The symptoms of hyperandrogenism are a common presenting feature and can usually be improved by simple treatments along with weight reduction.
- Infertility is a frequent concern resulting from the anovulation caused by the hormonal imbalance of PCOS. In the majority of women this can be improved by weight reduction alone.
- Chronic anovulation is a risk factor for endometrial hyperplasia and cancer, and requires management with cyclical or continuous progestogen therapy, preferably by using the LnG-IUS.
- All women presenting with PCOS require a psychological assessment and support as appropriate.
- PCOS is a long-term condition requiring regular monitoring to prevent the consequences of insulin resistance, i.e. cardiovascular disease and diabetes.

Case Scenario: Shazia

Shazia, a 27-year-old classroom assistant, attends the primary care clinic concerned about her inability to conceive over the previous 18 months. She has one child, Asha, who is now aged three, from her first and only pregnancy. Her husband, Asif, a bus driver, is the father of her daughter.

On further questioning Shazia reports that she is distressed about a change to her periods, which have become less frequent and this has added more upset because she is ready to have another baby. The gap between her periods is now between two and six months. She does frequent home pregnancy tests in the hope that the delayed period is caused by pregnancy.

Introduction

Polycystic ovary syndrome (PCOS) is a complex, long-term condition which has metabolic, reproductive and psychological sequelae. This condition requires a holistic approach to management.

The commonest endocrine disorder affecting women of reproductive age, PCOS is characterized by a variable presentation, which includes hyperandrogenism, ovulatory dysfunction and polycystic ovarian morphology. Estimates of prevalence vary, but PCOS may affect between 10–20% of women of reproductive age in the UK [1].

PCOS was first described by Stein and Leventhal in 1935 when they published a case series of seven patients with amenorrhoea, hirsutism and bilateral polycystic ovaries. This condition was initially known as the Stein–Leventhal syndrome [2].

After years of debate to establish criteria to diagnose PCOS, a consensus workshop was held in Rotterdam in 2004. This workshop, supported by the European Society of Human Reproduction and Embryology (ESHRE) and American Society of Reproductive Medicine (ASRM), led to what has become known as the Rotterdam criteria for the

Table 14.1 Diagnosing polycystic ovary syndrome: The Rotterdam criteria [3]

The diagnosis of PCOS can be made on the basis of two out of three of the following:
- Clinical and/or biochemical signs of hyperandrogenism (acne, hirsutism or elevated testosterone)
- Oligo- or anovulation (infrequent menstrual cycles)
- Polycystic ovaries on ultrasound scan: ovarian volume > 10 cm^3 or more than 12 peripheral follicles of 2–9 mm in diameter

And exclusion of other causes (i.e. congenital adrenal hyperplasia; androgen-secreting tumours; Cushing's syndrome)

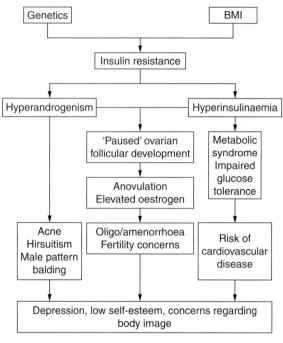

Figure 14.1 Causes and consequences of PCOS.

diagnosis of PCOS. The consensus criteria require two of the three key features: oligo- or anovulation, clinical and or biochemical hyperandrogenism and polycystic ovaries on ultrasound (Table 14.1) [3].

Whilst women with PCOS have traditionally been referred to gynaecology clinics, because the underlying cause was believed to be due to the abnormal ovarian function, the pathophysiology of this complex condition is now understood to be due to an endocrine abnormality resulting from insulin resistance. Insulin resistance is exacerbated by weight gain, which in turn exacerbates the clinical, reproductive and metabolic features of PCOS. The majority of care for this long-term condition should be provided in the primary care clinic with specialist referral for specific indications as required.

The clinical features of women with PCOS include:

- Endocrine (hyperandrogenism; acne, hirsutism, male pattern balding)
- Reproductive (anovulatory infertility)
- Metabolic (insulin resistance, impaired glucose tolerance, adverse cardiovascular risk profile)
- Psychological (increased anxiety, depression and reduced quality of life).

This condition requires a holistic life course approach with hyperandrogenic symptoms and infertility being more problematic in younger women and the metabolic features becoming more significant later. This does differ on an individual basis, and is dependent on other features, such as BMI and ethnicity (Figure 14.1 and Table 14.2).

Pathophysiology of PCOS [4]

The current understanding of the physiology of PCOS is summarized below:

- Insulin resistance caused by genetic factors and obesity results in hyperinsulinaemia.

- Hyperinsulinaemia causes overproduction of the gonadotrophin luteinizing hormone (LH), preventing the midcycle LH surge which is required for ovulation.

- The persistent high levels of LH antagonize the action of follicle-stimulating hormone (FSH), preventing the increase in FSH necessary for normal cyclical ovarian follicular development. The numerous small antral follicles produced are 'paused follicles', which have reduced cell growth and reduced cell death. These follicles typically arrest growth at 7 mm, which is an insufficient size for ovulation to occur.

- Ovarian follicles consist of two layers: an outer thecal layer and an inner granulosa cell layer.

Table 14.2 Consequences of PCOS

• Multiple peripheral ovarian cysts	• Insulin resistance	• Depression
• Menstrual irregularity	• Diabetes mellitus	• Endometrial hyperplasia and malignancy
• Subfertility	• Hyperlipidaemia	
• Mood disturbance	• Non-alcoholic steatohepatitis	
• Hyperandrogenism	• Adverse risk profile for CVD	
• Obesity		
• Sleep apnoea		
• Acne		
• Hirsutism		

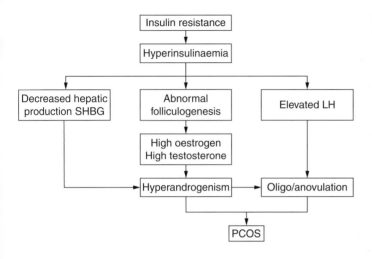

Figure 14.2 Hormonal influences on the development of PCOS.

- For normal development, the inner granulosa cells require FSH to synthesize and secrete oestradiol, whereas the thecal cells depend on LH to stimulate secretion of androgens, which are, in turn, converted into oestrogen in the granulosa cells.
- The ovary requires insulin to act as a co-factor to augment the LH-induced thecal cell androgen secretion. Women with insulin resistance produce excessive amounts of insulin in an attempt to promote glucose uptake in muscle and fat tissues. The ovary remains sensitive to insulin growth factor effects and the resultant hyperinsulinaemia causes more androgens to be produced.
- Anovulatory cycles lack the development of the corpus luteum, which produces progesterone necessary to induce secretory endometrial changes and subsequent endometrial shedding.
- Sex hormone binding globulin (SHBG) is the circulating protein which binds to and inhibits the effects of oestrogen and testosterone. In healthy women, 80% of circulating testosterone is bound to SHBG, 19% is bound to albumin and 1% circulates freely. It is the unbound (free) testosterone which is metabolically active.
- SHBG is inversely related to weight, so that overweight individuals produce less SHBG and have more circulating free androgens and oestrogen. As weight decreases, this effect reduces.
- Insulin is an anabolic hormone and has a role in energy storage. High insulin levels usually mean easier weight gain, which aggravates the symptoms and consequences of PCOS.

- Increased ovarian androgen production is caused by any, or a combination, of: increased LH, hyperinsulinaemia and obesity. In obese women, insulin resistance drives the hyperandrogenism, whereas in slender women elevated LH is the main cause. There is, however, significant overlap between these distinct types of PCOS, such that 10% of slender women with LH-driven PCOS will have impaired glucose tolerance.

Case Scenario

As the consultation with Shazia unfolds she becomes tearful. She knows she is putting on weight and has started shaving her upper lip and chin to try and hide the excessive hair growth she is bothered by.

Symptoms of PCOS

The initial concerns which the majority of women bring to their primary care clinician are consequences of the hyperandrogenism caused by PCOS.

Hirsutism is present in 60–80% of women with PCOS. It may be difficult to differentiate from idiopathic hirsutism, but the hirsutism secondary to excessive androgen production is found in a male pattern hair distribution. The Ferriman and Gallwey score [5] is the most commonly used objective grading, scoring 11 different body areas (upper lip, chest, chin, lower back, upper back, lower abdomen, upper abdomen, forearm, arm, thigh and lower leg). Each area is scored 0–4 with a total score of 8 or more defining hirsutism.

Androgenic alopecia (male pattern hair loss), whilst bothersome for some, is not a common feature of PCOS.

Acne is a less specific marker of hyperandrogenism as it is a common occurrence in teenage women, but new onset acne in adults is highly predictive of PCOS.

If there are signs of overt virilization, including voice deepening, increased muscle bulk and clitoral hypertrophy, then investigations including serum testosterone levels and an adrenal and ovarian ultrasound scan are essential to exclude an androgen-secreting tumour or late-onset congenital adrenal hyperplasia.

Acanthosis nigricans is also commonly found with PCOS and is dependent on the presence of insulin resistance. This skin condition is characterized by darkened velvety plaques most commonly occurring in the side of the neck, skin folds of the axilla and groin and on pressure bearing surfaces such as the elbows.

Other symptoms patients with PCOS complain of are related to their menstrual dysfunction. The most common complaint is of oligo- or amenorrhoea secondary to oligo- or anovulation. Oligomenorrhoea is defined as less than eight cycles per year with a cycle length of greater than 35 days.

The prevalence of depression and anxiety is higher in women with PCOS than in the general population. Concerns about body image and appearance due to the hyperandrogenic features can lead to eating disorders, and psychosexual and relationship problems, which can all be aggravated by the stress and upset associated with subfertility.

Case Scenario

On examination Shazia is noted to have acne and hirsutism, but no other obvious signs of virilization. She has a Ferriman and Gallwey score of 10. She has dark pigmentation in the nape of her neck and the skin folds of her axilla. Her BMI is 37 kg/m².

The diagnosis of PCOS can be made from her history and clinical examination as she has two of the three findings to fulfil the requirements of the Rotterdam criteria; clinical signs of hyperandrogenism and oligomenorrhoea.

Shazia is informed of her diagnosis and provided with the patient information leaflet downloaded from the resource www.patient.info. She is also advised to consult the Verity website at www.verity-pcos.org.uk [6]. This UK charity is for women whose lives are affected by polycystic ovary syndrome (PCOS) and is a useful resource for Shazia to understand the lifestyle changes she should make.

Examination

Examination is guided by the symptoms, but must also include blood pressure monitoring, body mass index and ideally a waist measurement (a value of > 80 cm indicating increased risk of metabolic complications). It is important to remember that many women with PCOS find examination, and particularly waist measurement, embarrassing.

Assessment of mood by commonly used scoring assessments can improve the identification and grading of psychological features and is an important part of every consultation.

Investigations

The diagnosis of PCOS is usually made from history and clinical examination, however, it is important to exclude other conditions such as hypothyroidism, hyperprolactinaemia and premature menopause.

Investigations could include serology for thyroid function, prolactin, FSH and LH levels. Ideally an FSH level should be taken during days 2–5 of the menstrual cycle. If this is not possible because of her long or absent menstrual cycles, a random sample repeated in six weeks is often the best possible option.

The expectation in PCOS is that the LH:FSH ratio is greater than 2:1.

Testosterone testing is complex as total testosterone levels do not demonstrate much variation, due to the low circulating testosterone usually found in women. However, serum total testosterone level can be useful to exclude an androgen-secreting tumour, as a level of <5.0 nmol/L is usually consistent with mild hyperandrogenism and hence PCOS, whereas a testosterone level of >5.0 nmol/L is more likely to be due to an adrenal or ovarian tumour, congenital adrenal hyperplasia or Cushing's syndrome, and requires further investigations.

Testing SHBG allows measurement of the more reliable free androgen index (FAI).

$$FAI = total\ testosterone/SHBG \times 100.$$

Other investigations include a pelvic and transvaginal ultrasound scan (TVUS). The TVUS allows more detailed examination of ovarian pathology, particularly in women who are obese, but may not be acceptable to all women, especially those who have never been sexually active.

The ultrasound findings which confirm PCOS are the presence of more than 12 follicles in each ovary, measuring 2–9 mm in diameter and/or increased ovarian volume (>10 cm^3). The follicles tend to be peripherally sited and provide a characteristic 'string of pearls' effect. The prevalence of endometrial hyperplasia and cancer is increased in obese women with oligo/anovulation caused by their elevated and unopposed circulating oestrogen levels [7]. TVUS findings of a thickened or cystic endometrium indicate that more detailed assessment by pipelle sampling or hysteroscopy is required.

Other investigations are indicated following a cardiovascular risk assessment. An HbA1C is indicated at the time of diagnosis and on an annual basis. Other investigations should include lipid levels, renal and liver function tests, as routine for assessment of women with a high risk of developing diabetes and non-alcoholic fatty liver [8].

Case Scenario

Shazia's main concern on this occasion is her inability to conceive. As she also has concerns about her appearance, these problems should also be addressed during the management discussions.

Management

The management of PCOS is aimed at:

- Helping to manage the short-term problems of hyperandrogenism, mood disturbance and fertility.
- Helping to reduce the long-term consequences of insulin resistance and endometrial hyperplasia.

The most important aspect of management must be aimed at weight reduction by a combination of good nutrition and exercise. This will reduce insulin resistance, reduce androgen levels and the systemic effects of ovarian dysfunction, resulting in improvement of symptoms, fertility and reduction of long-term consequences.

Other treatments should be individualized to provide appropriate symptom control. The symptoms of hyperandrogenism can be improved by any treatment to reduce circulating free androgens. Weight reduction will achieve this by increasing levels of SHBG and so will treatment with ethinyl-oestradiol, by use of any combined hormonal contraceptive, after a risk assessment.

Oral anti-androgen therapies such as cyproterone acetate, either alone or in combination with 35 mcg ethinyl-oestradiol, as Dianette®, are an alternative. Yasmin®, a combination of ethinyl-oestradiol and the anti-androgen drosperinone, may also be helpful in the treatment of some women with acne. Patients must be encouraged to continue with their medication because it may take up to nine months before they see significant improvement. The use of these treatments must be balanced against the risk of potential complications, particularly thrombo-embolic events in women with a BMI greater than 35 kg/m^2.

In those who have contraindications for the use of combined hormonal contraception, such as high BMI, focal migraine or other thrombotic or cardio-vascular conditions, then the usual treatments for acne, such as long-term oral or topical antibiotics, may be used. Roaccutane treatment, under specialist supervision, is also an option.

Once recruited, hair follicles remain active and long-term treatment for hirsutism may be required. Weight reduction and the use of anti-androgenic oral contraceptives will provide some improvement, but other women require additional symptomatic managements including: eflornithine cream, Vaniqa® or physical hair removal treatments such as shaving, waxing, electrolysis and laser treatments.

It is important for patients with PCOS to reduce weight to a BMI less than 30 kg/m^2 prior to conception because of the complications of pregnancy and poorer foetal outcomes which are associated with maternal obesity. Gestational diabetes mellitus (GDM) is the most frequently occurring problem, but others include: pregnancy-related hypertension, pre-eclampsia, placental abruption and thrombo-embolic events [9]. Reliable contraception should be provided, as recommended by the Endocrine Society guideline, until the appropriate BMI, blood pressure and glycaemic control is achieved to reduce these risks [10].

When couples present with fertility concerns, it is essential to consider other possible causes for their problem in addition to the PCOS and investigate following standard practice. Weight reduction may be sufficient to increase the chance of conception, but other investigations, including a semen analysis, should be performed [11].

Table 14.3 Management of women with PCOS

Problem	Management options
Obesity	Weight reduction including: • Diet/exercise • Medication • Bariatric surgery
Hirsutism	Physical therapies including shaving, waxing, electrolysis, laser treatments. Eflornithine cream Combined hormonal contraception including ethinyl-oestradiol and cyproterone acetate or drosperinone Other anti-androgenic treatments: spironolactone and cyproterone acetate
Acne	Combined hormonal contraception Topical or systemic antibiotics
Oligo or amenorrhoea	Levo-norgestrel intrauterine system Combined hormonal contraception Cyclical or continuous progestogens including medroxy-progesterone acetate
Infertility	Baseline investigations, including semen analysis Specialist management in line with local guidelines

Insulin resistance, metabolic syndrome and cardiovascular disease	Optimize cardiovascular risk factors including:
	• Smoking cessation
	• Managing abnormal factors:
	  · BP
	  · HbA1C
	  · Lipid profile

Depression and psychosexual problems	Improve emotional wellbeing: • Support • Antidepressants • Counselling, including relationship counselling

The role of metformin is controversial, due to lack of evidence of benefit. The current recommendation for use in primary care is only as treatment for those women with established type 2 diabetes. Metformin may also be used in conjunction with clomifene citrate, for ovulation induction, in specialist fertility units, as recommended by NICE [12].

Specialist Fertility Treatments

Initial fertility advice and management is standard practice for all couples referred to specialist services and follows NICE recommendations [12].

This includes lifestyle advice for both partners including:

• Weight optimization
• Smoking cessation

• Alcohol and reduction of other non-prescribed medication
• Regular unprotected penetrative sexual intercourse
• Stress management.

Further intervention is not indicated until the woman achieves her recommended BMI of <30 kg/m^2. Semen analysis and tubal patency tests are required, but, once other causes of infertility are excluded, ovulation induction treatment should be considered.

Clomifene citrate is the first-line recommended pharmacological therapy for ovulation induction. Clomifene is a selective oestrogen receptor modulator with both oestrogenic and anti-oestrogenic properties. It acts by inhibiting oestradiol receptor binding in the hypothalamus and pituitary, thereby blocking negative inhibition. This allows the hypothalamus to increase gonadotrophin-releasing hormone causing an increase in FSH production which promotes follicular growth necessary for ovulation.

Treatment with clomifene requires careful dose titration in a specialist unit, with regular ultrasound scanning to monitor ovarian stimulation, to reduce the risk of hyperstimulation and multiple pregnancy. In patients who achieve ovulation with clomifene, pregnancy rates are around 40% by the sixth cycle. If pregnancy is not achieved after nine ovulatory cycles, assisted conception should be considered.

NICE guidelines recommend that metformin may be added as adjuvant therapy to clomifene-resistant women with PCOS because combined therapy may improve pregnancy rates [12].

Patients who fail to ovulate using clomifene and metformin should be offered laparoscopic ovarian drilling (LOD). The aim of LOD is to destroy ovarian androgen-producing tissue which can:

• Reduce intraovarian androgen production causing a reduction in circulating androgens.
• Cause an indirect modulating effect on the pituitary gland. LH concentrations decrease and FSH increases which leads to a recruitment of a new set of follicles and resumption of normal ovarian function.

This is unsuccessful in less than 50% of women, who may then require additional ovulation induction [13].

Gonadotrophins are an alternative treatment option if clomifene fails to induce ovulation. Low-dose regimens are used to reduce rates of ovarian hyperstimulation and multiple pregnancy.

> **Case Scenario**
>
> The next time Shazia attends clinic she seems low and anxious. She discloses that her husband has commented on her weight and facial hair. She has continued to gain weight and now has a BMI of 39 kg/m². She is reluctant to socialize normally with family and friends and has started spending time and money on make-up and hair removal treatments.

The psychological features of PCOS are often overlooked, but the impact of subfertility and low self-esteem with negative body image often cause depression, anxiety and relationship problems, including sexual dysfunction.

Supporting women with psychological and psychosexual concerns is an important aspect of the holistic care required. Screening should be performed at an early stage so that support can be offered. Other managements, including anti-depressants and counselling, as well as relationship counselling, should be provided as usual for any patient seen in the primary care setting.

The lifestyle changes that are essential to reduce obesity are difficult to sustain for individuals who lack self-confidence and motivation. Addressing the psychological issues can empower women to comply with the weight reduction required to reverse the metabolic and endocrine problems.

Long-Term Monitoring and Management Requirements

Women with PCOS are at increased risk of cardio-vascular disease because of their obesity, hyperandrogenism, hyperlipidaemia and hyperinsulinaemia [14].

In summary these women require:

- Screening for cardio-vascular disease:
  - Conventional cardiovascular risk calculators have not been validated for patients with PCOS. But as 70% of women with PCOS have a dyslipidaemia and between 33–47% have metabolic syndrome the Androgen Excess and Polycystic Ovary Syndrome Society recommend that women with PCOS should have their blood pressure, waist circumference and BMI checked regularly and a lipid profile determined every two years [14].
- Screening for diabetes:
  - In view of the insulin resistance associated with PCOS an HbA1C should be performed at diagnosis and then on annual or biannual basis, dependent on their risks: BMI, ethnicity, FH, history of GDM.
- Screening and prevention of endometrial hyperplasia:
  - Women with PCOS who have oligo- or amenorrhoea are predisposed to developing endometrial hyperplasia and endometrial carcinoma due to the prolonged exposure to unopposed oestrogen.
  - Endometrial protection can be provided by:
    - Levonorgestrel-IUS
    - combined hormonal contraception, following risk assessment
    - induced withdrawal bleeds using intermittent progestogen therapy, usually medroxyprogesterone acetate 10 mg daily for 14 days or twice daily for 7–10 days every three to four months.

Summary

PCOS is a complex, life-long endocrine condition caused by insulin resistance. There are short- and long-term problems associated with this condition that require appropriate understanding, management and monitoring.

Patient education, psychological support and weight reduction are important elements of management that can and should be done in primary care.

Further Reading

cks.nice.org.uk/polycystic-ovary-syndrome#! topicsummary (accessed September 2016).

PCOS Australian Alliance. Assessment and management of polycystic ovary syndrome: summary of an evidence-based guideline. www.mja.com.au/journal/ 2011/195/6/assessment-and-management-polycystic-ovary-syndrome-summary-evidence-based (accessed September 2016).

Royal College of Obstetricians and Gynaecologists. Polycystic ovary syndrome, long-term consequences.

Green-top Guideline No. 33. www.rcog.org.uk/en/guidelines-research-services/guidelines/gtg33/ (accessed September 2016).

References

1. March WA, Moore VM, Willson KJ, *et al*. The prevalence of polycystic ovary syndrome in a community sample assessed under contrasting diagnostic criteria. *Hum Reprod* 2010;25(2):544–551.

2. Stein I, Leventhal M, Amenorrhoea associated with bilateral polycystic ovaries. *Am J Obstet Gynecol* 1935;29:181–189.

3. Rotterdam ESHRE/ASRM–sponsored PCOS Consensus Workshop Group. Revised 2003 consensus on diagnostic criteria and long-term health risks related to polycystic ovary syndrome. *Fertil Steril* 2004;81:19–25.

4. Duncan WC, A guide to understanding polycystic ovary syndrome (PCOS). *J Plann Reprod Health Care* 2014;40:217–225.

5. Ferriman DM, Gallwey JD, Clinical assessment of body hair growth in women. *J Clin Endocrinol* 1961; 21:1440–1447.

6. Verity PCOS charity. www.verity-pcos.org.uk (accessed September 2016).

7. Haoula Z, Salman M, Atiomo W, Evaluating the association between endometrial cancer and polycystic ovary syndrome. *Hum Reprod* 2012;27:1327–1331.

8. Shaw LJ, Bairey Merz CN, Azziz R, *et al*. Postmenopausal women with a history of irregular menses and elevated androgen measurements at high risk for worsening cardiovascular event-free survival: results from the National Institutes for Health – National Heart, Lung, and Blood Institute sponsored Women's Ischaemia Syndrome Evaluation. *J Clin Endocrinol Metab* 2008;93:1276–1284.

9. Qin JZ, Pang LH, Li MJ, *et al*. Obstetric complications in women with polycystic ovarian syndrome: a systematic review and meta-analysis. *Reprod Biol Endocrinol* 2013;26:11–56.

10. Wild RA, Carmina E, Diamanti-Kandarakis E, *et al*. Assessment of cardiovascular risk and prevention of cardiovascular disease in women with the polycystic ovary syndrome: a consensus statement by the androgen excess and polycystic ovary syndrome (AE-PCOS) society. *J Clin Endocrinol Metabol* 2010; 95(5):2038–2049.

11. Balen AH, Anderson RA, Impact of obesity on female reproductive health: British Fertility Society, Policy and Practice Guidelines. *Hum Fertil* 2007;10(4): 195–206.

12. NICE. Fertility: Assessment and treatment for people with fertility problems. NICE guidelines CG156. 2013. https://www.nice.org.uk/guidance/CG156 (accessed September 2016).

13. The Thessaloniki ESHRE/ASRM-Sponsored PCOS Consensus Workshop Group. Consensus on infertility treatment related to polycystic ovary syndrome. *Hum Reprod* 2008;23(3):462–477.

14. Fauser BC, Tarlatzis BC, Rebar RW, *et al*. Consensus on women's health aspects of polycystic ovary syndrome: The Amsterdam ESHRE/ASRM – sponsored 3rd PCOS Consensus Working Group. *Fertil Steril* 2012;97:28–38.

Management of Premature Ovarian Insufficiency in Primary Care

Henny Lukman, Amanda Hillard and Timothy Hillard

Key Points

- Consider POI in young women presenting with more than three months of amenorrhoea.
- Elicit family history of early menopause, autoimmune conditions, fragile X syndrome.
- Untreated premature ovarian insufficiency increases the risk of osteoporosis, cardiovascular disease, dementia, cognitive decline and parkinsonism.
- Treatment should be with HRT or COCP until at least the average age of menopause at 51.
- Emphasize the importance of long-term replacement and that benefits far outweigh any risks.
- Risks of cancer and stroke quoted for HRT treatment for 'normal' menopausal women do not apply to younger women.
- Spontaneous POI is associated with 5–10% pregnancy rate. Contraception may be needed.
- Advise weight-bearing exercise, limiting caffeine and alcohol intake, smoking cessation and maintaining healthy body weight.
- Be aware of the psychological impact and provide appropriate support.

Introduction

Premature menopause is a potentially life-changing condition which is often under-recognized and incompletely managed. Premature ovarian failure (POF), premature menopause, premature ovarian insufficiency (POI) and premature ovarian senescence are all terms that have been used to describe a syndrome consisting of amenorrhoea, sex steroid deficiency and menopausal levels of gonadotrophins (LH and FSH) in a woman more than two standard deviations below the mean age at menopause [1]. It is not a homogeneous condition; for some there is a genetic or congenital cause such as Turner's syndrome, congenitally absent or infantile ovaries, whilst for others, it is cessation of hormone production and reproductive function at an early age due to cancer treatments, surgery or an autoimmune disorder. In the majority of cases the aetiology is unknown.

The study of this condition is complicated by its low incidence, lack of agreed nomenclature and agreed diagnostic criteria. The management of this group of women can be complex and made difficult by the paucity of research studies in this area.

Definition and Nomenclature

The nomenclature in this area is confusing and the terms and definitions are applied inconsistently. The median age of menopause in the Western world is 51. Approximately 5% of women will undergo menopause at the age of 40–45. This is often referred to as 'early menopause'. Premature menopause is usually reserved for women who undergo menopause before 40. This condition affects about 1 in 100 women under 40, 1 in 1000 women under the age of 30 and 1 in 10,000 women under the age of 20 [2]. It accounts for 10–28% of women with primary amenorrhoea and 4–18% of those with secondary amenorrhoea. However, with the number of survivors from childhood cancers increasing, these traditional figures may be an underestimate.

The term 'menopause' denotes an irreversible condition. However, in women with spontaneous onset of POF, there may be some return of ovarian function and even pregnancies achieved so the term premature menopause is best avoided. The terms premature ovarian failure (POF) and premature

Women's Health in Primary Care, edited by Anne Connolly and Amanda Britton. Published by Cambridge University Press
© Cambridge University Press 2017

Table 15.1 Known causes and risk factors for POI

Primary	Examples
Congenital	Absent/infantile ovaries
Chromosome abnormalities	Turner's, Fragile X, Down's syndrome
Other genetic cause	FSH receptor gene mutations, BRCA1
Enzyme deficiency	Galactosaemia
Autoimmune diseases	Thyroid, Addison's
Family history of early menopause	Inheritable genetic cause of premature ovarian aging
Secondary	
Chemotherapy and radiotherapy	
Surgical removal of ovaries	
Previous hysterectomy	
Uterine artery embolization	
Severe endometriosis	
Infections	Mumps, tuberculosis

ovarian insufficiency (POI) are most frequently used, but the former may have negative connotations for some so the recommended nomenclature, which is used in this chapter, is POI.

Causes and Risk Factors

The aetiology of premature ovarian ageing remains elusive, despite the numerous conditions that are associated with POI (Table 15.1). A genetic aetiology will be identified in approximately 5% and autoimmune in up to 30% [3]. In women presenting with spontaneous POI, no cause will be found in up to 90% of the cases. With improvement in cancer therapy, there is an increasing number of young women with iatrogenic POI. Management of POI in this group of patients is an important cancer survivorship issue that is often overlooked.

Presentation

POI commonly presents with amenorrhoea and symptoms of oestrogen deficiency, such as hot flushes and night sweats, vaginal dryness, low libido, low energy levels, sleep disturbance, lack of concentration, stiffness, skin/hair changes and mood swings. Other more subtle presentations which may be missed include pubertal delay, oligomenorrhoea, menstrual

dysfunction and infertility. However, these symptoms may be atypical and presenting in a younger woman may not automatically be considered to be menopausal. Sexual dysfunction, fertility concerns and psychological problems are the issues that disturb women the most [4].

Diagnosis

A comprehensive gynaecological and obstetrics history, including surgery and family history of autoimmune diseases and early menopause, should be elicited. A full family history is important as many cases of spontaneous POI appear to be inherited; estimates vary from 4% to 31% [5]. An autoimmune aetiology may be suspected from a family history of autoimmune diseases. A detailed contraceptive history should be taken, as combined pill use, for example, usually produces a regular cycle and could mask evidence of POI that may have occurred some years earlier. In young women and adolescents, physical examination should be performed to confirm normal secondary sexual characteristics and breast development.

There are no definitive diagnostic criteria for POI. The most commonly used definition is four to six months of amenorrhoea, with serum FSH levels of greater than 40 IU/L on two occasions taken four to six weeks apart [6,7]. Other studies have used levels of FSH greater than 40 IU/L and oestradiol levels below 50 pmol/L [8]. Other initial investigations should include measurement of serum oestradiol, prolactin, androgens and thyroid function tests. The diagnosis of POI is frequently delayed as it often presents a fluctuating clinical picture with ovarian dysfunction preceding failure.

Once POI is suspected, further tests may include karyotyping, genetic studies, autoimmune antibodies, pelvic ultrasound and DEXA scan for bone mineral density. There is no role for tests of ovarian reserve in primary care. These tests are expensive, unreliable and need cautious interpretation.

Consequences

POI and early menopause, whether spontaneous or induced, are associated with significant long-term health risks, mainly associated with oestrogen deficiency. Oestrogen replacement mitigates some, but not all, of these consequences [9]. Untreated POI is associated with a 50% higher mortality than woman who undergo menopause at a normal age [10]. There are also significantly increased risks of cardiovascular disease (80%), dementia, cognitive decline and parkinsonism [7,11]. Prolonged premature oestrogen deficiency has a potentially devastating effect on bone, with a reduction in bone mineral density at an early age, osteoporosis and an increased risk of fracture. Individual long-term strategies for the monitoring and prevention of osteoporosis should be established with the patient.

Menopausal symptoms can have a profound effect on a woman's quality of life and self-esteem at any age, but this may be particularly pronounced in the younger age group. These women may also suffer significant psychosexual dysfunction and mood disorders.

In some with autoimmune-associated POI, thyroid and rarely adrenal dysfunction can develop [3], however POI is also associated with a reduction in the risk of breast cancer [12].

Published evidence in this area is derived mainly from cohort studies of women with surgical menopause [11]. There is very little known about the long-term outcome of spontaneous POI or the effect of hormone replacement in this group of women.

Fertility

For many women, the loss of fertility that comes with a diagnosis of POI can be devastating. However, unless they have had a bilateral oophorectomy, women with POI should not automatically be considered infertile. In 50% of women with spontaneous POI there is some background ovarian activity with a 5–10% pregnancy rate [13]. Unfortunately it is not possible to predict the likelihood of a pregnancy in individuals; therefore if pregnancy is not desired, contraceptive use is essential. The use of the combined oral contraceptive pill (COCP) as replacement treatment will be useful as HRT is not contraceptive. Conversely for those who do wish a pregnancy, referral to fertility services is recommended. The use of assisted reproductive techniques does not improve the conception rate in this group of women [14], thus the only realistic treatment option is *in vitro* fertilization with donor oocytes and her partner's sperm. There are many psychological and ethical implications involved, and appropriate counselling before embarking on such treatment is mandatory. The availability and costs of such treatment vary widely, although it is being used more in Europe. Prior cryopreservation of oocytes is an option if a woman is about to lose her ovaries through surgery or radiotherapy. For women with POI as the result of cancer treatment, pregnancy may carry increased risk of preterm deliveries, intrauterine growth retardation and miscarriages. Other options such as adoption should also be discussed.

Counselling/Emotional Support

POI can be a very difficult diagnosis for a woman to accept. The impact of such a diagnosis on a young woman's view of her sexuality, femininity and self-image can be devastating. The resulting infertility can be the hardest aspect to come to terms with, and this doesn't necessarily depend on whether or not she already has children.

Women with POI have an increased incidence of sexual dysfunction, depression and a sense of isolation [4,15]. The younger the woman, the more likely she is to have psychosexual problems. These women need holistic care and specialized support, ideally from a multidisciplinary team, which includes counselling and support from professionals with experience in POI. They need adequate information which is given in a sensitive way and they should be encouraged to seek additional support through national support groups such as the Daisy Network (www.daisynetwork.org .uk).

Specific genetic counselling may also be needed, depending on the aetiology of the POI.

Hormone Replacement

POI is an endocrine condition of oestrogen deficiency and the appropriate treatment is replacement of the missing hormones. Thus oestrogen or hormone replacement therapy (HRT) is recommended to treat the symptoms of POI and prevent the long-term adverse effects of oestrogen deficiency. This is the recommendation from all national and international menopause societies and the NICE guidance [4,7,16,17]. HRT should be continued at least until the natural age of menopause at around 51. Other treatments such as SSRIs have much poorer efficacy, offer no long-term protections for cardiovascular and bone health and are not recommended unless there is evidence of clinical depression [7,18]. Long-term use of bisphosphonates in young women for prevention of bone loss has not been studied, may be harmful and is not recommended.

There is relatively little research done on the optimal treatment of POI. Currently most clinics use oestradiol-based HRT (with a progestogen if the uterus is present) or the COCP as replacement therapy. There is emerging evidence that oestradiol-based HRT may give superior long-term benefits when compared to synthetic-oestrogen-containing COCP. However, in this group of women, where long-term replacement is necessary, compliance is important and the COCP may be a better choice. It is very popular among the younger patients as it is a medication that they and their peers are familiar with and it does not carry the negative association with menopause.

Specific Considerations

Women with POI who take HRT often need a higher dose of oestrogen to control their symptoms than women in their fifties; 100 mcg transdermal oestradiol or 3–4 mg oral oestradiol or even higher doses maybe necessary. Specialist help should be sought if symptoms prove hard to control. Although these doses may seem high, it should be remembered that with fully functioning ovaries the circulating oestradiol levels would be much higher through the cycle. Vaginal oestrogens may be needed in addition to systemic HRT to control symptoms of uro-genital atrophy.

Women with POI may report reduced libido or sexual function, despite apparently adequate doses of oestrogen replacement. This is more common in oophorectomized women. The use of testosterone should be considered in such cases [7].

There are very few absolute contraindications to HRT in young women with POI. For the vast majority, the benefits of oestrogen replacement will outweigh any risks. The use of HRT does not increase risk of breast cancer when compared to normally menstruating women. Some of the negative publicity around HRT in recent years has resulted in some women being worried or anxious about taking HRT. They should be specifically reassured that any such concerns do not apply to women with POI who are simply replacing the hormones they would have produced if their ovaries had still been functioning.

Women with POI should be reviewed annually and advised to lead a healthy lifestyle to improve cardiovascular and bone heath. These include weight-bearing exercise, limiting caffeine and alcohol intake, smoking cessation and maintaining healthy body weight.

Conclusion

POI is a devastating diagnosis for a young woman. It has wide-ranging implications for her physical and mental health. Its treatment and management is long term. HRT or the COCP are the mainstays of treatment up until the age of natural menopause, but the risks and sequelae of POI may be lifelong. Although some of aspects of the care will require specialist medical, diagnostic and counselling input, the role of the general practitioner is central to the overall management of such a long-term condition. The general practitioner is ideally placed to provide ongoing support for the woman and her family, and monitoring for associated morbidity such as subsequent development of osteoporosis and autoimmune diseases.

References

1. Rees M, Stevenson J, Hope S, Rozenberg S, Palacios S, Premature ovarian failure. In: *Management of the Menopause: The Handbook, 5th edn.* Royal Society of Medicine Press Ltd. 2009: 147–156.

2. Coulam CB, Adamson SC, Annegers JF, Incidence of premature ovarian failure. *Obstet Gynecol* 1986;67(4): 604–606.

3. Bakalov VK, Vanderhoof VH, Bondy CA, Nelson LM. Adrenal antibodies detect asymptomatic auto-immune adrenal insufficiency in young women with spontaneous premature ovarian failure. *Hum Reprod* 2002;17(8):2096–2100.

4. Singer D, Mann E, Hunter MS, Pitkin J, Panay N, The silent grief: psychosocial aspects of premature ovarian failure. *Climacteric* 2011;14(4):428–437.

5. Van Kasteren YM, Hundscheid RD, Smits AP, *et al.* Familial idiopathic premature ovarian failure: an overrated and underestimated genetic disease? *Hum Reprod* 1999;14(10):2455–2459.

6. Sassarini J, Lumsden MA, Critchley HO, Sex hormone replacement in ovarian failure: New treatment concepts. *Best Pract Res Clin Endocrinol Metabol* 2015; 29(1):105–114.

7. NICE. Menopause: diagnosis and management. NICE guidelines NG23. 2015.

8. Vujovic S, Brincat M, Erel T, *et al.* EMAS position statement: Managing women with premature ovarian failure. *Maturitas* 2010;67(1):91–93.

9. Shuster LT, Rhodes DJ, Gostout BS, Grossardt BR, Rocca WA, Premature menopause or early menopause: long-term health consequences. *Maturitas* 2010;65(2): 161–166.

10. Ossewaarde ME, Bots ML, Verbeek AL, *et al.* Age at menopause, cause-specific mortality and total life expectancy. *Epidemiol* 2005;16(4):556–562.

11. Rocca WA, Bower JH, Maraganore DM, *et al.* Increased risk of cognitive impairment or dementia in women who underwent oophorectomy before menopause. *Neurol* 2007;69(11):1074–1083.

12. Titus-Ernstoff L, Longnecker MP, Newcomb PA, *et al.* Menstrual factors in relation to breast cancer risk. *Cancer Epidemiol Biomarkers Prevent.* 1998;7(9): 783–789.

13. Bidet M, Bachelot A, Touraine P. Premature ovarian failure: predictability of intermittent ovarian function and response to ovulation induction agents. *Curr Opin Obstet Gynecol* 2008;20(4):416–420.

14. Van Kasteren YM, Schoemaker J. Premature ovarian failure: a systematic review on therapeutic interventions to restore ovarian function and achieve pregnancy. *Hum Reprod Update.* 1999;5(5):483–492.

15. Liao KL, Wood N, Conway GS. Premature menopause and psychological well-being. *J Psychosom Obstet Gynecol* 2000;21(3):167–174.

16. Panay N, Hamoda H, Arya R, Savvas M. The 2013 British Menopause Society and Women's Health Concern recommendations on hormone replacement therapy. *Menopause International.* 2013 May 23: 1754045313489645.

17. De Villiers TJ, Pines A, Panay N, *et al.* Updated 2013 International Menopause Society recommendations on menopausal hormone therapy and preventive strategies for midlife health. *Climacteric* 2013;16(3): 316–337.

18. Rees MCP, Panay N. Alternatives to HRT for the management of symptoms of the menopause. RCOG Scientific Advisory Committee Opinion Paper 6, 2nd edn. Royal College of Obstetricians and Gynaecologists. 2010.

Chapter 16

Premenstrual Disorders PMD
A Practical Approach in Primary Care

Carolyn Sadler

Key Points

- The diagnosis should be made by analyzing the patient's daily recordings of the frequency and severity of symptoms over two cycles.
- A woman may be suffering from core premenstrual disorder or one of its variants.
- All women should be advised of general lifestyle changes that could improve symptoms.
- Cognitive behavioural therapy has been shown to be effective in the treatment of PMD
- Agnus castus is a recommended treatment. Other complementary therapies for which there is some evidence of effectiveness include calcium and vitamin D, isoflavones, pollen extract and ginko biloba.
- Evidence-based therapies include combined third-generation pills, transdermal oestradiol, selective serotonin reuptake inhibitors (SSRIs) and GnRH analogues.
- Progestogens and progesterone can induce symptoms in sensitive women.
- Any specific treatment may take up to three months to be effective. If a woman's symptoms are severe, the more aggressive treatment options should be started earlier rather than later.
- Hysterectomy and bilateral oopherectomy can be offered in severely resistant cases.
- The National Association for Premenstrual Syndrome provides support for sufferers, their personal carers and the health professionals who care for them.

'It's like somebody else has taken over my body, mind and soul. There is a demon spirit inside me, telling me to do inappropriate things, prompting me to say hurtful, offensive words, urging me to be the meanest bitch that ever walked the earth.'

Quote from *The Twenty-Eighth Day* by Catherine Barry, an Irish poet and novelist, portraying the experience of a PMS sufferer. Published by the National Association for Premenstrual Syndrome.

Introduction

Most women are aware of physical and/or psychological changes during their menstrual cycle. For a significant number, these symptoms are troublesome and impact their daily activities. A cross-sectional survey of 974 women in Southampton, aged between 19 and 34, who completed a six-week prospective symptom diary, found a 24% prevalence of premenstrual symptoms [1]. It is estimated that between 5% and 8% of women in the reproductive age group suffer severely, and that this group may fulfil the American Psychiatric Association criteria for premenstrual dysphoric disorder, as detailed in the Diagnostic and Statistics Manual, Version 1V [2].

There have been many different definitions and terms used to describe this cyclical menstrual disorder, namely premenstrual syndrome, premenstrual tension and premenstrual dysphoric disorder. During 2008, a group of international experts (the International Society for Premenstrual Disorders or ISPMD) attended a series of meetings in Montreal, Canada. Their aim was to reach a consensus on the definition of premenstrual disorders and the criteria for their diagnosis. They hoped their work would lead to the development of a consistent approach to diagnosis and treatment, and aid research in the field. Together they produced what is now termed the Montreal Consensus [3,4], which defined 'core premenstrual disorder' (akin to premenstrual syndrome), and four other variants (Figure 16.1 and Table 16.1).

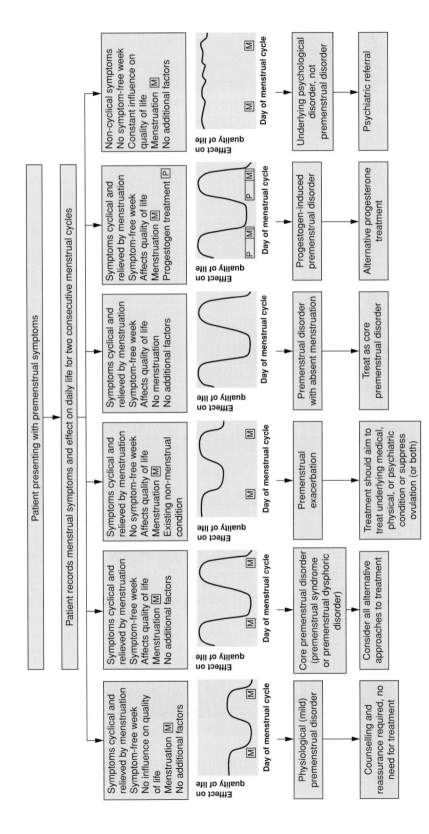

Figure 16.1 Schematic representation of daily record of severity of problems charts obtained on patients presenting with a presumed diagnosis of premenstrual disorder.

Table 16.1 Possible diagnoses in women presenting with premenstrual symptoms.

Diagnosis	Cyclical symptoms	Symptoms in luteal phase	Symptoms in follicular phase	Impairment	Comment
Physiological premenstrual symptoms[a]	Present	Present	Absent	None	Although symptoms are cyclical and there is a symptom-free week, they are of insufficient severity to cause serious impairment
Core premenstrual disorder[a]	Present	Present	Absent	Present	This is the typical or core premenstrual disorder: symptoms are cyclical, relieved by the end of menstruation with a follicular phase symptom-free week; they cause serious impairment
Premenstrual exacerbation	Present	Present	Remain high, but reduced compared with luteal phase	Present	Symptoms are cyclical, cause serious impairment, but are only partially alleviated by menstruation because of an underlying psychological, physical or medical condition
Premenstrual disorder, menstruation absent[a]	Present	Present	Absent	Present	Essentially the same as core premenstrual disorder, but without menstruation as a reference event as a result of iatrogenic amenorrhoea (hysterectomy with ovarian conservation, endometrial ablation, levonorgestrel intrauterine system)
Progestogen-induced premenstrual disorder[b]	Present	Present during progestogen treatment	Absent during progestogen-free phase of HRT or variably during exposure to hormonal contraceptives	Present	Symptoms are generated without ovulation by the cyclical administration of progestogen for therapeutic (HRT) or contraception purposes
Mis-attribution	Absent	Present	Present	Present	Although symptoms may be severe they are non-cyclical; this suggests the presence of a continuous and serious psychological disorder

[a] Symptoms probably result from ovulation and endogenous progesterone or its metabolites.
[b] Symptoms are iatrogenic and result from treatment with exogenous progestogens.
HRT = hormone replacement therapy.

Core Premenstrual Disorder

Definition: Symptoms occur regularly in ovulating women during the luteal phase of the cycle, resolve by the end of menstruation, and are followed by a symptom-free interval. Substantial impairment of daily activities at work or school, social activities and hobbies, and interpersonal relationships is a key feature.

About 200 possible physical and psychological symptoms have been described, but the diagnostic criteria do not require specific symptoms to be present. The most frequently encountered physical symptoms are breast tenderness, bloating and headaches. Anxiety, depression and mood swings are the commonest psychological symptoms.

Core premenstrual disorder is akin to definitions for premenstrual syndrome.

Premenstrual Exacerbation of an Underlying Physiological or Medical Condition

Physical conditions, such as asthma and epilepsy, and psychological conditions, such as depression and anxiety, can all worsen premenstrually.

Premenstrual Symptoms in the Absence of Menstruation

This may happen when amenorrhoea has been induced by insertion of a progestogen-releasing intrauterine system (IUS), following an endometrial ablation or hysterectomy with conservation of the ovaries.

Progestogen-Induced Premenstrual Syndrome

In susceptible women, giving cyclical progestogen in the form of sequential HRT or combined hormonal contraceptives can induce symptoms.

Non-Ovulatory Premenstrual Disorders

This disorder is poorly understood but it is thought that, in some women, follicular activity can precipitate symptoms even if ovulation does not occur.

Aetiology

The aetiology of premenstrual disorders is still uncertain, but is thought to be due to a combination of physiological, psychological and social factors in susceptible women. A genetic predisposition has also been postulated.

One suggested physiological factor is hormonal change at the time of ovulation, affecting the neurotransmitters serotonin and gamma-amino butyric acid (GABA) in the brain.

This theory is supported by the observation that women can expect a welcome relief of symptoms during pregnancy and after their menopause.

Women who suffer with a premenstrual disorder also have a higher prevalence of postnatal depression and low mood during their menopause transition.

Guidelines reviewing the diagnosis and management of premenstrual disorders are available from the Royal College of Obstetrics and Gynaecology (RCOG), [5]. The National Association for Premenstrual Syndrome (NAPS) guidelines are also available to download from its website [6].

Diagnosis of Premenstrual Disorders

Case History 1

Rachel is 34 years old. She is married to Tom and has two children: Bethany, aged six, and Charlie, aged four. She works part-time as a saleswoman for a greetings card company. Her work involves regular visits to local retailers to present the company's products and secure business deals. Tom is a self-employed joiner.

She attends surgery and at the start of the consultation bursts into tears saying that she cannot cope. On questioning, she explains that she has been suffering with symptoms of anxiety, low mood,

emotional lability and has been having difficulty concentrating. She reports that the symptoms start about a week before her period is due and she usually feels better one to two days after her bleeding starts.

During this time her symptoms are so severe that she occasionally has to cancel some of her appointments at work. She has a good relationship with her husband, but when she has symptoms she finds fault, and arguments follow.

As her GP I will now describe the different ways I can provide support for Rachel and the different treatments that I could offer. Throughout, I will indicate three levels of evidence available to support the different treatment recommendations.

In summary:

Level 1: Well-conducted trials or systematic reviews support using this treatment
Level 2: Some evidence from research trials supports the use of this treatment
Level 3: There is little evidence from research trials to support the use of this treatment but consensus of medical opinion supports its use.

With the exception of the progesterone pessaries (Cyclogest), none of the products mentioned are licensed for the treatment of premenstrual disorders.

The Initial Consultation

I would ask Rachel about the nature and severity of her symptoms and the degree to which they impact her relationships at work and at home. I would assess her physical health, significant past medical history and current regular medication, including contraceptive use. I would also ask about lifestyle factors, including diet, level of exercise, alcohol intake, smoking status and level of stress. Not easy (or possible) in 10 minutes!

Case History 1

On questioning, Rachel describes moderately severe anxiety for about 10 days leading up to her period and for the first two or three days of bleeding. She has no features of an endogenous depression or suicidal intent. She eats a healthy, balanced diet, but, a few days before her period, craves chocolate. She drinks about 20 units of alcohol a week and does find that she uses alcohol as a way of 'unwinding' after the children have gone to bed. She enjoys exercise and tries to go to the gym about three times a week, but sometimes this is not possible due to work and family commitments. Her BMI is 29. She has no significant past medical history, has never smoked and uses condoms for contraception.

Making the Diagnosis

It is important to try and secure the diagnosis at an early stage, before specific treatments are initiated. The best way to do this is by asking the patient to prospectively record the frequency and severity of the symptoms on a daily basis over two cycles. Retrospective recording is unreliable. I would recommend using either the Daily Record of Severity of Problems [7] or the menstrual chart, available to download on the NAPS website [8].

During the first consultation, I would inform Rachel that I believe that she is suffering from PMD, and I would suggest that she complete a prospective symptom diary over two cycles.

I would discuss with her the benefits of a healthy lifestyle (Level 2 evidence) including good nutrition, regular exercise, avoiding sleep deprivation, moderating her alcohol intake and minimizing stress where possible. With respect to diet I would advise regular meals and snacks with low glycaemic index (unrefined starchy foods), to avoid the effects of low blood sugars. The diet should be low in fat and refined carbohydrate, and high in fruit and fibre.

I would direct her to the NAPS website where she could find details of the various treatment options available, their guidelines and a free menstrual diary to download [6,8] (Figure 16.2).

Case History 1

Rachel returns two months later. She has completed a menstrual chart, which shows a pattern typical of core premenstrual disorder. She has made some lifestyle modifications and has noticed a slight improvement in her symptoms, but is still not coping with work and family commitments. She has read the NAPS guidelines and wants to know which complementary therapies I would recommend. She is not keen on taking anti-depressants or hormone treatment.

Treatment of Premenstrual Disorders

Cognitive Behavioural Therapy (Evidence Level 1 [9])

Cognitive behavioural therapy, including relaxation, stress management and assertiveness training has been shown to be effective.

The availability of psychological services varies from area to area, but women could also be directed to internet-based resources and reading material.

Complementary Therapies

It is difficult to assess the true value of the following interventions. They are freely available with little regulation. Research studies are limited and side effects and interactions are underestimated.

Reflexology and Acupuncture (Evidence Level 2 [10])

Some studies have shown benefit from these interventions.

Calcium and Vitamin D (Evidence Level 2 [11])

Some evidence suggests that they are useful in menstrual migraine. A dietary assessment should be made and levels checked prior to treatment.

Agnus Castus (Evidence Level 1 [12])

In a systematic review into herbal remedies for PMD, four of the trials supported the use of Vitex agnus castus. It comes from the fruit of the chaste tree and contains a mixture of iridoids and flavonoids.

- It should not be used with SSRIs
- Adverse effects: low
- Recommended dose: 20–40 mg/day, depending on product.

Isoflavones (Evidence Level 2 [13])

Early studies have shown a possible benefit in menstrual migraine.

- Adverse effects: low
- Recommended dose: red clover isoflavones, 40–80 mg/day, depending on product.

Vitamin B6 (Evidence Level 3 [14])

Studies have shown mixed results:

Treatment guidelines for PMS

Nick Panay BSc MRCOG MFSRH

Chairman of the National Association for Premenstrual Syndrome, Director of West London Menopause & PMS Centre, Consultant Gynaecologist Imperial College Healthcare NHS Trust & Chelsea and Westminster NHS Foundation Trust, Honorary Senior Lecturer, Imperial College London

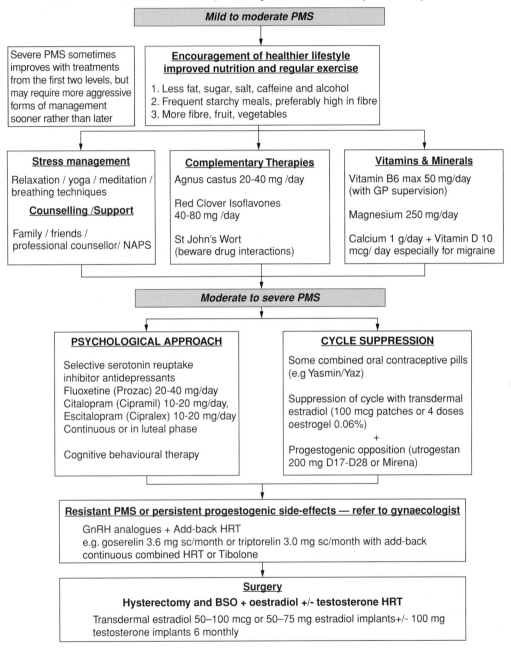

Figure 16.2 Treatment guidelines for PMS.

- It is often used to treat PMD with little evidence for its effectiveness
- Adverse effects: risk of peripheral neuropathy with higher doses
- Recommended dose: The Department of Health and Maternal and Child Health advises that the daily dose should not exceed 10 mg (recommended dietary allowance is around 2 mg/day).

Evening Primrose Oil (Evidence Level 2 [15])

Some studies have shown that it may alleviate symptoms of breast tenderness, but that it is not helpful for other premenstrual symptoms.

Others

Research has also been carried out on ginkgo biloba, pollen extract, magnesium supplements and St John's Wort (caution is needed because of interactions with conventional medicines), but further work needs to be undertaken before recommendations can be made.

Case History 1

Rachel decides to take Agnus Castus. She comes back three months later. Again, she has noticed some improvement in her symptoms and reports that she is much calmer and less confrontational with her husband. However, she is still having problems with anxiety. Having read about the different treatment options, she would like to try a selective serotonin reuptake inhibitor (SSRI). She expresses two concerns about starting an SSRI. Firstly, she is not keen to take it all the time when she only is symptomatic for part of the month. Secondly, she and her husband are considering having another baby and she asks whether taking an SSRI has been shown to be harmful in early pregnancy.

Selective Serotonin Reuptake Inhibitors (Evidence Level 1 [16])

There is a good body of evidence for the use of SSRIs in the treatment of PMD.

In addition, studies have suggested some benefit with serotonin and noradrenaline reuptake inhibitors (SNRIs) as well.

It has also been shown that SSRIs can be helpful in PMD if they are only taken during the time that a woman is symptomatic in the luteal phase of the cycle. Symptoms may improve within 48 hours of starting treatment.

All the SSRIs appear to be equally effective.

There is some concern that the use of SSRIs in early pregnancy may increase the risks of cardiac and other congenital defects. It is possible that the reported risk is also driven by other confounding factors, but when possible SSRIs should be discontinued prior to and during pregnancy [5].

There is not one SSRI that is safer than another, but perinatal psychiatrists favour sertraline because of its low secretion into the breast milk and fluoxetine because of the amount of data available about its use.

- Adverse effects:
  - Initially: nausea, exacerbation of anxiety, fatigue, sweating
  - Ongoing: loss of libido, flattening of mood
- Recommended doses:
  - Fluoxetine: 20–40 mg/day
  - Citalopram: 10–20 mg/day
  - Sertraline: 50–100 mg/day

Conclusion

Rachel could be advised to start the SSRI at symptom onset, or 24–48 hours beforehand through to day 3 of her next cycle, when her symptoms would usually resolve. Gradual withdrawal is unnecessary if treatment is with low-dose luteal phase and side effects are less common. She will need to make an informed choice about taking the treatment, however, given the potential risks.

Case History 2

Karen is 42 years old. She attends the surgery for advice about contraception. She has been divorced for two years and her ex-husband had had a vasectomy. She has just entered into a new relationship and is very worried about becoming pregnant. On questioning, she explains that her cycle has become more irregular recently and her periods heavier. She reports that for years she has noticed that she is more emotionally labile a few days before her period, but that she has not felt the need to seek help for this. In recent months this problem has

---

worsened and she is having difficulty coping with daily activities in the days leading up to her period. She has also noticed occasional hot flushes and night sweats. She has no significant past medical history and has never smoked. She has a BMI of 22. Her mother went through the menopause at the age of 40, but she has no other family history of note.

The Initial Consultation and Diagnosis

As her GP, I would take a full history and counsel Karen about dietary and lifestyle changes that could improve her symptoms.

It is likely that Karen is starting to go through the menopause transition, a time during which premenstrual symptoms can worsen. Even though Karen's fertility will be declining, she still requires contraception until two years after her last natural period.

I would discuss Karen's contraceptive options with her, focussing on treatment regimes that may also alleviate her premenstrual and menopausal symptoms.

Combined Hormonal Contraceptives (Evidence Level 1 [17])

Early studies showed mixed results with respect to the effect of the combined pill on PMD. Combined hormonal methods do suppress ovulation, but symptoms can be induced by exogenous hormones (such as the second-generation progestogens norethisterone and levonorgestrel) and can be precipitated by fluctuations in hormone levels around the time of the hormone-free interval.

Further research has focussed on some of the newer combined pills, in particular those pills containing the progestogen drospirenone, which has anti-mineralocorticoid and anti-androgenic properties. Pills containing 20 and 30 mcg ethinylestradiol are available. A combined pill containing 20 mcg of ethinylestradiol and 3 mg of drospirenone is licensed in Europe and the USA for women with premenstrual dysphoric disorder who also require contraception.

There is evidence to support the use of extended regimes, reducing the pill-free interval. In one study the participants took an ethinylestradiol/drospirenone pill on a 168-day regime. There was a significant reduction in premenstrual symptoms compared with the standard 21/7 regime.

A combined pill in an extended regime would be an option for Karen, as she has no contraindications to its use. In addition, treating her with oestrogen may also help her mild menopausal symptoms.

Progestogens and Natural Progesterones: Do They have a Role in the Treatment of Premenstrual Disorders?

There is insufficient data to recommend the routine use of progestogens or natural progesterone in the treatment of PMD [18]. Indeed, in sensitive women, progestogens may precipitate and worsen symptoms.

However, two observational studies [1,19] have shown a lower prevalence of premenstrual symptoms in women using injectable progestogens.

Natural progesterone may have anxiolytic and mild diuretic effects. Cyclogest (a progesterone pessary) is the only product licensed for treatment of PMD in the UK.

Non-Oral Oestradiol with Progestogenic Opposition (Evidence Level 1 [20])

Even though these regimes suppress ovulation, it is not recommended that they be relied upon for contraception, except when the IUS is used.

There is no data on the safety of these regimes with respect to the long-term effects on breasts and endometrium. However, it is reassuring that when the cycle is adequately suppressed, oestradiol levels should be no higher overall than the expected levels during a woman's natural menstrual cycle.

- This treatment should be initiated with the support of specialist advice
- Evidence-based regimes:

  · Oestradiol patches: 75–100 mcg patch, twice weekly
  · Progestogens and natural progesterones that provide endometrial protection and minimize side effects given for a minimum of 12 days per 28-day cycle:

    – The progestogen releasing intrauterine system (IUS)
    – Natural progesterone utogestran: 200 mg a day either orally or per vagina.

- – Vaginal progesterone gel, crinone 8%: One applicator/alternate days for 12 days/28 day cycle i.e. six applications
- – Cyclogest pessaries 400 mg a day: One/day for 12 days/28 day cycle. Usually used vaginally but use rectally if vaginal infection, postpartum or using barrier contraception.

Danazol (Evidence Level 1, for Breast Tenderness [21])

Studies have shown the benefit of danazol for breast tenderness. However its use is restricted because of potential irreversible virilizing effects and teratogenicity. For these reasons it should only be used under the supervision of a specialist. It is not a contraceptive.

Recommended dose: 200 mg twice daily.

GnRH Analogues and Hysterectomy and Bilateral Oophorectomy (Evidence Level 1 [22])

In the most resistant and severe cases of PMD, referral to a specialist is indicated and consideration can be given for treatment with GnRH analogues. GnRH analogues cause profound cycle suppression and elimination of premenstrual symptoms. A lack of effectiveness when using this treatment would challenge the accuracy of the diagnosis rather than the efficacy of the medical treatment.

To reduce the loss of bone mineral density, treatment should be combined with hormone replacement therapy (continuous combined therapy or tibolone in preference to a cyclical progestogen therapy, to minimize progestogen intolerance). Women on long-term treatment should have bone densitometry on an annual basis.

Hysterectomy and removal of the ovaries is occasionally performed, but only after very detailed counselling [23]. It should always be preceded by a course of GnRH analogues to confirm the diagnosis. HRT, including consideration of testosterone therapy, is needed after the operation, as premenstrual symptoms are often replaced with menopausal symptoms.

Adverse effects: induces a hypo-oestrogenic state, which can cause hot flushes, night sweats and an increased risk of osteoporosis.

Conclusion

Transdermal oestradiol and an IUS would be a good treatment option for Karen.

The two case histories illustrate features of core premenstrual disorder. The same treatment options can be applied to any of the variant premenstrual disorders. When severe psychopathology is suspected, it is important to consider incorporating the support of local psychiatric services.

It is appropriate for most women to be managed in a primary care setting, but women at the severe end of the spectrum should be preferentially referred into specialist hospital services with a multidisciplinary team. This team should include a psychologist, dietitians and a gynaecologist with expertise in the management of this common and at times challenging medical condition.

The National Association for Premenstrual Syndrome, pms.org.uk

This is a charitable organisation, which supports sufferers, their carers and health professionals. Guidelines and other relevant articles are available to download. Members can seek help through an e-mail enquiry service, which is manned by experts in the field.

The charity organizes, on average, two national conferences a year, which cover a full spectrum of women's health topics.

References

1. Sadler C, Smith H, Hammond J, *et al.* Lifestyle factors, hormonal contraceptives, and premenstrual symptoms: The UK Southampton Women's Survey. *J Womens Health* 2010;19(3):1–6.

2. American Psychiatric Association. Premenstrual dysphoric disorder. In *Diagnostic and Statistical Manual of Mental Disorders, 4th edn.* American Psychiatric Press. 2000:771–774.

3. O'Brien PMS, Backstorm T, Brown C, *et al.* Towards a consensus on diagnostic criteria, measurement and trial design of the premenstrual disorders: the ISPMD Montreal consensus. *Arch Womens Ment Health* 2011; 14:13–21.

4. O'Brien PMS, Rapkin A, Dennerstein L, Nevatte T. Diagnosis and management of premenstrual disorders. *BMJ* 2011;342:1–10.

5. RCOG Green Top Guideline No 48 Premenstrual Syndrome Management 2016. www.rcog.org.uk.

6. National Association for Premenstrual Syndrome. Treatment guidelines for premenstrual syndrome. www.pms.org.uk/support/ (accessed September 2016).

7. Endicott J, Nee J, Harrison W. Daily Record of Severity of Problems: reliability and validity. *Arch Womens Ment* 2006;9(1):43.

8. National Association for Premenstrual Syndrome. Support/menstrual diary. www.pms.org.uk/ (accessed September 2016).

9. Hunter M, Ussher J, Cariss M, et al. Medical (fluoxetine) and psychological (cognitive behavioural therapy) treatment for premenstrual dysphoric disorder: A study of treatment processes. *J Psychosom Res* 2002;53:811–817.

10. Guo S, Sun Y. Comparison of therapeutic effects of acupuncture and medicine on premenstrual syndrome. *Chinese Acupunct Moxib* 2004;24(1):29–30.

11. Thys-Jacobs S, Starkey P, Bernstein D, Tian J. Calcium carbonate and the premenstrual syndrome: Effects on premenstrual and menstrual symptoms. *Am J Obstet Gynecol* 1998;179(2):444–452.

12. Dante G, Facchinetti F. Herbal treatments for alleviating premenstrual symptoms: a systematic review. *J Psychosom Obstet Gynaecol* 2011;32(1):42–51.

13. Burke B, Olson R, Cusack B. Randomized controlled trial of phytoestrogen in the prophylactic treatment of menstrual migraine. *Biomed Pharmacother* 2002;56:283–288.

14. Wyatt K, Dimmock P, Jones P, O'Brien P. Efficacy of vitamin B6 in the treatment of premenstrual syndrome: Systematic review. *BMJ* 1999;318:1375–1381.

15. Khoo s, Munro C, Battistutta D. Evening primrose oil and the treatment of premenstrual syndrome. *Med J Aust* 1990;153(4):189–192.

16. Marjoribanks J, Brown J, O'Brien P, Wyatt K. Selective serotonin reuptake inhibitors for premenstrual syndrome and (review). *Cochrane Database Syst Rev* 2013;(6):CD001396.

17. Lopez L, Kaptein A, Helmerhorst F. Oral contraceptives containing drospirenone for premenstrual syndrome. *Cochrane Database Syst Rev* 2012;(2):CD006586.

18. Wyatt K, Dimmock P, Jones P, Obhrai M, O'Brien P. Efficacy of progesterone and progestogens in management of premenstrual syndrome: Systematic review. *BMJ* 2001;323:1–8.

19. Hourani L, Yuan, Bray R. Psychosocial and lifestyle correlates of premenstrual symptoms among military women. *J Womens Health* 2004;13:812–821.

20. Naheed B, Uthman O, O'Mahony F, Kiuper J, O'Brien P. Non-contraceptive estrogen containing preparations for controlling symptoms of premenstrual syndrome. *Cochrane Database Syst Rev* 2014;(9):CD010503.

21. O'Brien P, Abukhalil I. Randomized controlled trial of the management of premenstrual syndrome and premenstrual mastalgia using luteal-phase only danazol. *Am J Obstet Gynecol* 1999;180:18–23.

22. Wyatt K, Dimmock P, Ismail K, Jones P, O'Brien P. The effectiveness of GNRHa with and without 'add back' therapy in treating premenstrual syndrome: a meta-analysis. *BJOG* 2004;111:585–593.

23. Cronje W, Vashisht A, Studd J. Hysterectomy and bilateral oopherectomy for severe premenstrual syndrome. *Hum Reprod* 2005;19:2152–2155.

Non-Menstrual Vaginal Bleeding Management in Primary Care

Clare Spencer and Jackie Tay

Key Points

- Post-coital bleeding is a symptom of cervical cancer, but most causes are benign.
- A cervical ectropion can cause abnormal bleeding, but does not require treatment if asymptomatic.
- In young women with post-coital bleeding always exclude sexually transmitted infections.
- Women under the age of 25 years with abnormal bleeding do not need a smear, but should always be examined and investigated.
- A transvaginal pelvic ultrasound scan is a useful investigation if routinely referring a woman with intermenstrual bleeding.
- Consider exogenous hormones as a cause of abnormal vaginal bleeding in women of reproductive age.
- Women with postmenopausal bleeding should be referred urgently to gynaecology to exclude malignancy.
- Fluctuations in endogenous hormones can cause non-menstrual bleeding, but pathology must be excluded.

Box 17.1 Causes of Non-Menstrual Vaginal Bleeding

- Physiological
- Hormonal contraception (all routes)
- Pelvic inflammatory disease
- Cervix – benign lesions – cervical ectropion, polyps
  - pre-malignancy – CIN
  - malignancy
- Endometrium – benign lesions – endometrial polyps, endometrial hyperplasia
  - malignancy
- Vaginal and vulval benign lesions – including dermatoses
- Vaginal and vulval malignancy
- Trauma
- Bleeding disorders
- Retained tampon
- Sexually transmitted infections

Vaginal bleeding that is not related to menstruation is a common symptom presenting to general practice. It causes concern as gynaecological malignancy can present with abnormal bleeding, but often fluctuations in endogenous hormones are the cause. The age of the patient and an accurate history will determine the relevant investigations to arrange.

The causes of non-menstrual vaginal bleeding are listed in Box 17.1.

Case Scenario 1

Anna is a 22-year-old student who attends clinic in a routine slot. She has been bleeding after sex and is worried about it. She stopped taking the combined pill six months ago at the end of a relationship. She has a new partner and is currently using condoms for contraception. She is otherwise well.

History

Sensitive and careful history-taking is important. Post-coital bleeding can be a symptom of gynaecological malignancy and patients are often very anxious about their symptoms. Box 17.2 outlines the important points in the history. As Anna is young she should also be asked her history of human papilloma virus (HPV) vaccination. See Box 17.3 for more information.

Women's Health in Primary Care, edited by Anne Connolly and Amanda Britton. Published by Cambridge University Press
© Cambridge University Press 2017

Box 17.2 Non-Menstrual Vaginal Bleeding: History Points

- Menstrual history
  · Timing, duration and frequency of abnormal bleeding
  · Last menstrual period date
- Exogenous hormone therapy (combined hormone contraception, progesterone-only contraception)
- Other contraceptive use
- Dyspareunia
- Sexual history and any recent STI screening of patient and partner
- Unusual vaginal discharge
- Pelvic pain
- Cervical smear history
- Bladder symptoms
- Bowel symptoms
- Symptoms suggesting bleeding disorders
- Past gynaecological and obstetric history
- Ask about any treated gynaecological premalignant and malignant lesions
- Past medical history
- Family history including history of cancers
- Drug history
- Social history – including smoking and alcohol

Box 17.3 Notes on HPV Vaccination

HPV is an important risk factor for cervical cancer [1]. It is a double-stranded DNA virus which infects the basal cells of the squamous epithelia. There is no national screening programme in the UK, but there has been a vaccination programme since 2008, aiming to vaccinate girls before they become sexually active [2]. HPV is one of the most common infections in the world, the lifetime cumulative risk being greater than 80% [3]. Most infections are transient, but persistent infection with HPV-16 and HPV-18 is associated with 70% of all invasive cervical cancer. Cervarix® vaccine was initially used, protecting against HPV16 and HPV18. Gardasil® has been used since 2011 and is a quadrivalent vaccine, protecting against HPV16, HPV18, HPV6 and HPV11. HPV 6 and 11 cause the majority of genital warts, so Gardasil® protects against them also [4]. Gardasil® has been shown to be over 99% effective in preventing precancerous lesions associated with HPV16 or 18 in young women and this is likely to be maintained for at least 10 years. Condoms reduce, but do not completely prevent, the transmission of HPV.

Box 17.4 Examination

- *General inspection:*
  · Abdominal palpation: Assess for areas of tenderness in the iliac fossae, any pelvic masses and distension
  · Vulval: Trauma, skin changes, inflammation, scarring, discolouration, ulceration/fissuring
- *Pelvis:*
  · Cuscoes speculum: Inspect the vaginal wall, noting the colour, any lesions and any prolapse
  · Inspect the cervix, noting any ectropion or contact bleeding. Take a cervical smear test if due
  · Assess any discharge and take the appropriate swabs
  · Look for blood and where it may be coming from
  · Bimanual examination:
    – Palpate the cervix and assess the uterine size and adnexal regions
    – Check for cervical excitation by gently moving the cervix.

Examination

Examination requirements are listed in Box 17.4. These can inform investigations and referral. Knowing what is normal is imperative. In the case of Anna, it is particularly important to fully visualize her cervix.

Investigations should include swabs to check for sexually transmitted infection (STIs) during the pelvic examination [5]. As Anna has symptoms which could be due to genital infection she requires: a high vaginal swab (HVS) to check for *Candida*, *Trichomonas vaginalis*, bacterial vaginosis and anaerobes; a cervical or vaginal nucleic acid amplification test (NAAT) swab for chlamydia and gonorrhoea and an endocervical charcoal swab if gonorrhoea is suspected clinically, as this will allow culture for sensitivities. Urine testing for chlamydia is not as sensitive as taking a cervical or vaginal swab, or using a self-taken vaginal swab [6]. All women of reproductive age require a pregnancy test if there is any possibility of pregnancy.

Management

Management depends on the findings. In this age group, checking for STIs and excluding pregnancy and cervical pathology are the main priorities.

If the cervix has an abnormal appearance or if there is an ectropion with contact bleeding, she requires an urgent fast-track referral to gynaecology. Colposcopy and a cervical biopsy should be performed to exclude cervical intraepithelial neoplasia (CIN) and cervical malignancy [7]. It is inappropriate to perform a cervical smear first. The NHS Cervical Screening Programme recommends screening between the ages of 25 and 64 [8]. The number of women who develop cervical cancer aged 20–24 years is fewer than 50 cases per year, whilst it has been estimated that 1500–7500 women will present to the GP with abnormal vaginal bleeding each year [9]. The rate of false positive smears in the under 25s is high, as the cervix is still developing, causing the immature cell structure to confuse the cytologist [10]. This can lead to unnecessary investigation and anxiety when the majority of the changes will revert to normal with time. Screening women under 25 has little or no effect on the incidence of cervical cancer.

Gynaecological malignancies are rare in young women, but may arise from any part of the genital tract and may cause abnormal bleeding. Cervical carcinoma is the most common malignancy in women aged under 35, although the incidence has decreased since the roll out of the cervical screening programme [11]. There are two age-related incidence peaks: the first in women aged 30–34 (20 per 100,000 women) and the second in women aged 80–84 (13 per 100,000 women) [11]. The earlier peak has been caused by women becoming infected with HPV when they become sexually active in their late teens/early 20s, but should reduce as the cohort of women reaching this age have been immunized against HPV.

The prevalence of postcoital bleeding among women with cervical cancer has been reported as being up to 39%.

Benign Cervical Pathology

A cervical ectropion is a common finding as the cause of postcoital bleeding. It occurs where the dark red vascular columnar epithelium of the endometrium is found on the surface of the cervix. This area would usually be covered with the paler squamous epithelium of the vagina. The squamous epithelium usually becomes columnar at a transformation zone within the endocervical canal. In high oestrogen states associated with puberty, pregnancy or with anovulation, the transformation zone everts to be found on the

> **Box 17.5** Symptoms and Signs of Pelvic Inflammatory Disease
>
> - *Symptoms*
>   - Lower abdominal pain – usually bilateral
>   - Abnormal vaginal bleeding – can be intermenstrual, postcoital or menorrhagia
>   - Abnormal vaginal discharge – can be purulent
>   - Deep dyspareunia
> - *Signs*
>   - Fever
>   - Lower abdominal tenderness
>   - Cervix motion tenderness (cervical excitation)
> - Adnexal tenderness on bimanual pelvic examination

external surface of the cervix (ectocervix). An ectropion is a common finding and occurs after puberty. Unless it causes symptoms such as postcoital bleeding, it does not require treatment. However, the columnar cells can bleed and are also more prone to infection. If the ectropion is symptomatic, symmetrical and even, a routine referral to gynaecology can be made. The ectropion can be 'removed' with cryotherapy or electrocautery in the outpatient setting. In primary care, prior to referral, a cervical smear should be taken if due and infection should be excluded. If there is any doubt about its benign nature, a fast-track referral for colposcopy should be made as it can be difficult to visually differentiate between a benign ectropion and CIN.

A cervical polyp may also cause postcoital bleeding. These may be twisted off in primary care or referred for removal in an outpatient setting, or they sometimes require removal with loop diathermy. The polyp must be sent for examination, but will usually have benign histology.

Anna is at risk of an STI because of a recent change in partner. STIs can cause bleeding by causing cervicitis and/or endometritis. The clinical features are listed in Box 17.5. If there is strong suspicion of an STI and the patient has other symptoms of pelvic inflammatory disease she should be treated empirically after swabs have been taken. Delay in treatment can increase the risk of tubal damage and, subsequently, ectopic pregnancy, infertility and chronic pelvic pain. Antibiotic regimes should be according to The British Association for Sexual Health and HIV [5]. Treatments include a combination of ceftriaxone for possible gonorrhoea and doxycycline for chlamydia. Metronidazole is included in some regimens as anaerobes are of relatively greater importance in patients with severe

PID. Quinolone-resistant gonorrhoea in the UK is becoming an increasing problem and quinolone should therefore be avoided in areas where >5% of PID is caused by quinolone-resistant *Neisseria gonorrhoeae*.

Occasionally, chronic yeast infection or eczema-like dermatoses can cause fissures and inflammation that can bleed during or after sex as a result of friction. Treatment with soap substitutes and anti-fungal therapy can help with chronic yeast infections. Eczema and dermatitis are treated with emollients and topical steroids.

Management Summary

The examination of Anna demonstrated a normal appearing cervix, with a small central ectropion. Her swab results were normal and she had no further episodes of bleeding.

The bleeding is presumed to be due to a physiological cause and she is reassured.

She is advised to return if she has any further postcoital bleeding because even with a normal appearance of the cervix she would need to be referred to the colposcopy clinic for further examination if this recurred.

Case Scenario 2

Helen is a 44-year-old-health care assistant who attends an appointment. She has noticed bleeding in between her periods for the last four months. It is light and she finds it more of a nuisance than anything else. She has two children and her family is complete.

History

The history of her bleeding problem is important, refer to Box 17.1.

As Helen is of reproductive age, it is important to ask about any use of contraception, pregnancy risk or change in sexual partner, as well as assessing her risk of cervical or endometrial malignancy.

Examination

Pelvic and speculum examination are required with screening for STIs as in Case Scenario 1 and Box 17.4. Careful examination of her cervix is essential,

---

Box 17.6 'Red Flag' Symptoms for Gynaecological Malignancy to Consider Alongside Clinical Judgement and Examination Findings [7]

- Alterations in menstrual cycle
- Intermenstrual bleeding
- Postcoital bleeding
- Vaginal discharge
- Postmenopausal bleeding not on HRT
- Persistent postmenopausal bleeding after stopping HRT
- Postmenopausal bleeding in women taking tamoxifen.

---

remembering that there are similar causes of post-coital and intermenstrual bleeding [12].

It is important to note her BMI as obese women have increased risk of developing endometrial hyperplasia and malignancy as a result of their increased exposure to oestrogen. Adipose tissue is the major site of conversion of androstenedione to oestrone, and plasma levels of sex hormone binding globulin (SHBG), which binds oestradiol (E2), are lower in obese women, so higher levels of serum oestradiol and oestrone are available to target sensitive tissues such as the endometrium.

Investigations

In planning investigations and management, exclusion of malignancy is a consideration. The incidence of endometrial cancer starts to gradually increase after the age of 40 and in the UK, between 2009 and 2011, almost 75% of endometrial cancers were diagnosed in women aged between 40 and 74 [13].

The risk of cervical cancer is low, as long as the patient has adhered to the national screening programme and previous smears have been normal. Other gynaecological malignancies are rare in this age group [13].

If there are abnormal findings in the history and examination that increase the suspicion of malignancy she requires a two-week wait referral as per NICE guidelines [7]; for example, if she also has postcoital bleeding, a change in her menstrual pattern, is grossly obese or has an abnormal-looking cervix on speculum examination. See Box 17.6 for 'red flag symptoms'. If she is bleeding after a diagnosis of premature ovarian insufficiency she should be urgently investigated in the same way as for a presentation of postmenopausal bleeding.

Blood Tests

Bleeding disorders usually present with menorrhagia, but some women can also experience intermenstrual bleeding [14]. These disorders may be related to platelet number (for example idiopathic thrombocytopenic purpura) or function (for example Von Willebrand disease). A full blood count and coagulation screen are recommended if the history is suggestive of a clotting disorder with a discussion with a haematologist if abnormalities are found.

If there are symptoms and signs suggestive of ovarian cancer in particular ascites or a pelvic/abdominal mass or other suspicious symptoms as discussed in Chapter 26, a CA125 blood test should be taken [15].

Pregnancy Test

Helen is still fertile and pregnancy-related bleeding must be excluded. Early pregnancy bleeding is very common and if the pregnancy test is positive she needs a referral to an early pregnancy assessment unit.

Transvaginal Ultrasound (TVUS)

Transvaginal ultrasound scanning is a safe and cheap test to organize. This will provide information on pelvic structures and endometrial thickness, and may pick up benign endometrial pathology, including submucosal fibroids, endometrial polyps or endometrial hyperplasia. It is appropriate to request an ultrasound scan (USS) before routine referral to gynaecology. In menstruating women, the endometrial thickness varies throughout the cycle and can measure up to 16 mm in the secretory phase. Therefore, the endometrial thickness measurement guidelines used in postmenopausal women do not apply (see Case Scenario 3).

If the USS shows any benign pathology she requires a routine referral for hysteroscopic examination. This referral is also necessary with normal USS findings if she continues to experience intermenstrual bleeding. Hysteroscopy is the 'gold-standard' investigation allowing direct visualization of the endometrium, including any endometrial or endocervical polyps not seen on USS, and any suspicious looking lesions can be biopsied. Small polyps may also be removed in the outpatient hysteroscopy clinic with larger lesions requiring removal under general anaesthesia.

The USS may indicate endometrial thickening or abnormal cystic appearances suggestive of endometrial hyperplasia. This is caused by greater than normal proliferation occurring during the menstrual cycle. It is confirmed from an endometrial biopsy sample. Endometrial histology can be benign proliferative, secretory or atrophic. There may also be hyperplasia with or without atypia, or endometrial adenocarcinoma.

Endometrial hyperplasia is associated with increased unopposed oestrogen stimulation of the endometrium, e.g. in women who are obese, or have long episodes of amenorrhoea from their polycystic ovary syndrome, or in women taking unopposed systemic oestrogen-only HRT.

Hyperplasia is classified according to the presence of atypia by the histopathologists. For hyperplasia without atypia, the risk of progression to carcinoma is less than 5% and these patients can be managed medically with high-dose oral or intrauterine progestogens to maintain a thin endometrium [16]. The risk of progression to carcinoma in women with hyperplasia with atypia is around 30% [16] and is usually managed surgically because of the higher risk of endometrial malignancy.

Exogenous Hormones

In the case of Helen, she could be using hormonal contraception as she is of reproductive age and not wanting more children. Exogenous hormones influence endometrial pathology. Although not fully understood, there may be changes in blood vessel fragility and other factors that influence bleeding [17]. Frequent and irregular bleeding are common in the first three months after starting any hormonal method of contraception.

Irregular bleeding is more likely if pills are not taken consistently. Bleeding with the combined contraceptive pill may result because of insufficient sex-steroid concentrations to maintain the endometrium and may require dose adjustment if continuing after the initial three months. Bleeding with the progestogen-only pill may result from partial suppression of ovulation and is unpredictable and often difficult to improve.

If a woman has experienced a regular bleeding pattern whilst using a form of contraception and is taking it regularly, any change in bleeding pattern should be investigated.

Hormonal contraception reduces the risk of endometrial cancer, but not completely. An endometrial biopsy should always be performed in women over the aged of 45 with persistent intermenstrual bleeding using hormonal contraception and in women under the age of 45 with severe or persistent symptoms and/or risk factors for endometrial cancer [18].

Physiological Causes

If all investigations are normal, there may be a physiological explanation for intermenstrual bleeding. During the normal menstrual cycle, oestradiol levels increase in the follicular phase and result in endometrial proliferation. Progesterone secretion in the luteal phase is anti-oestrogenic, inhibiting endometrial growth and glandular differentiation. Withdrawal of both hormones results in menstruation. If there is an excessive fall in oestrogen after the follicular phase peak there is premature shedding of the endometrium, causing intermenstrual bleeding. As the corpus luteum forms, oestrogen and progesterone levels rise again and so bleeding stops. This is most common in younger women. In this situation, cyclical progesterones or the combined oral contraceptive may be considered if management is required.

Summary

Helen has a BMI of 34 kg/m^2, she is up to date with her cervical screening and infection was excluded. She has not been using any contraception as her long-standing partner had a vasectomy five years previously.

There were no abnormal findings on speculum or pelvic examination so a TVUS was organized.

The TVUS reported an area of thickened endometrium at the fundus, suggestive of an endometrial polyp and she was referred to the local gynaecology department for hysteroscopy.

Case Scenario 3

Clare is a 65-year-old woman who attended for her annual diabetic review appointment with the nurse and mentioned that she had experienced some vaginal bleeding. She is now very anxious as she has waited in surgery to be seen in an extra urgent appointment.

History

As previously the history is important to determine what exactly she means by 'bleeding' (refer to Box 17.1). In the postmenopausal age group, a possible malignancy should be in the forefront of diagnosis and risk factors for gynaecological malignancy, in addition to her age, should be considered.

After 50 years of age, cervical screening is performed every five years. Over 65 years routine screening stops and should only be performed for women not screened since age 50 or who have recently had abnormal results [8].

Important risk factors for endometrial cancer include obesity, diabetes mellitus, previous atypical endometrial hyperplasia, past ovarian or breast cancer and hereditary non-polyposis colorectal cancer (Lynch syndrome).

Other possible causes of postmenopausal bleeding to consider include the use of hormone replacement therapy – previous, ongoing or recent changes. As with any exogenous hormone use, bleeding irregularity can be experienced following change to dose or formulation of the treatment. Additionally, the use of sequential combined HRT for more than five years is associated with a small increase in risk of endometrial cancer, whereas continuous combined HRT is associated with a small decrease in risk [19].

Other medication to consider is the use of tamoxifen, which has anti-oestrogenic effects on breast tissue but oestrogenic effects on the endometrium, causing an increase in risk of endometrial cancer using this. Overtreatment with warfarin can also cause unexpected vaginal bleeding.

A postmenopausal woman is also at risk of developing ovarian cancer and important points in the history must include any change in appetite, weight loss, feeling bloated or changes in bowel habit, along with questions about any significant family history [20].

Examination

A pelvic examination is essential, as in Box 17.4, even if it is limited by patient tolerance. Vulval examination includes looking for ulcers and skin changes. Atrophic labia are thin and may be pale or inflamed in patches. Lichen sclerosus can cause pale white scarring and labial fusion. Vulval intraepithelial neoplasia (VIN) may result in lesions that are white, red, grey or raised.

If she can tolerate a speculum examination this should be performed. Atrophic vaginal skin can look thin and dry with tiny clusters of blood vessels resulting in patchy redness. Stretching of tight skin can cause fissures that can bleed during examination. Vaginal cancer is rare, but lesions are most commonly found in the posterior wall of the upper third of the vagina.

Cervical and a bimanual pelvic examination are important to determine whether a referral for assessment of cervical, endometrial or ovarian pathology is indicated, to avoid potential diagnostic delay.

Management

In postmenopausal women, exclusion of cancer is the primary objective, so referral must be made to gynaecology on a two-week wait, as per local guidelines and NICE recommendations [7]. Endometrial cancer incidence increases with age to a peak at 70–74 years, after which the incidence declines [13]. The absolute risk of endometrial cancer in non-users of HRT who present with post-menopausal bleeding ranges from 5.7% to 11.5% [21]. The risks of cervical and ovarian malignancies are lower, but not insignificant.

A one-stop service in secondary care will offer a pelvic ultrasound scan examination followed by hysteroscopy if indicated by the history and/or endometrial thickness measurement.

A general rule is the thicker the endometrium of a postmenopausal woman on ultrasound, the higher the likelihood of endometrial cancer being present. The threshold for concern about endometrial thickness varies, dependent on local criteria in the UK, ranging from 3–5 mm; a thickness of greater than 5 mm gives 7.3% likelihood of endometrial cancer and direct visualization by hysteroscopy is required [22].

The pelvic ultrasound scan will also examine the ovaries. Ovarian volume is reduced in the menopause. If there are any concerns about the ovarian appearance on USS, or there are symptoms and signs suggestive of ovarian cancer, then CA125 requires testing [23]. Ovarian malignancies that secrete oestrogen, such as granulosa cell tumours, can result in vaginal bleeding.

Women with suspected vulval and vaginal cancer should be referred for colposcopic examination on a two-week fast-track form [7].

Atrophic changes are the commonest cause of postmenopausal bleeding, but the diagnosis cannot be made until other more serious causes are excluded.

Atrophic vaginitis can be managed in primary care. This occurs due to lack of oestrogen, most commonly after the menopause, but can also occur after oophorectomy and with some drugs, i.e. depo-provera, GnRH analogues. A lack of oestrogen causes thinning of the vaginal epithelium and can lead to an overgrowth of Gram-negative bacteria, e.g. *Escherichia coli*, which can cause urinary tract infections. Atrophic vaginitis can be treated with topical oestrogens in the form of pessaries, rings or cream, or systemic HRT, or a combination if required. Long-term data show that there are no adverse effects on the endometrium from topical oestrogens [24], as systemic absorption is very low, with plasma levels not exceeding normal postmenopausal levels, so no endometrial protection is required, even with long-term use. In women who have had oestrogen-dependent malignancies and other contraindications to oestrogen therapy, advice should be taken from breast surgeons and gynaecologists. Non-hormonal vaginal moisturizers and lubricants can also be used, either with or independently of hormonal treatment.

Summary

Clare presented with a history of vaginal bleeding which had lasted for three days and required her to use a sanitary towel. She had also noticed a similar episode two weeks previously, but this has settled after 24 hours so she had not felt this was significant.

Examination had revealed a dry atrophic vagina with a normal postmenopausal cervix. Bimanual examination was normal. Clare was referred to the gynaecology department using the fast-track form. She was seen in the one-stop hysteroscopy service within 10 days and had a reassuringly normal TVUS which demonstrated a thin endometrium of 3 mm. She was reassured of the findings and returned to the clinic for discussion about the use of vaginal oestrogens a few days later.

She was prescribed a course of vagifem with the understanding that she could continue to use this on a long-term basis if she wanted to.

Conclusion

Non-menstrual bleeding is a common presentation in primary care. A logical approach to history-taking, examination, investigations and management is required using the clinical findings and risk assessment on an individualized basis.

References

1. Goodman, A, HPV testing as a screen for cervical cancer. *BMJ* 2015;350:h2372.

2. Public Health England Human papillomavirus (HPV) vaccine coverage in England, 2008/09 to 2013/14. A review of the full six years of the three-dose schedule. 2015. https://www.gov.uk/government/uploads/system/uploads/attachment_data/file/412264/HPV_Vaccine_Coverage_in_England_200809_to_201314.pdf (accessed September 2016).

3. Dunne EF, Unger ER, Sternberg M, *et al*. Prevalence of HPV infection among females in the United States. *JAMA* 2007;297:813–819.

4. Dochez C, Bogers JJ, Verhelst R, *et al*. HPV vaccines to prevent cervical cancer and genital warts: an update. *Vaccine* 2014;32:1595–1601.

5. Clinical Effectiveness Group British Association for Sexual Health and HIV UK national guideline for the management of pelvic inflammatory disease. 2011 (updated June 2011). www.bashh.org/documents/3572.pdf (accessed September 2016).

6. Schachter J, McCormack WM, Chernesky MA *et al*. Vaginal swabs are appropriate specimens for diagnosis of genital tract infection with Chlamydia trachomatis. *J Clin Microbiol* 2003;41(8):3784–3789.

7. NICE. Referral guidelines for suspected cancer NICE guidelines, CG27. 2005. (http://guidance.nice.org.uk/CG27 (accessed September 2016).

8. Public Health England. Cervical screening: programme overview. 2015. www.gov.uk/guidance/cervical-screening-programme-overview (accessed September 2016).

9. NHS. Clinical practice guidance for the assessment of young women aged 20–24 with abnormal vaginal bleeding. 2010. www.gov.uk/government/uploads/system/uploads/attachment_data/file/436924/doh-guidelines-young-women.pdf (accessed September 2016).

10. Public Health England. Cervical cancer consultation Q&A. legacy.screening.nhs.uk/cervicalcancer-qa (accessed September 2016).

11. Cancer Research UK. Cervical cancer incidence statistics. 2016. http://www.cancerresearchuk.org/health-professional/cancer-statistics/statistics-by-cancer-type/cervical-cancer/incidence#heading-One (accessed September 2016).

12. Connolly A, Jones, S, Nonmenstrual vaginal bleeding in women under 40 years of age. *TOG* 2004;6:153–158.

13. Cancer Research UK. Uterine cancer statistics. 2016. http://www.cancerresearchuk.org/health-professional/cancer-statistics/statistics-by-cancer-type/uterine-cancer/incidence#heading-One (accessed September 2016).

14. Ray S, Ray A, Non-surgical interventions for treating heavy menstrual bleeding (menorrhagia) in women with bleeding disorders. *Cochrane Database Syst Rev* 2014;11:CD010338.

15. NICE Ovarian cancer: recognition and initial management guidelines, CG122. 2011. https://www.nice.org.uk/guidance/cg122 (accessed September 2016).

16. Lacey JV Jr, Sherman ME, Rush BB, *et al*. Absolute risk of endometrial carcinoma during 20-year follow-up among women with endometrial hyperplasia. *J Clin Oncol* 2010;28(5):788–792.

17. Smith OP, Critchley HO, RSRH vascular change with hormone contraception: Progestogen only contraception and endometrial breakthrough bleeding. *Angiogenesis* 2005;8:117–126.

18. Faculty of Sexual & Reproductive Healthcare Clinical Effectiveness Unit Clinical Guidance: Problematic bleeding with hormonal contraception. 2015. www.fsrh.org/standards-and-guidance/documents/ceuguidanceproblematicbleedinghormonalcontraception/ (accessed September 2016).

19. Panay N, Hamoda H, Arya R, Savvas M, The 2013 British Menopause Society & Women's Health Concern recommendations on hormone replacement therapy. *Menopause Int* 2013;19(2):59–68.

20. Early Breast Cancer Trialists' Collaborative Group (EBCTCG) Effects of chemotherapy and hormonal therapy for early breast cancer on recurrence and 15-year survival: an overview of the randomised trials. *Lancet* 2005; 365(9472):1687–1717.

21. Gredmark T, Kvint S, Havel G, Mattsson LA, Investigation of Post-Menopausal Bleeding. SIGN Publication No. 61, 2002.

22. Smith-Bindman R, Weiss E, Feldstein V, How thick is too thick? When endometrial thickness should prompt biopsy in postmenopausal women without vaginal bleeding. *Ultrasound Obstet Gynecol* 2004;24(5):558–565.

23. NICE. Ovarian cancer: recognition and initial management guidelines, CG122. 2011. https://www.nice.org.uk/guidance/cg122 (accessed September 2016).

24. Kalentzi, T, Panay N, Safety of vaginal oestrogen in postmenopausal women. *TOG* 2005;7:241–244.

Chapter 18

Management of the Patient with Suspected Endometriosis in Primary Care

Keith A. Louden

Case Scenario

Vicky presents as a 25-year-old complaining of painful periods and pain with sexual penetration. She has been married for two years and says that she is unable to have intercourse with her husband. She has tried a variety of different simple analgesics, which have been ineffective.

Introduction

Endometriosis is a common benign condition affecting women in their reproductive years, and is defined by the presence of endometrial glands and stroma outside the uterus.

Prevalence is difficult to establish because only laparoscopy with direct visualization and histological confirmation is reliable, but may be as high as 10% in the community [1], and 35–50% in women with chronic pain and infertility [2], peaking between 25 and 35 years of age.

Risk is increased in first-degree relatives, with early menarche and late menopause, with delayed first pregnancy and with some congenital abnormalities which prevent menstrual outflow. Half of the variation in endometriosis risk is inherited [3].

Symptoms include dysmenorrhoea, dyspareunia and dyschezia (rectal pain), along with infertility, leading to adverse effects on personal relationships, quality of life and work productivity [4].

There are three recognized morphological lesions, superficial peritoneal implants, ovarian endometriomas ('chocolate cysts') and deep infiltrating lesions (DIE) affecting the rectum, bladder and uterosacral ligaments. Pathogenesis remains unclear, with competing theories involving retrograde menstruation, impairment of the immune system, enhanced angiogenesis and metaplasia of normal tissues.

The major challenge in general practice is the timing of the referral decision. There is international evidence of unacceptable diagnostic delay of eight to twelve years (especially in teenagers) from the onset of symptoms to laparoscopic diagnosis [5], yet the prevalence of simple dysmenorrhoea amongst healthy young women is high, and there is considerable symptomatic overlap between endometriosis and other causes of pelvic pain, such as irritable bowel syndrome (IBS). A UK study of primary care [6] found that women with endometriosis were 3.5 times more likely to have had an initial diagnosis of irritable bowel syndrome and 6.4 times more likely to have had a diagnosis of pelvic inflammatory disease compared with controls. One-third of patients consulted their GP six times or more before referral. Earlier diagnosis and treatment is likely to be the best way to

Women's Health in Primary Care, edited by Anne Connolly and Amanda Britton. Published by Cambridge University Press
© Cambridge University Press 2017

prevent severe and debilitating disease and protect fertility. If this diagnostic delay is to be avoided, consideration should be given to referral criteria for suspected endometriosis. These criteria encompass symptoms, physical signs, and imaging findings.

Case Scenario

Vicky's pain history reveals a story of painful periods dating back to menarche. She was prescribed the OCP in cyclical fashion with a monthly withdrawal bleed, but it didn't make much difference. She lost time from school, and her exam results were disappointing. She experienced pain at mid-cycle, but was reassured that this was natural.

Pain is the most likely presenting symptom, and a detailed pain history is particularly important. Dysmenorrhoea is the most common symptom of endometriosis, but is described by 50–75% of healthy nulliparous women. The index of suspicion of underlying endometriosis is raised when simple treatment strategies using the combined oral contraceptive pill (OCP) and non-steroidal anti-inflammatory drugs (NSAIDs) such as mefenamic acid have been unsuccessful. There is little advantage to be gained by swapping one OCP or NSAID for another unless there is a problem with tolerability. These treatment strategies would be expected to be effective in perhaps 90% of women with dysmenorrhoea, so a failure of conservative treatment should lead to active consideration of endometriosis as the underlying diagnosis.

The patient's description of pain may also help. The timing of the pain offers important clues. Whilst patients with simple dysmenorrhoea describe pain with the onset of menstrual flow, or perhaps a few hours beforehand, endometriosis patients often describe premenstrual pain for days or even a week or more before menstruation. Mid-cycle pain is also common. The timing of the pain may reflect the underlying anatomical pathology. For example, if an ovary is adherent to the lateral pelvic sidewall secondary to the inflammatory nature of endometriosis with its propensity for scarring and adhesions, then the description of mid-cycle pain around the time of ovulation can be understood. Peritoneal lesions in the pouch of Douglas become more florid during the luteal phase, as both the normal endometrium and the endometriotic deposits undergo cyclical proliferation, and this is consistent

with the description of premenstrual pain symptoms. Over years, symptoms may change from the obviously cyclical to a more chronic and less cyclical or indeed acyclical pattern. This may reflect the chronic inflammatory changes in the pelvis, with the development of adhesions, scarring and deep nodular disease, which can ultimately result in a 'frozen pelvis'. In a situation with a fixed retroverted uterus, bilateral endometriotic cysts kissing in the midline, and obliteration of the pouch of Douglas, then pain may be relatively constant.

Endometriosis may be found in the rectovaginal septum, infiltrating the wall of the rectum or sigmoid colon, or invading the bladder. Unsurprisingly, these relatively uncommon manifestations of endometriosis may present with specific and anatomically understandable symptoms. The most important of these is cyclical dyschezia, the description of rectal pain during defaecation at the time of menstruation. This pain is often described as knife-like, and can be very severe and debilitating. It may, however, be a symptom which the patient does not disclose unless directly questioned.

In the context of the cyclical changes in endometriotic lesions, the symptom is easily understood at the time of surgery when a thick-walled inflammatory lesion of the anterior rectum has caused narrowing of the lumen. A rectal nodule which extends through into the mucosa of the bowel has the potential for cyclical rectal bleeding, but this bleeding pattern is also not uncommonly observed with simple internal haemorrhoids.

Similarly, endometriotic lesions within the bladder wall may cause cyclical dysuria, and sometimes cyclical haematuria if the nodule is full thickness and reaches the bladder mucosa.

There is a common theme here, in that any pain or non-menstrual bleeding which is cyclical in nature may represent underlying endometriosis. Patients occasionally present with cyclical pain in the region of hernial orifices or the tip of the shoulder, reflecting endometriosis within a small hernial sac, or on the peritoneum of the subdiaphragmatic space. Cyclical blue-black swelling or even bleeding from the umbilicus or a lump in a Pfannenstiel or episiotomy scar is caused by endometriosis. Even recurrent respiratory symptoms such as pneumothorax and haemoptysis can be attributed to endometriosis, but the crucial aspect of diagnosis is the recognition that the symptoms are cyclical.

Endometriotic lesions are most commonly found in the pouch of Douglas, affecting the peritoneal surfaces, the uterosacral ligaments and the ovaries. It is little surprise then, that deep dyspareunia may occur, because of the intimate anatomical relationship between the posterior fornix of the vagina and the peritoneum of the pouch of Douglas. This also explains why some women will describe deep dyspareunia, but find that they can sometimes ameliorate this symptom by changing sexual position.

Whilst considering symptoms, if the patient presents with heavy and painful periods, and the uterus is a little enlarged and tender, then there may be underlying adenomyosis, i.e. endometrial glands and stroma within the myometrium. This condition is often difficult to diagnose because ultrasound findings may be subtle. There may be evidence of small myometrial areas of cystic change, and the myometrium may be described as inhomogenous. MRI can be helpful in making the diagnosis. The condition may occur alongside endometriosis, and the levonorgestrel-releasing intrauterine system (IUS) may be helpful.

> **Box 18.1 Symptoms Associated with Endometriosis**
>
> - Dysmenorrhoea
> - Deep dyspareunia
> - Cyclical/mid-cycle/premenstrual pain
> - Cyclical bowel and bladder symptoms of pain or bleeding
> - Infertility
> - Family history of endometriosis

> **Case Scenario**
>
> The notes show that Vicky has not had a vaginal examination. She is very reluctant to be examined, and becomes tearful and withdrawn. She discloses that she loves her husband, but cannot tolerate any sexual penetration. She has stopped taking the OCP because she wants to start a family, and is very upset that she is unable to tolerate intercourse. There are no other psychological or relationship problems.

Perhaps surprisingly, there is no correlation between the severity of pain symptoms and the reported stage of endometriosis using the Revised American Fertility Society (RAFS) score [7], although deeper lesions are more painful. This may be explained by the method used to calculate the stage of endometriosis in this scoring system, which weighs heavily towards the effect of endometriosis on fertility rather than pain. Alternative staging systems for endometriosis which attempt to focus more towards pain symptoms than fertility concerns have been suggested, but not widely adopted. Patients with DIE can describe very high pain scores, and an appreciation of the subjective intensity of pain symptoms is another opportunity to consider the diagnosis.

Although non-specific, living with chronic pain is exhausting, and endometriosis patients will commonly complain of tiredness. The impact of endometriosis may be reflected by time off school or work, with reduced exercise and social activity. The condition may be challenging both to work performance and personal relationships. These factors are of major importance to patients, over and above specific pain and fertility issues.

The limitations of pelvic examination in terms of diagnosis for ovarian cysts, for example, are well known. However, in the context of a patient in whom endometriosis is suspected, important diagnostic information may be revealed. Most obviously, pelvic tenderness may be demonstrated, but additionally, the location of endometriotic deposits and the consequent chronic inflammatory changes with scarring and nodule formation in the pouch of Douglas may allow these lesions to be detected, or at least suspected on bimanual examination. The uterus may be in a position of fixed retroversion, with reduced mobility of the tissues. There may be palpable tender nodularity of the uterosacral ligaments. Occasionally, a deep deposit of rectovaginal endometriosis may be palpable in the posterior fornix of the vagina, and may even be visible as a blue-black lesion penetrating the vaginal mucosa. A pelvic mass may be apparent if there is an endometrioma present. Abnormal vaginal examination findings should lead to further investigation with transvaginal ultrasound, and prompt referral to secondary care.

> **Case Scenario**
>
> An attempt at vaginal examination fails because of pain and apparent vaginismus. A scan is requested. This has to be by the transabdominal route as the patient is unable to consent to the preferred transvaginal route. The result is normal, with no abnormality demonstrated.

There is often a reluctance to consider referring teenagers when endometriosis is suspected, because the incidence of primary dysmenorrhoea is so high, and it might seem inappropriate to consider early laparoscopy. It should be remembered that endometriosis does affect teenagers; the long diagnostic delays which patients experience often extend back to their teenage years. Failure of conservative management should prompt referral, even though management strategies in secondary care are likely to be more conservative in this age group. Younger women often present with widespread peritoneal lesions at laparoscopy. The natural history of these lesions is unclear, and under these circumstances hormonal cycle suppression may be preferred to surgical excision.

In terms of investigations, serum CA125 measurement has been suggested as a potential screening tool, but has been found to be of no clinical value, even though levels can be elevated with endometriosis, particularly with endometrioma formation. Transvaginal ultrasound is the imaging modality of choice for suspected endometriosis, as ovarian endometriomas have a characteristic ground glass appearance. It may be difficult to make the diagnosis between a small corpus luteum haemorrhagic cyst and a small endometrioma, but a rescan three months later allows time for a corpus luteum cyst to resolve, whilst an endometrioma will remain. Aside from the finding of an endometrioma, a normal transvaginal ultrasound does not exclude the diagnosis of endometriosis, as peritoneal and uterosacral disease may escape detection. In specialist centres, there is some evidence that transvaginal ultrasound may be able to predict severe disease with rectal involvement [8], although this level of discrimination has not been validated in routine clinical practice. Further imaging with MRI or CT may be undertaken in secondary care in an attempt to map the disease before surgery.

For each individual patient, there will come a time when an initial problem-solving approach with pragmatic choices about initial symptom-based treatment may need to shift towards referral. Of course, in general practice, the definitive diagnosis will not have been made because laparoscopy is required to make that diagnosis. Hence treatment efforts focus on the practical management of a patient with a set of symptoms which may or may not reflect underlying endometriosis, but might also reflect IBS, pelvic inflammatory disease, primary dysmenorrhoea, interstitial cystitis or chronic pelvic pain.

Case Scenario

There are no symptoms suggestive of IBS, and Vicky describes normal bowel and bladder function. Her pain symptoms are severe and she is clearly distressed. She is referred to the local endometriosis clinic in secondary care.

If symptoms are mild to moderate, and there are no obvious physical signs of endometriosis to suggest nodular DIE or an endometrioma, then a three to six month trial of blind medical treatment may be indicated when endometriosis is suspected [9]. However, some patients may wish to have a definitive diagnosis, particularly if there is associated infertility.

Choice of analgesia usually rests with paracetamol and NSAIDs; there is very little specific research concerning the best analgesia for endometriosis. Opiates may be required, but with symptoms of this severity, then referral should be considered.

Beyond analgesia, medical strategies involve hormonal suppression of the cyclical ovarian activity which causes the cyclical proliferative changes in the endometriotic implants, hence relieving symptoms. The combined OCP and progestogens are most commonly employed, with no clear superiority of one treatment over the other. A principle of treatment, however, is that cycle suppression should aim for amenorrhoea, so the OCP should be used continuously, as long as breakthrough bleeding allows. Unfortunately, the usefulness of this strategy is limited by moderate to severe side effects in 14% of women [10].

The progesterone-only pill or the subcutaneous progestogen-releasing implant are often used, although there are no studies demonstrating effectiveness in endometriosis patients. Similarly, depot provera and oral progestogens such as medroxyprogesterone acetate have been employed; 100 mg of medroxyprogesterone acetate daily was associated with side effects of acne and fluid retention.

The IUS has been found to be effective in the treatment of endometriosis, and is an obvious choice in women presenting with dysmenorrhoea, as long as contraception is welcome. The IUS may also offer benefit in those women with underlying adenomyosis, and is also an effective treatment for primary dysmenorrhoea. Furthermore, the IUS will commonly be offered to patients as an adjunct to surgical treatment.

The use of gonadotrophin-releasing hormone analogues, which are effective at suppressing ovarian activity, is limited by the side effects of vasomotor symptoms and bone demineralization with prolonged use. The use of add-back hormone replacement therapy greatly increases tolerability and reduces the risk of bone demineralization, but long-term studies are lacking.

The limitations of medical therapy include the side effect profile, the associated contraception, which may or may not be wanted, and the duration of treatment. It is also clear that whilst medical treatment can suppress the cyclical activity of individual lesions, it is unable to resolve issues of the formation of chronic inflammatory nodules, with the associated scarring and adhesions which result. Whilst success in terms of reduction of pain symptoms is similar to that of a surgical approach, the practical difficulty of maintaining cycle suppression and amenorrhoea in the long term is considerable. When hormonal therapy is discontinued, the endometrial deposits become active again, and symptoms usually recur. When helping patients to choose between hormonal medical treatment and surgical treatment (or a combination of both), it is important that the relative merits and problems with each strategy are considered. Hormonal treatment of endometriosis is not only contraceptive in nature during treatment, but is not associated with improved fertility outcomes thereafter.

If symptoms are severe, if hormonal treatment is unsuccessful or contraception is not wanted, or there is the suggestion of severe disease, then referral is indicated. Similarly infertile patients with endometriosis symptoms require referral. Ideally such a referral should be made to a local specialist endometriosis or fertility clinic.

Box 18.2 Indications for referral

- Failure of conservative treatment
- Pelvic mass
- Endometrioma on transvaginal ultrasound
- Physical signs of endometriosis, e.g. palpable nodularity in the pouch of Douglas
- Severity of pain symptoms

In secondary care, patients should be offered laparoscopy to make the diagnosis and assess the stage of disease, and consider treatment. This procedure should be undertaken by a surgical team who are able to offer a 'see and treat' approach for mild to moderate disease, following appropriate preoperative

counselling [11], whilst accepting that unexpectedly severe disease such as a rectovaginal nodule, diagnosed at initial laparoscopy, may require repeat surgery after further counselling. The concept of the 'diagnostic laparoscopy' without the facility for treatment is no longer acceptable.

The surgical principle for the management of endometriosis-related pain is the surgical excision of all disease, almost invariably by laparoscopy. The aim is to be as conservative as possible to maintain pelvic organ function. Peritoneal and uterosacral disease is excised. Endometriomas are separated from their attachments to the lateral pelvic sidewall, opened, drained and the cyst lining carefully stripped. Simple fenestration is insufficient because of high recurrence rates. Great care must be taken to minimize ovarian injury because of the associated risk of reduced ovarian function, hence surgical accuracy and the avoidance of excessive diathermy are important. DIE is a common finding in association with an endometrioma, hence these patients may be best managed in a specialist centre.

The British Society for Gynaecological Endoscopy (BSGE) have established centres of excellence for the surgical treatment of DIE, ensuring appropriate caseload, audit and multidisciplinary teams for complex cases involving the rectum and the bladder. The most severe cases may involve surgical 'shaving' of a deep nodule off the anterior surface of the rectum, and the excision of full thickness lesions from the posterior fornix of the vagina or bladder. Disc resection of the rectum or even segmental resection may be needed. Ureteric lesions may require excision and reanastomosis. Hence there is a requirement for multidisciplinary teamworking in the BSGE centres.

The surgical management of endometriosis in patients suffering with infertility is contentious. There is some evidence that the surgical treatment of even minimal and mild endometriosis may improve pregnancy outcomes, but it has been estimated that 24 women would need to be treated to result in one extra pregnancy [12]. Surgical treatment to an endometrioma may successfully treat pain symptoms, but can reduce ovarian function. Excision of DIE may not improve fertility outcome.

Surgery for moderate to severe disease yields spontaneous pregnancy rates of 52–69% compared with no treatment [13]. However, many fertility specialists will recommend assisted reproductive techniques. Such decisions are made on an individual basis, taking into account the relevant importance of infertility and pain symptoms.

A difficulty may commonly arise when a patient has a laparoscopy for suspected endometriosis and only minor disease is found. It is known that there is a poor correlation between the stage of endometriosis and the severity of pain symptoms, yet the surgical results for the treatment of mild disease is very poor. Endometriosis may be asymptomatic, and the excision of minor peritoneal disease may yield little benefit, but the patient may interpret these events as the revelation of a long sought for explanation for her symptoms. There may be brief symptomatic improvement as a consequence, with a placebo-type effect, followed by return of symptoms which the patient may interpret as recurrent endometriosis. It is important, therefore, to be careful and cautious in the postoperative interpretation of the surgical treatment of mild endometriosis, as sequential laparoscopic treatments for minor disease should be avoided.

Case Scenario

In secondary care, Vicky is first seen by a specialist registrar, who recommends referring the patient for psychosexual counselling. She appears depressed, and is wearing shapeless black clothing. She is exhausted and fears for her marriage. She has lost her job because of repeated absences from work. The consultant in the endometriosis clinic recommends day-case admission for examination under anaesthetic, and laparoscopy with a view to excision of any endometriosis found, explaining that the findings may be normal.

It is unfortunate that such a common and important condition is not more widely understood and recognized. Patients have often never heard of endometriosis, and it does not feature prominently in the media. More information is available online through Endometriosis UK (www.endometriosis-uk.org), the Royal College of Obstetricians and Gynaecologists (www.rcog.org.uk/globalassets/documents/patients/endometriosis.pdf) and NHS Direct (www.nhs.uk/conditions/endometriosis/Pages/Introduction.aspx). Specialist endometriosis clinics are few, and recognition that treatment of endometriosis in secondary care has become an increasingly specialist area has been slow. The BSGE project to create specialist centres for the surgical treatment of DIE is an important step forward, but such centres are not evenly distributed across the UK. The key to improving outcomes for endometriosis patients is through earlier suspicion of the diagnosis and referral to secondary care, ideally to an endometriosis clinic, with links to a BSGE centre for the most severe cases.

Case Scenario

At laparoscopy, the patient has extensive nodular endometriosis within both uterosacral ligaments, and both ovaries are adherent to the lateral pelvic sidewalls. There is a full thickness vaginal nodule penetrating from the pouch of Douglas, where the rectum has been pulled up onto the back of the cervix. The endometriotic tissue is excised, the ovaries released and the vaginal defect sutured, leaving no visible or palpable endometriosis remaining. Vicky describes an 80% improvement in her pain, and is able to enjoy comfortable sexual intercourse. She goes on to complete her family with two normal pregnancies.

References

1. Eskanazi B, Warner ML, Epidemiology of endometriosis. *Obstet Gynecol Clin N Am* 1997;24(2):235–258.

2. Ozkan S, Murk W, Arici A, Endometriosis and infertility: epidemiology and evidence based treatments. *Ann NY Acad Sci* 2008;1127;92–100.

3. Treoar SA, O'Connor DT, O'Connor VM, Martin NG, Genetic influences on endometriosis in an Australian twin sample. *Fertil Steril* 1999;71:701–710.

4. DeGraaff AA, D'Hooghe TM, Dunselman GA, *et al.* The significant effect of endometriosis on physical, mental and social wellbeing: results from an international cross-sectional survey. *Hum Reprod* 2013;28:2677–2685.

5. Ballard K, Lowton K, Wright J, What's the delay? A qualitative study of women's experiences of reaching a diagnosis of endometriosis. *Fert Steril* 2006;86: 1296–1301.

6. Pugsley Z, Ballard K, Assessment of endometriosis in general practice: the pathway to diagnosis. *Br J Gen Pract.* 2007:57(539):470–476.

7. Gruppo Italiano per lo Studio dE. Relationship between stage, site and morphological characteristics of pelvic endometriosis and pain. *Hum Reprod* 2001;16(12):2668–2671.

8. Holland TK, Yazbek J, Cutner A, *et al.* Value of transvaginal ultrasound in assessing severity of pelvic

endometriosis. *Ultrasound Obstet Gynaecol* 2010;36(2):241–248.

9. Dunselman G, Vermeulen N, Becker C *et al.* ESHRE guideline: management of women with endometriosis. *Hum Reprod* 2014;29(3):400–412.

10. Vercellini P, Frontino G, De Giorgi O, *et al.* Continuous use of an oral contraceptive for endometriosis-associated recurrent dysmenorrhoea that does not respond to a cyclic pill regimen. *Fertil Steril* 2003;80(3):560–563.

11. Duffy JMN, Arambage K, Correa FJS *et al.* *Laparoscopic Surgery for Endometriosis.* The Cochrane Library. Issue 4. John Wiley and Sons Ltd. 2014.

12. Jacobsen TZ, Duffy JM, Barlow D, *et al.* Laparoscopic surgery for subfertility associated with endometriosis. *Cochrane Database Syst Rev* 2010;(1):CD001398.

13. Vercellini P, Fedele L, Aimi G, *et al.* Reproductive performance, pain recurrence and disease relapse after conservative surgical treatment for endometriosis: the predictive value of the current classification system. *Hum Reprod* 2006;21:2679–2685.

Chapter 19

Management of the Patient with Heavy Menstrual Bleeding in Primary Care

Helen Barnes

Key Points

- Heavy menstrual bleeding affects around 25% of women aged 30–50 years old. It can have a considerable effect on quality of life.
- All women presenting with HMB should have a full blood count.
- An endometrial biopsy should be considered in women with risk factors for endometrial hyperplasia/malignancy which include age >45 years, PCOS and obesity.
- Women without risk factors for structural or histological abnormalities should be offered medical treatment for the HMB at their initial assessment.
- NICE recommend the LNG-IUS as first-line treatment for HMB in women without significant structural or histological pathology to whom hormonal treatment is acceptable.
- Endometrial ablation is less invasive and lower risk than a hysterectomy, but has less quality of life years (QALYs) than a hysterectomy.
- Newer, less invasive treatment options are now available for fibroids, including medical management, transcervical resection of fibroids and uterine artery embolization for women wanting fertility-sparing treatments.

Case Scenario

Lisa attends the surgery complaining of worsening heavy menstrual bleeding (HMB). Lisa is a 42-year-old flight attendant and mother to 10-year-old Thomas and 12-year-old Emily. Her periods are regular, and tend to last six days and are particularly heavy for the first four days when she experiences clots and flooding. It is having a significant impact on her quality of life, affecting her work and her ability to enjoy her children.

Introduction

Background

Heavy menstrual bleeding (HMB) is defined clinically as excessive menstrual blood loss, interfering with a woman's physical, social, emotional and/or material quality of life. It can occur alone or in combination with other symptoms [1].

HMB affects around 25% of women aged 30–50 years old. It can have a considerable effect on quality of life, and many women will see their GP for help and advice. It is estimated, in England and Wales, that 80,000 women are referred to secondary care annually for HMB [2], with around 30,000 women undergoing surgical treatment each year [3].

There has been a significant change in how HMB is managed over the last 25 years, with the introduction of the levonorgestrel-releasing intrauterine system, endometrial ablation and uterine artery embolization. In the early 1990s it was estimated that at least 60% of women presenting with HMB went on to have a hysterectomy. The most recent NICE guidelines were published in 2007, a NICE quality statement was published in 2013 and an updated guideline was published in August 2016.

Aetiology

In 2011 the International Federation of Gynaecology and Obstetrics (FIGO) published a classification system for the causes of abnormal uterine bleeding (AUB) [4]. They include the term heavy menstrual bleeding within the umbrella of AUB, thus encouraging us not to consider HMB in isolation from other forms of AUB. The FIGO classification system for AUB is

Women's Health in Primary Care, edited by Anne Connolly and Amanda Britton. Published by Cambridge University Press
© Cambridge University Press 2017

Table 19.1 Causes of heavy menstrual bleeding

Structural	Non-Structural
Polyps	Coagulopathy
Adenomyosis	Ovulatory disorder
Leiomyoma	Endometrial
Malignancy or hyperplasia	Iatrogenic
	Not yet classified

named PALM–COEIN. This classification system can be applied when considering causes of HMB.

Structural Causes

Around 40–60% of women with HMB will have no structural cause.

Approximately 30% of women with HMB will be found to have leiomyoma (fibroids), 10% endometrial polyps and 5% adenomyosis [5]. However, in many women, these structural pathologies are asymptomatic. Although adenomyosis, polyps or fibroids may be present, they may not always be implicated in the cause of a woman's HMB. With regards to fibroids, it is generally accepted that intracavity fibroids, or those fibroids which contain a submucous component, are the most likely to contribute to the genesis of heavy or abnormal bleeding [4].

Endometrial Hyperplasia and Malignancy

Endometrial hyperplasia is the proliferation of glands making them irregular in size and shape, with an increase in glands-to-stroma ratio. Hyperplasia is classified into hyperplasia with or without atypia. Hyperplasia without atypia has a 1–3% risk of becoming malignant if left untreated, compared with hyperplasia with atypia having a progression rate to endometrial carcinoma of 30–60% [6].

The incidence of endometrial hyperplasia and malignancy increases with age. It is also associated with conditions resulting in higher circulating levels of oestrogen (e.g. obesity and polycystic ovarian syndrome (PCOS)), which causes over-proliferation of the endometrium. Although hyperplasia is not a common cause of HMB, it is an important consideration as the consequences of a missed or delayed diagnosis could be catastrophic for the patient.

The likely rates of endometrial carcinoma per 10,000 consultations for HMB in primary care are [1]:

- Age 35–39 years: 1 per 10,000 consultations

- Age 40–44 years: 3 per 10,000 consultations
- Age 45–49 years: 8 per 10,000 consultations.

Risk factors for endometrial hyperplasia and malignancy include:

- Age over 45 years
- Obesity
- Diabetes
- Polycystic ovarian syndrome (unopposed estrogens from anovulatory cycles)
- Nulliparity
- Unopposed oestrogen therapy in an intact uterus
- Tamoxifen in postmenopausal women
- Endogenous oestrogens, e.g. ovarian granulosa cell neoplasm
- Family history of breast or endometrial cancer, or colonic cancer.

Non-Structural Causes

- The term coagulopathy encompasses the many disorders of systemic haemostasis which may contribute to HMB.
- Ovulatory dysfunction can result in unpredictability of the timing of menstrual cycles, which can contribute to HMB.
- The endometrial category in the PALM-COEIN system refers to disorders of the mechanisms controlling local endometrial haemostasis, for example inhibited production of local vasoconstrictors or accelerated clot lysis due to excessive production of plasminogen activator.

Initial Assessment

To determine the likely cause of Lisa's HMB, and to formulate an appropriate management plan, a thorough initial assessment needs to be undertaken.

History

The history should identify symptoms suggestive of structural causes for HMB and any risk factors for malignancy, it should also determine the effect of the HMB on Lisa's life.

Important aspects to clarify include:

- How is this heavy bleeding affecting her physically, emotionally and socially?
- Does she have any intermenstrual or postcoital bleeding?

- Is she experiencing dysmenorrhoea or pelvic pain?
- Does she need contraception?
- Has she completed her family?
- Is she up to date with her cervical screening?
- Does she have a history suggestive of a clotting disorder?
- Does she have any significant family history?

Although gynaecological malignancy is rare in premenopausal women such as Lisa, it is crucial to be aware of it as a possibility and to act on any red flag symptoms appropriately. Postcoital bleeding and persistent intermenstrual bleeding are symptoms which can warrant a two-week rule referral for possible malignancy.

Examination

Women presenting with HMB should have a body mass index recorded. Obesity is an important risk factor for endometrial hyperplasia and malignancy.

The purpose of a physical examination is to detect underlying pathology to inform a further management plan, including investigations and treatment options. Many women presenting with HMB will not have a structural or histological cause for their symptoms. The NICE guidelines therefore advise it is not necessary to do a physical examination in women whereby the history does not suggest a structural or histological abnormality. However, women who are not up to date with their cervical screening should have their cervix examined. The NICE guidelines do advise a physical examination in all women who choose the levonorgestrel-releasing IUS as their preferred treatment. Women should also have a physical examination before any referral for further investigations or specialist assessment.

Case Scenario

As Lisa has no symptoms or risk factors to suggest a structural or histological abnormality it would be reasonable not to examine her at the initial appointment. Should she have had a history suggestive of a structural or histological abnormality, for example intermenstrual bleeding or dysmenorrhoea, then an abdominal examination, speculum examination and bimanual examination would be an important part of the initial assessment.

Blood Tests

A full blood count is recommended in all women presenting with HMB and should be performed (or requested) at the initial assessment [1]. If iron deficiency anaemia is present, treatment for this should be provided in parallel with the treatment planned for Lisa's HMB.

Thyroid function testing is not recommended in the absence of other signs or symptoms of thyroid disease. Hormone testing is not indicated in women with isolated HMB, with no associated menstrual irregularity. Testing for disorders of coagulation is only recommended in women who report having HMB since menarche and have a personal or family history suggestive of a clotting disorder.

Further Investigations

Women who are identified from the history or examination as being at risk of structural causes including hyperplasia/malignancy should have further investigations as outlined below. Additionally those for whom initial medical management of HMB has failed, or those who are considering surgical management, should also have further investigations.

Investigations for Structural Pathology

The first-line investigation for the assessment of structural causes of HMB is a pelvic ultrasound; preferably a transvaginal ultrasound (TVS), if this is appropriate and acceptable to the patient. Ultrasound can identify structural causes, including submucous fibroids, adenomyosis and endometrial pathology. TVS is more acceptable to women, more accurate and less costly than other methods (including MRI, saline infusion sonography and hysteroscopy) [1].

NICE recommend hysteroscopy should only be used as a diagnostic tool when ultrasound results are inconclusive. This may include, for example, the need to determine the location of a fibroid prior to planning surgical treatment.

Investigations for Histological Pathology

Histological assessment is most commonly undertaken as a blind pipelle endometrial biopsy. A pipelle biopsy is a simple outpatient procedure, whereby a small sampling tube is passed through the cervix and a sample of endometrium is obtained by suction. The overall sensitivity for pipelle endometrial sampling is from 70% to 90%, and specificity is 100% [1].

The NICE guidelines advise an endometrial biopsy should be undertaken in women with persistent intermenstrual bleeding or in women aged over 45 years old in whom first-line medical treatment has failed or been ineffective. However, more recent guidance suggests endometrial biopsy should be considered in all women over 45 years old, and additionally in those whom other risk factors for hyperplasia exist (see section 'Endometrial Hyperplasia and Malignancy' above) [7]. Combining TVS with pipelle endometrial sampling in high-risk women gives improved sensitivity for detecting endometrial hyperplasia/malignancy [1].

Case Scenario

As Lisa has no risk factors for structural or histological pathology, she does not require any further investigations at this stage.

Management

Medical Management

Women without risk factors for structural or histological abnormalities should be offered medical treatment at their initial assessment (the initial assessment may require more than one appointment in primary care). Those who are being referred on for further investigations, or to secondary care, should be offered treatment with tranexamic acid or a non-steroidal anti-inflammatory drug (NSAID) whilst they are waiting for their definitive treatment plan.

Non-Hormonal Treatment

Tranexamic Acid

Tranexamic acid is an anti-fibrinolytic drug. The mode of action is inhibition of the breakdown of fibrin in preformed clots in the spiral endometrial arterioles. Whilst it inhibits factors associated with coagulation, it does not affect coagulation within healthy blood vessels. Studies have shown no overall increase in the rate of thrombosis in those taking tranexamic acid compared with those not taking it [1]. The dose for HMB is 1 g three to four times daily from the onset of the heavy bleeding for a maximum of four consecutive days. Trials have shown tranexamic acid can reduce menstrual blood loss (MBL) by 29–58% [1]. It has no

effect on dysmenorrhoea or cycle regularity and is less cost effective than the levonorgestrel-releasing IUS.

NSAIDs

NSAIDs affect prostaglandin synthesis. Prostaglandins are involved in the local pathways affecting both uterine bleeding and uterine cramps, as well as generalized pain pathways. They should be taken regularly from the onset of the bleeding until the bleeding has settled. NSAIDs are less effective at reducing MBL when compared with tranexamic acid (reductions of 20–49%), but have the advantage of being effective at treating dysmenorrhoea [1]. NICE guidelines advise that when dysmenorrhoea is present NSAIDS should be used in preference to tranexamic acid. NSAIDs should not be used if it is suspected that the HMB is related to a coagulopathy.

Hormonal Treatments

Levonorgestrel-Releasing Intrauterine System

The levonorgestrel-releasing intrauterine system (LNG-IUS) is licensed for contraception as well as the treatment of HMB and the progesterone component of HRT. The LNG-IUS releases 20 mcg of levonorgestrel daily, this acts locally to prevent proliferation of the endometrium, thicken cervical mucus and, in some women, prevent ovulation. It is licensed for five years and is required to be inserted and removed by a qualified practitioner.

The LNG-IUS may take up to six months to reach full effect and over that time women can experience some unscheduled bleeding which is usually light, but may be persistent. Systemic absorption of progesterone from the LNG-IUS is minimal, but can incur hormonal side effects in some women. These undesirable effects can include acne, breast tenderness, headache and mood changes; however, they tend to be mild and transient, decreasing with duration of use [8].

RCTs have demonstrated the reduction in MBL with an LNG-IUS to be between 71% and 96% [1]. It is the most cost-effective pharmaceutical treatment option and is recommended by NICE as the first-line treatment for HMB in women without significant structural or histological pathology to whom hormonal treatment is acceptable.

Combined Oral Contraceptives

Combined hormonal contraceptives (COCs) contain oestrogen and progesterone and act on the hypothalamic-pituitary axis to suppress ovulation.

In doing this they also prevent proliferation of the endometrium. COCs are usually taken as a 21-day treatment cycle followed by a seven-day break during which a withdrawal bleed occurs.

COCs can also be taken in extended regimens, including both shorter breaks and tri-cycling regimens with a seven-day break once every 63 days. These extended regimens potentially eliminate or reduce the frequency of the withdrawal bleed and any related symptoms, which may theoretically be helpful in women experiencing painful or heavy periods. However, these extended regimens are off licence and there is currently insufficient data to recommend one regimen over another [9]. Additionally, extended regimens can lead to unscheduled bleeding in some women.

An RCT looking at standard-strength second-generation COCs taken in 21-day treatment cycles found a reduction in menstrual blood loss of 43% [1].

Oral High-Dose Progestogens

Norethisterone 15 mg daily given from days 5 to 26 of the cycle has been found to reduce MBL by up to 83%. However, this has a low satisfaction rate (22%), probably due to the progestogenic side effects of such a regimen. High-dose norethisterone given just in the luteal phase for 7–10 days has been found to be ineffective at reducing menstrual blood loss [1].

At doses of 5 mg or more, norethisterone and norethisterone acetate are partly metabolized to ethinylestradiol (EE). The conversion equates to an oral dose of 4 mcg of EE per 1 mg of norethisterone, thus therapeutic doses of norethisterone (15 mg daily) should be viewed similarly to a combined oral contraceptive pill with regards to the risks of venous thrombo-embolism (VTE) [10]. When considering prescribing high-dose norethisterone, clinicians should elicit any additional risk factors for VTE which may render this regimen too high risk.

Medroxyprogesterone acetate is not metabolized to EE and therefore may be a suitable alternative for the treatment of HMB, with a usual dose of 10 mg once daily (cyclically as above). The dose can be increased to 20–30 mg daily if not effective at the standard 10 mg/day dose. Medroxyprogesterone acetate may be as effective as norethisterone, but supporting data is not available.

Progesterone-Only Injectable Contraceptive

There is no evidence directly assessing the use of injected progestogens for HMB. However, the

Table 19.2 Efficacy of pharmaceutical treatments [1]

Method	Percentage decrease in menstrual blood flow
LNG-IUS	70–100%
Oral progesterone high dose	83%
COC	43%
Tranexamic acid	29–58%
NSAIDs	20–49%

contraceptive injection, depot medroxyprogesterone acetate (DMPA) is likely to induce amenorrhoea as a side effect and thus may be a suitable treatment for HMB if this is something the patient wishes to consider. DMPA is not as effective, or as cost-effective as the LNG-IUS, and is more likely to incur progestogenic side effects, including weight gain, breast tenderness, acne and mood changes [1,11].

Oral Desogestrel and the Progesterone Contraceptive Implant

Both the progesterone-only pill containing desogestrel 75 mcg and the progesterone contraceptive implant act to inhibit ovulation. As a result of this, a proportion of women will become amenorrhoiec with these methods. However, both these methods can also be associated with variable unpredictable bleeding, which may be frequent or prolonged [12,13]. Neither method has any supporting evidence for use in managing women with HMB and neither method is included in the NICE guidelines.

Medical Management Summary

Pharmaceutical treatment should be considered in women without structural or histological abnormalities, or for women with fibroids smaller than 3 cm which are causing no distortion of the uterine cavity.

NICE guidelines recommend if either hormonal or non-hormonal treatments are acceptable they should be considered in the following order:

1. Levonorgestrel-IUS (provided treatment is wanted for at least one year)
2. Tranexamic acid or NSAIDs, or the COC
3. Norethisterone 15 mg daily from days 5 to 26 of the menstrual cycle (taking note of the above effect on VTE risk) or injectable long-acting progestogens.

Case Scenario

Lisa requires contraception and is interested in managing her HMB medically, initially. Having outlined the available treatment options to Lisa she is keen to consider these and discuss them with her husband. You provide her with a patient information leaflet on HMB and the treatment options. You also issue her with a prescription for tranexamic acid to try in the interim.

Lisa returns to you having decided she would like a LNG-IUS. You examine her and find no abnormalities and as a trained coil fitter you counsel her fully regarding the procedure and arrange this for her.

Surgical Management

For women who have had unsuccessful medical treatment, or for women who choose not to have medical management, surgical treatment may be an option. Surgical management includes endometrial ablation, hysterectomy and surgical treatment of fibroids.

Endometrial Ablation

For women who have a normal-sized uterus, or small uterine fibroids, endometrial ablation or resection can be offered as an initial treatment option, or as an option for women who have had failed attempts at medical management. Endometrial ablation is a less invasive procedure than a hysterectomy and associated with fewer complications, and can now be performed under local anaesthetic.

The principle of endometrial ablation or resection is to destroy or remove the endometrium along with the superficial myometrium resulting in the destruction of most or all of the glands from which the endometrium develops. There are several different ablation methods available and these will depend on local secondary care provision.

It is important to note that endometrial ablation (or resection) is not a fertility-conserving treatment. Women who undergo endometrial ablation must be advised to use adequate contraception to avoid a subsequent pregnancy. Pregnancy following endometrial ablation or resection can have life-threatening consequences for both fetus and mother. In some cases it is appropriate to consider tubal sterilization at the time of ablation. All women considering endometrial ablation should be counselled about their contraceptive options in parallel to discussing surgical treatment for HMB.

The short-term effectiveness of endometrial ablation is high, with up to 35% of women being amenorrhoeic at 24 months following the procedure and 90% of women being satisfied. However, longer-term follow-up (five years) finds that around 20–30% of women will either be dissatisfied or require additional treatment [5].

Hysterectomy

Hysterectomy is defined as the surgical removal of the uterus. There are different methods available, including abdominal hysterectomy, vaginal hysterectomy and laparoscopic hysterectomy, all considered to be major surgery and require considerable physical recuperation. NICE guidelines state hysterectomy should not be used as a first-line treatment solely for HMB, but should be considered only when:

- Other treatment options have failed, are contraindicated or declined
- There is a wish for amenorrhoea
- The woman (who has been fully informed) requests it
- The woman no longer wishes to retain her uterus and fertility.

Women considering hysterectomy should be fully informed of the risks and complications of surgery. Their expectations should be fully explored and all other treatment options should be discussed.

A recent cost-effective analysis looking at meta-analyzed data found that although hysterectomy is more expensive than endometrial ablation, it does produce more QALYs for women with HMB and is thus a more cost-effective treatment than endometrial ablation [14].

Treatment of Uterine Fibroids

For women with large fibroids (>3 cm in diameter) and HMB which is having a severe impact on quality of life, interventions for the treatment of uterine fibroids can be considered. The type of treatment offered to women with large fibroids should take into account the location of the fibroid, the number of fibroids and whether women wish to conserve their fertility.

Myomectomy may be offered for treatment of large focal fibroids and can be hysteroscopic (a transcervical resection of fibroid, TCRF), laparoscopic or open. A TCRF can be offered to women with fibroids which contain a significant submucosal element. Laparascopic or open myomectomy can be undertaken for women with intramural or subserosal fibroids; however, it should be noted these may not produce a significant effect on their bleeding if they are not distorting the endometrial cavity. Although myomectomy can be considered a fertility-sparing option, it is important to note the risk of bleeding and subsequent hysterectomy as a complication when undertaking a myomectomy. In women who wish to maintain fertility, the benefits versus risks of any surgery on the uterus need to be carefully considered and discussed with the patient.

For women who have HMB related to fibroids and have completed their family, a hysterectomy is a curative treatment option for women to consider.

Uterine artery embolization is a radiological technique performed under local anaesthetic. It can be offered to women who wish to retain their uterus and can be effective for multiple fibroids. Particles are used to block the uterine arteries; this causes the fibroids to shrink, but is believed to have no permanent effect on the rest of the uterus.

Ulipristal acetate (Esmya®) is a selective progesterone receptor modulator which has a license to treat moderate to severe symptoms of fibroids in women of reproductive age. This can be provided as intermittent treatment, taking 5 mg daily for three months, with repeated courses or more definitive treatment by TCRF if chosen [15].

Case Scenario

Unfortunately, after 12 months of use, the LNG-IUS is not successful in treating Lisa's HMB. Given medical management has failed she does now require further investigations. An ultrasound shows no structural cause for her HMB. Lisa is keen for a definitive treatment as she has completed her family and potentially has over a decade of menstrual cycles ahead of her. She is therefore referred to secondary care. Following a discussion regarding the risks and benefits of endometrial ablation versus laparoscopic hysterectomy she elects to go ahead with the latter procedure, thus providing a curative treatment for her HMB.

Conclusion

Heavy menstrual bleeding is a common problem which can have a considerable effect on a woman's quality of life. A careful history of the problem and examination, where appropriate, helps determine whether further investigations are required.

Following NICE guidance on HMB [1] allows primary care clinicians a logical evidence-based pathway of care, the majority of which can be provided in a primary care setting.

References

1. National Institute for Clinical Excellence (NICE). Heavy menstrual bleeding. Clinical guidelines No. 44. 2007. www.nice.org.uk/guidance/cg44 (accessed January 2017).

2. Royal College of Obstetricians and Gynaecologists, London School of Hygiene & Tropical Medicine, Ipsos MORI. National heavy menstrual bleeding audit: First annual report. 2011. www.rcog.org.uk/en/guidelines-research-services/audit-quality-improvement/national-hmb-audit/ (accessed September 2016).

3. Royal College of Obstetricians and Gynaecologists, London School of Hygiene & Tropical Medicine, Ipsos MORI. National heavy menstrual bleeding audit: final report. 2014. www.rcog.org.uk/en/guidelines-research-services/audit-quality-improvement/national-hmb-audit/ (accessed September 2016).

4. Munro, M, Critchley HO, Broder MS *et al*. FIGO classification system (PALM-COEIN) for causes of abnormal uterine bleeding in nongravid women of reproductive age. *Int J Gynaecol Obstet* 2011; 113(1):3–13.

5. Royal College of Obstetricians and Gynaecologists. Abnormal uterine bleeding: stratog online learning module. 2014. stratog.rcog.org.uk/tutorial/abnormal-uterine-bleeding (accessed September 2016).

6. Kurman RJ, Carcangiu ML, Herrington CS, Young RH (editors), *WHO Classification of Tumours of Female Reproductive Organs, 4th edn*. IARC. 2014.

7. Royal College of Obstetricians & Gynaecologists. Advice for heavy menstrual bleeding services and commissioners. 2014. https://www.rcog.org.uk/globalassets/documents/guidelines/research–audit/advice-for-hmb-services-booklet.pdf (accessed September 2016).

8. Faculty of Sexual and Reproductive Healthcare. Intrauterine contraception. 2015. www.fsrh.org/pdfs/CEUGuidanceIntrauterineContraception.pdf (Accessed 1 August 2015).

9. Faculty of Sexual and Reproductive Healthcare. Combined hormonal contraception. 2011. www.fsrh.org/pdfs/CEUGuidanceCombinedHormonalContraception.pdf (accessed September 2016).

10. Mansour, D. Safer prescribing of therapeutic norethisterone for women at risk of venous thromboembolism. *J Fam Plann Reprod Health Care* 2012; 38:148–149.

11. Faculty of Sexual and Reproductive Healthcare. Progesterone-only injectable contraception. 2014. www.fsrh.org/pdfs/ CEUGuidanceProgestogenOnlyInjectables.pdf (accessed September 2016).

12. Faculty of Sexual and Reproductive Healthcare. Progesterone-only implants. 2014. www.fsrh.org/pdfs/ CEUGuidanceProgestogenOnlyImplants.pdf (accessed September 2016).

13. Faculty of Sexual and Reproductive Healthcare. Progesterone-only pills. 2015. www.fsrh.org/pdfs/ CEUGuidanceProgestogenOnlyPills.pdf (accessed September 2016).

14. Roberts, TE, Tsourapas A, Middleton LJ, *et al.* Hysterectomy, endometrial ablation, and levonorgestrel releasing intrauterine system (Mirena) for treatment of heavy menstrual bleeding: cost effectiveness analysis. *BMJ* 2011; 342:d2202.

15. Donnez J, Hudecek R, Donnez O, *et al.* Efficacy and safety of repeated use of ulipristal acetate in uterine fibroids. *Fertil Steril* 2015; 103(2):519–527.

Management of the Patient with Continence Problems in Primary Care

Victoria Corkhill

Key Points

- Urinary incontinence is a debilitating, chronic condition of multiple aetiologies. It can affect a patient's quality of life, sexuality and relationships.
- The prevalence of urinary incontinence is increasing alongside our rising ageing population, making it essential for clinicians to understand the impact of the condition and management in both primary and secondary care settings.
- Urinary incontinence can be classified into three main types: stress, urge and mixed urinary incontinence.
- Pelvic floor muscle training and surgical interventions (tension-free vaginal tapes) are the mainstay treatments for stress urinary incontinence symptoms.
- Behavioural, lifestyle and pharmacological therapies are the basis of treating urge urinary incontinence symptoms
- Multidisciplinary teams, including community-based continence teams, general practitioners and urogynaecologists play an invaluable role in treating patients with urinary incontinence.

Case Scenario

Jane is a 52-year-old who complains that every time she coughs, laughs or does any exercise she leaks small volumes of urine. She states she has reduced her activities to reduce the amount of 'accidents' she has on a daily basis. She also complains of urinary urgency and frequency up to six times during the day and three times at night.

Jane has had three vaginal deliveries (one forceps delivery) and no other medical problems or current medication. She has a BMI of 39 and smokes 10 cigarettes/day.

Introduction

Urinary incontinence (UI) is a common yet debilitating problem that affects about 50% of women at some point in their lives [1].

The prevalence of UI peaks at 45–55 years of age, plateaus or falls between 50–70 years old, and then steadily increases thereafter. This pattern relates to variations in types of UI. Stress UI incidence decreases after the age of 55, but there is an increasing incidence of overactive bladder (OAB) over the age of 60 [2].

UI is defined by the International Continence Society as 'the complaint of any involuntary leakage of urine' and is broadly subcategorized as:

- *Stress urinary incontinence (SUI)* – involuntary urine leakage on effort or exertion, sneezing or coughing. It can be associated with bladder neck weakness, obesity, poor pelvic floor muscle strength or nerve damage [3].
- *Urgency urinary incontinence (UUI)* – involuntary urine leakage accompanied by or immediately preceded by urgency (a sudden compelling desire to urinate that is difficult to delay).
- *Mixed urinary incontinence (MUI)* – involuntary urine leakage associated with urgency *and* exertion, coughing or sneezing.
- *Overactive bladder (OAB)* – urgency symptoms usually with frequency and nocturia. It can be subclassified as 'OAB wet' and 'OAB dry',

Women's Health in Primary Care, edited by Anne Connolly and Amanda Britton. Published by Cambridge University Press © Cambridge University Press 2017

depending on whether or not the urgency is associated with incontinence. These combinations of symptoms are suggestive of the urodynamic finding of detrusor overactivity (DO) [4].

- *Functional* (unable to reach toilet in time), *overflow* (bladder outlet obstruction from uterine prolapse or previous surgery) and *true incontinence* (due to fistulas) are rare types of UI which need excluding.

Stress UI appears to be the most common UI type and overall 50% of incontinent women in the EPINCONT survey [2] reported this as their only symptom; 11% described only urgency UI and 36% reported mixed UI [2,4].

Treatment options are varied and specific to the pattern of symptoms, type of UI and its specific pathophysiology.

Social and Financial Implications of UI

The impact of UI is considerable for both the patient and the NHS as a whole. The total annual service costs in the UK have been estimated at over £230 million [5]. The psychosocial impact of UI to a woman includes feelings of shame, low self-esteem, depression, social withdrawal, concerns over sexuality and strained personal relationships [6]. On average, a woman will have experienced UI for six to nine years before seeking medical help [7].

Initial Assessment

The vast majority of patients will fall into three categories of UI and therefore the aim of the initial clinical assessment is to classify the woman's UI as either:

- Stress UI
- Mixed UI (MUI)
- Urgency UI/OAB.

The National Institute for Health and Care Excellence (NICE) recommends starting initial treatment on this basis. For a mixed UI picture, the advice is to direct treatment towards the predominant symptom [4]).

Co-Existing Conditions

It is very important to take a comprehensive medical history when diagnosing patients with urinary incontinence. Co-existing conditions and medications need

Table 20.1 Main symptoms of the different types of UI in women

Stress urinary incontinence	Urge urinary incontinence/OAB
• Urinary leakage on: · Coughing · Exercising · Sneezing · Lifting heavy weights	• Frequency • Urgency • Urge incontinence • Nocturia
Worse when bladder full	Urgency is the main symptoms of OAB

Mixed urinary incontinence can have a mixture of symptoms

to be optimized as a priority to aid UI symptom control, as many routine medications can alter bladder function or create fluid shifts, such as diuretics.

Predisposing Conditions

- Poorly controlled diabetes significantly increases urine output.
- Respiratory conditions causing chronic cough symptoms predispose patients to pelvic organ prolapse (POP) and UI symptoms.
- Neurological conditions such as multiple sclerosis, Parkinson's disease, cerebrovascular accident and Alzheimer's diseases are important to note as they can affect nerve stimulation to the bladder [3] as well as causing mobility issues.
- Recurrent urinary tract infections (UTI) are also important to note as this may significantly worsen any UI symptoms.
- Bowel symptoms, including constipation, can weaken pelvic floor muscles and predispose a patient to UI and POP [8,9].

Lifestyle choices such as alcohol, caffeine, fluid intake and smoking tend to worsen UI symptoms.

Occupations involving heavy lifting can worsen Stess UI symptoms.

Past Medical History

Obstetric and gynaecological risk factors for UI include:

- Parity
- Mode of delivery (assisted vaginal deliveries, i.e. forceps)
- Gynaecological procedures, in particular vaginal hysterectomy
- Menopausal status.

Any previous urological investigations, surgery and nocturnal enuresis as a child (associated with detrusor overactivity) are also very important to note [8].

Quality-of-Life Assessment (QoL)

In order to gain a detailed insight of the psychosocial burden associated with a patient's UI, it is vital to ask about the restrictions that her symptoms put on the patient's daily functions and how they cope with these restrictions, such as only shopping in areas with readily accessible toilets.

QoL questionnaires are a useful adjunct in assessing the impact that incontinence and bladder dysfunction have on a woman's life.

NICE recommends eight QoL questionnaires, which have shown the highest validity and reliability including: International Consultation on Incontinence Questionnaire (ICIQ); Bristol Female Lower Urinary Tract Symptoms (BFLUTS); Incontinence Quality of Life (I-QoL) [4]. ICIQ-SF has only four questions and is a good screening tool (Figure 20.1).

Bladder Diaries

These are a method of quantification of urinary frequency, diurnal variations, nocturia, voided volumes, functional bladder capacity, severity of incontinence episodes and fluid input/output [8]. NICE recommends the use of bladder diaries for a minimum of three days spanning over work and leisure days in the initial assessment of women with UI [4].

These diaries enhance the clinical assessment regarding excessive fluid consumption, normal consumption at inappropriate times (e.g. bedtime) or an excessive intake of alcohol or caffeinated drinks.

Physical Examination

A physical examination is required in the assessment of a woman presenting with UI. This assists the diagnosis and management of UI, excludes other related conditions and should routinely include:

- BMI.
- Abdominal and pelvic examination to assess for masses, a palpable bladder, atrophic vaginitis and pelvic organ prolapse (POP), and should include a cough stress test to demonstrate SUI.
- Digital assessment of pelvic floor contractions before commencement of supervised pelvic floor muscle training for the treatment of SUI/MUI is

recommended by NICE [4]. The strength of the contraction is graded from no contraction to strong contraction and its duration.

- If there are symptoms that suggest a neurological cause, it is important to perform a screening neurological exam with emphasis on the sacral roots S2–4 (main innervation of muscarinic receptors of the bladder):
  - Deep tendon reflexes (Achilles – S1)
  - Abduction and dorsiflexion of toes (S3)
  - Sensory innervation at:
    - Sole and lateral aspect of foot (S1)
    - Perineum (S3)
    - Perianal area (S4) [9].
- Assessment of cognitive impairment of women may be required.

Investigations

Urinalysis

Symptoms of detrusor overactivity overlap with those of UTI. The presence of a UTI will worsen irritative bladder symptoms and give false outcomes on any urodynamic investigations.

Women with symptoms of a urinary tract infection with or without a positive urine dipstick should have a mid-stream urine (MSU) sent for culture and consider empirical treatment if urine dip is positive.

If a woman is asymptomatic, but has a positive dipstick for leucocytes/nitrites, she should also have an MSU sent but await culture results before treatment [4].

Postvoid Residuals

Postvoid residual (PVR) is the volume of urine remaining in the bladder following micturition. It should be sought in women with symptoms suggestive of voiding dysfunction or recurrent UTI to assess if the patient is fully emptying the bladder.

Bladder scanning is recommended as a first-line measurement of PVR in view of acceptability and lower incidence of adverse events [4].

Ultrasound

Ultrasound assessment is not routinely recommended for the assessment of women with UI except for PVR measurements or ruling out pelvic masses in obese patients [4].

ICIQ-UI Short Form

CONFIDENTIAL

Initial number

DAY   MONTH   YEAR
Today's date

Many people leak urine some of the time. We are trying to find out how many people leak urine, and how much this bothers them. We would be grateful if you could answer the following questions, thinking about how you have been, on average, over the PAST FOUR WEEKS.

1   Please write in your date of birth:

DAY   MONTH   YEAR

2   Are you *(tick one)*:   Female ☐   Male ☐

---

3   How often do you leak urine? *(Tick one box)*

never ☐ 0
about once a week or less often ☐ 1
two or three times a week ☐ 2
about once a day ☐ 3
several times a day ☐ 4
all the time ☐ 5

---

4   We would like to know how much urine <u>you think</u> leaks.
How much urine do you <u>usually</u> leak (whether you wear protection or not)?
(Tick one box)

none ☐ 0
a small amount ☐ 2
a moderate amount ☐ 4
a large amount ☐ 6

---

5   Overall, how much does leaking urine interfere with your everyday life?
Please ring a number between 0 (not at all) and 10 (a great deal)

0   1   2   3   4   5   6   7   8   9   **10**
not at all   a great deal

ICIQ score: sum scores 3+4+5 ☐ ☐

---

6   When does urine leak? *(Please tick all that apply to you)*

never – urine does not leak ☐
leaks before you can get to the toilet ☐
leaks when you cough or sneeze ☐
leaks when you are asleep ☐
leaks when you are physically active/exercising ☐
leaks when you have finished urinating and are dressed ☐
leaks for no obvious reason ☐
leaks all the time ☐

Thank you very much for answering these questions.

Figure 20.1 ICIQ-UI SF Quality of life assessment tool. Reproduced with permission from Avery *et al.*, 2004 [10].

FULL NAME: Jane Smith   **Date of Birth** 1/1/63 **NHS No:** 123 456 7891

Figure 20.2 Bladder diary example.

	Time	DAY 1 DATE 1 Drinks	Urine	Wet	DAY 2 DATE 2 Drinks	Urine	Wet	DAY 3 DATE 3 Drinks	Urine	Wet
Morning	6 am		340						350	
	7 am							200		
	8 am	300			400	350		200		
	9 am		200						190	
	10 am	200	150		150	150				
	11 am			W		200		150		
Afternoon	12 md		200		200		W	400	200	
	1 pm	150			200	150			200	
	2 pm		175							
	3 pm				150			150		W
	4 pm	450	150			170				
	5 pm		100					200		
Evening	6 pm		100	W	400	130 200		300	100	
	7 pm	250	175		300	150			100	
	8 pm	200	50		500	200	W	400	200	W
	9 pm	100				50	W	200	50	BED
	10 pm	350	180	BED	150				250	
	11 pm					250	BED			
Night	12 mn									
	1 am		270					250		
	2 am	100					W		300	
	3 am		300			300				
	4 am									
	5 am									
	Totals	2100	2390		2450	2300		2450	1920	

Cystoscopy

Cystoscopy (direct visualization of bladder and urethra) is not recommended for the initial assessment of women with UI alone [4]. It is required in cases of haematuria (including persistent microscopic haematuria) and useful in cases of recurrent UTI or bladder pain to exclude bladder pathology or interstitial cystitis (see Table 20.2).

Urodynamics

Urodynamics aims to demonstrate an abnormality of urine storage or voiding via a combination of tests. It is more useful and accurate for diagnosis of lower urinary tract dysfunction than just symptoms alone [8] and also for selecting the most appropriate intervention to the underlying pathology.

- *Uroflowmetry* measures flow of urine over time. It aids diagnosis of voiding difficulties.
- *Cystometry* measures the pressure–volume relationship of the bladder during filling and voiding. The bladder is filled (through a catheter) with saline and the woman indicates her first and maximal desires to void. During the filling phase, tests to provoke the bladder for SUI and DO are performed.

Detrusor overactivity (DO) is diagnosed if there are spontaneous or provoked detrusor contractions.

A diagnosis of urodynamic stress incontinence (USI) is confirmed if leakage on coughing occurs, in the absence of detrusor contractions.

NICE found no evidence to support the use of urodynamics before starting conservative management or for women with 'pure' stress incontinence considering surgical intervention [4].

NICE recommend the use of preoperative urodynamics in cases where:

- Clinical diagnosis is not clear
- Symptoms of OAB lead to clinical suspicion of DO (e.g. frequency and urgency) as these patients have multiple symptoms
- Symptoms indicative of voiding dysfunction or anterior compartment prolapse with UI are present
- Initial surgical therapy for stress incontinence has failed.

Case Scenario

On examination by her GP, Jane was found to have a first-degree uterine descent with a moderate anterior vaginal wall prolapse. Cough test showed no leak and pelvic floor muscle tone was assessed as moderate (3/5 on the Oxford scale).

Jane's urine dipstick was negative.

Referral to Secondary Care

Table 20.2 Referral guidelines for women with urinary incontinence

When to refer a UI patient [2,4]
Urgent (possibly fast track) referral for:
• Microscopic haematuria in women aged 50 years and older
• Visible haematuria
• Recurrent or persisting UTI associated with haematuria in women aged 40 years and older
• Suspected malignant mass arising from the urinary tract
Consider urgent referral for:
• Pelvic pain
• Pelvic or vaginal mass
• Complex neurological symptoms
• Suspected urogenital fistulae
• Severe prolapse (at level of introitus or below)
Consider routine referral for:
• History of pelvic/previous continence surgery
• Previous pelvic radiation therapy
• Patients refractory to conservative or initial pharmacological therapy
• Voiding or postmicturition symptoms such as hesitancy, slow stream, intermittency, straining, incomplete bladder emptying sensation, postmicturition leakage, urinary retention and position-dependent micturition

Treatment Options for UI

Management of a patient with UI depends on the underlying diagnosis, with treatment options including conservative, medical and surgical methods.

Conservative and anti-muscarinic drug treatments will most commonly be offered within a primary and community care setting. If these treatments are unsuccessful, the next option for women would involve a surgical option or second-line agent and therefore most women would need to be referred from primary care to receive these interventions.

Conservative Management of UI

Conservative management steps should be used as a first-line approach to treating any patient with UI.

Lifestyle Advice

- NICE advise a trial of caffeine reduction in women with OAB as caffeine increases the irritability of the bladder. Alcohol should also be reduced or avoided [4].
- Modification of high and low fluid intakes to 1–1.5 litres per day will lessen the severity of OAB symptoms.
- Weight loss should be advised to BMI less than 30.
- Medication review is advised as various drugs such as diuretics and antipsychotics affect bladder function.
- Dietary advice to prevent constipation if needed.
- Smoking cessation advice to reduce the risk of a chronic cough and urgency episodes.

Behavioural Therapy

Bladder drill (retraining) is a behavioural modification used for overactive bladder syndrome (OAB) that involves timed voiding at incremental intervals (15–30 mins). The drill re-educates the bladder into holding increasing volumes of urine for longer periods of time, ultimately up to a desired interval of 3–4 hours [8].

Bladder training should be used for at least six weeks and is a first-line treatment for urgency or mixed UI. If a woman does not achieve satisfactory benefit from bladder training programmes, NICE recommend combining OAB drugs with bladder training, especially if frequency is a predominant symptom.

Biofeedback aims to teach the voluntary inhibition of detrusor contractions in DO and improve pelvic floor contraction in SUI [9]. The patient receives auditory, visual or tactile signals relaying information about these usually subconscious physiological processes. Initial cure/improvement rates of 80% have been quoted, but the relapse rate is high [8].

Hypnotherapy is used in cases where there are underlying psychological factors exacerbating OAB. Unfortunately relapse rates are high.

Acupuncture increases the level of encephalins in the CSF, which are thought to inhibit detrusor contractions. Studies have shown symptomatic improvement, but usually short-lasting effects.

Physical Therapy and Interventions

Pelvic floor muscle training (PFMT) results an increase in tone and strength of the pelvic floor muscles and an increased conscious awareness of the muscle groups.

NICE recommends PFMT as a first-line treatment for women with stress or mixed UI. The duration of exercises should be at least eight contractions (working up to an ideal duration of 10 seconds), three times a day for a minimum of three months. If benefit is found these exercises should be continued. PFMT requires high levels of motivation, education and is ideally performed under clinical supervision.

Women who are experiencing difficulty in performing PFMT may benefit from biofeedback or electrical stimulation, although NICE do not recommend this as a routine part of PFMT [4].

Vaginal cones act as a form of biofeedback by producing graded resistance levels applied to the pelvic floor muscles. These help to increase muscle strength and endurance of the pelvic floor muscles. A Cochrane review [14] concluded that cones are better than no treatment although not better than PFMT alone [14].

Electrical stimulation uses short pulses of current from a probe placed transvaginally. For DO, electrical stimulation inhibits detrusor contractions by the sensory feedback it produces. For SUI it directly stimulates the pelvic floor muscles. NICE found that study results were inconsistent and therefore electrical stimulation is not routinely recommended except in women who have either extremely weak contractions or are unable to produce a muscle contraction [4].

Alternative Physical Interventions

These include bladder catheterization, absorbent products and toileting aids.

NICE only recommend these as a coping strategy pending definitive treatment, as an adjunct to ongoing therapy or as a long-term management of UI, only after treatment options have been explored.

Bladder catheterization may be required in patients who suffer with persistent urinary retention causing incontinence, recurrent UTIs or those who have intractable incontinence and are not fit for other treatments.

Case Scenario

Jane's main complaints come initially from her stress UI symptoms so her initial management should target these, including lifestyle advice (weight loss, smoking cessation, caffeine reduction) and referral to the community-based continence team for PFMT. Alongside PFMT the specialist team should also commence bladder training in view of her frequency symptoms.

As a result of these conservative measures Jane reports an improvement in her symptoms and reduction in incontinence episodes to three times a week. However, she is still using sanitary pads on a daily basis and reports increasing awareness of urgency symptoms.

Pharmacological Treatment for UUI/OAB

Most women with DO will require drug therapy (Table 20.3). Before commencing any treatment, NICE recommends discussing with women:

- Likelihood of success
- Associated common adverse effects
- Best route of administration
- Duration of treatment needed to see full effects (commonly up to four weeks) [4].

NICE also recommends prescribing the lowest recommended dose when starting a new OAB medication and then alter according to side effects or efficacy.

If a patient is stable on long-term UI or OAB drug therapy, she should be reviewed annually if under 75 years old or every six months if over 75.

Alternative Pharmacological Agents for UUI/ OAB

Desmopressin or DDAVP is a long-acting synthetic analogue of vasopressin inhibiting diuresis and is effective in patients with nocturnal polyuria. However, it should be avoided in those with cystitic fibrosis or over 65 years old with cardiovascular disease. The main side effects are hyponatraemia and fluid retention.

Table 20.3 Pharmacological options for OAB/UUI

Drug	Dosage	Dose titration	Benefits	Side effects
First line (NICE 2013) [3, 4]				
Oxybutynin (immediate release)	2.5 mg once daily to 5 mg three times daily	Gradual increase	Immediate effect, can be used on a PRN basis Targets urgency and urge incontinence Low cost	Marked anti-cholinergic side effects[a,b] High discontinuation rate Not advised for frail older women
Tolterodine (Immediate release)	1–2 mg twice daily	Increase after four weeks if needed	High selectivity for bladder receptors thus less side effects Does not cross blood–brain barrier – less CNS effects[b] Dose can be titrated	Better tolerability than oxybutynin[a]
Darifenacin (Once daily)	7.5–15 mg once daily	After two weeks, reassess and increase dose if needed	High selectivity for bladder receptors thus fewer side effects No significant CNS effects[b] Extended release Titration of dose	
Second line				
Oxybutynin XL (Extended release)	5–15 mg once daily	Increase after four weeks if needed	Extended release Can reduce side effect profile	Better tolerability than oxybutynin immediate release[a,b]
Oxybutynin patches	3.9 mg/24 hours applied twice weekly	Nil	Extended release Avoids hepatic first pass	Better tolerability than oxybutynin immediate release[a,b] Skin irritation
Tolterodine (Extended release)	4 mg once daily		Extended release	Better tolerability than oxybutynin[a,b]
Solifenacin	5–10 mg once daily	Increase after four weeks if needed	Extended release Titration of dose Long half life – offering 24 hour control of bladder smooth muscle tone	Side effects well tolerated[a]
Trospium (Immediate release)	20 mg twice daily		Potent blocking action on detrusor contraction No CNS effects[b] – useful in treating elderly patients	Side effects[a]
Trospium (Extended release)	60 mg once daily			
Fesoterodine	4–8 mg once daily	Increase after four weeks if needed	Extended release Dose titration	Better tolerability than oxybutynin[a,b]
Propiverine	15 mg once daily to three times daily	Increase after four weeks if needed	Anti-muscarinic and calcium-channel blocking actions Improvement in frequency symptoms – useful in OAB dry Extended release	Side effects[a]
Third line				
Mirabegron	50 mg once daily	25 mg in renal or hepatic impairment	β-3-adrenoreceptor causing bladder relaxation Similar clinical effectiveness to anti-muscarinics Can be used when anti-muscarinic drugs are contraindicated, clinically ineffective or have unacceptable side effects	Hypertension, headache, painful micturition/ UTI, tachycardia and bowel dysfunction
Intravesical Botulinum toxin A	Botox 100–200 IU Dysport 250 IU		See text	

[a] Common anticholinergic side effects: dry mouth, blurred vision, tachycardia, constipation, dyspepsia.
[b] CNS side effects: disorientation, hallucinations, convulsions, cognitive impairment.
Contraindications: untreated narrow angle glaucoma, myasthenia gravis, bladder retention, bowel obstruction, severe ulcerative colitis.

Oestrogens are important in maintaining healthy lower genital and urinary tract tissues. NICE recommend the use of intravaginal oestrogens in postmenopausal women with OAB and vaginal atrophy. Systemic hormone replacement confers no extra benefit [4].

> **Case Scenario**
>
> Jane was commenced on oxybutynin immediate release (2.5 mg twice daily), but had to swap to a second-line anti-muscarinic in view of problematic side effects. Jane reports this change in medication gave her an acceptable reduction in frequency with manageable side effects.
>
> Twelve months after initial presentation, the patient reported her OAB symptoms to be well controlled, but the stress UI had returned. At this point Jane's GP referred her for secondary care assessment, including urodynamic investigation which confirmed mixed UI (stress UI and detrusor overactivity).

Pharmacological treatment for Stress Urinary Incontinence (SUI)

Duloxetine is the only drug therapy licensed for moderate to severe SUI. Duloxetine is a serotonin and noradrenaline reuptake inhibitor, which acts to increase pudendal nerve activity and ultimately increases urethral sphincter contraction and closure pressure.

A short-term study [15] suggests that the use of duloxetine is associated with a reduction in leakage episodes and improved quality of life in women with SUI or MUI, but it causes a high rate of gastrointestinal side effects (mainly nausea and vomiting) leading to a high rate of treatment discontinuation. Starting at a 20 mg BD dose for two weeks and increasing to 40 mg BD after that can reduce the incidence of side effects.

NICE recommends that duloxetine should only be offered as second-line therapy in women wishing to avoid surgery [4].

Surgical Management Options for Urinary Incontinence

Overactive Bladder/Detrusor Overactivity

Botulinum toxin A blocks the release of acetylcholine and can relax the overactive detrusor muscle when injected directly into it. In general, the injection would need to be repeated every 6–12 months.

NICE suggest offering bladder wall botulinum toxin A injections for OAB only in women who have proven detrusor overactivity, identified by urodynamic investigation, which has not responded to conservative or drug therapy and who are able and willing to intermittently self-catheterize (5–20% risk of urinary retention). Short-term data states a reduction in urinary frequency (by 25%), urgency (50%) and incontinence (33%) [16].

Percutaneous sacral nerve stimulation uses implantable electrical stimulation of the sacral (S3) reflex pathway to inhibit the reflex behaviour of the bladder and reduce detrusor overactivity. NICE recommend these treatments should only be offered to women if their OAB symptoms have not responded to conservative management, including drugs, or are unable to perform intermittent self-catheterization. Success rates are 55–65% for symptomatic improvement [3].

Adverse effects are pain at implant site, leg pain, disturbed bowel function, urinary retention, anal pain and skin irritation at implant site.

Stress Urinary Incontinence

Surgery is usually the most effective way of curing urodynamic stress incontinence, and a 90% cure rate can be expected for a primary procedure [17].

The main aims of the surgical interventions for SUI are to:

- augment urethral closure
- support or stabilize the bladder neck or urethra.

Synthetic mid-urethral tape (MUT) is the most common surgery to treat SUI. It provides tension-free support to the mid-urethra using non-absorbable polypropylene mesh. The tape is tension-free until the patient strains or coughs, which increases the tension, leading to a degree of obstruction of the urethra.

Complications for MUT include [4,8]:

- Bladder perforation (0.5–4.5%) [1]
- Postoperative voiding dysfunction (6%)
- Tape erosion
- *De novo* OAB symptoms (~10%)
- Groin pain.

As a result of the minimal access approach, the patient's hospital stay and morbidity are very much reduced and recovery is speedier than traditional open procedures [4].

Open colposuspension (Burch) is the 'gold standard' surgical treatment for SUI, however it involves an abdominal incision and carries a much higher morbidity risk. The success rate has been quoted at 85–90% at one year, which falls to 70% at five years [3].

Intramural urethral bulking agents are injected into the urethral submucosa at the bladder neck. This is thought to improve SUI symptoms by increasing resting tone and pressure of the sphincter. NICE advises that it should only be offered in those who are unfit for other surgical options.

Case Scenario

Jane was counselled about her options and chose to undergo a mid-urethral tape procedure and continue on with her anti-muscarinic therapy for treatment of her OAB symptoms. Her six-week postoperative check reported excellent results and Jane's quality of life had significantly improved.

Conclusions

Female urinary incontinence is a chronic, debilitating symptom that a GP will encounter frequently in their practice. The psychological impact of the condition is far reaching and patients need an empathic and caring approach to the management of their UI.

The aim is for a patient-centred treatment bundle, which educates and empowers women to self-care in adjunct to additional conservative, pharmacological and surgical treatments.

It is also important to engage multidisciplinary expertise using community-based continence teams and secondary care professionals in a stepwise approach.

References

1. Ford AA, Rogerson L, Cody JD, Ogah J, Mid-urethral sling operations for stress urinary incontinence in women. *Cochrane Database Syst Rev* 2015; (7):CD006375.

2. Hannestad YS, Rortveit G, Sandvik H, Hunskaar S, A community-based epidemiological survey of female urinary incontinence: the Norwegian EPINCONT study. Epidemiology of incontinence in the county of Nord-Trondelag. *J Clin Epidemiol* 2000;53:1150–1157.

3. Bedoya-Ronga A, Cheung WH, Clinical review of urinary incontinence: epidemiology, diagnosis and management. *GPonline* 2014. www.gponline.com/clinical-review-urinary-incontinence-epidemiology-diagnosis-management/genito-urinary-system/incontinence-nocturnal-enuresis-nocturia/article/1295578 (accessed September 2016).

4. National Institute for Health and Care Excellence. Urinary incontinence in women: the management of urinary incontinence in women. 2013. www.nice.org.uk/guidance/cg171/evidence/urinary-incontinence-in-women-full-guideline-191581165 (accessed September 2016).

5. Papanicolaou S, Pons M, Hampel C, *et al.* Medical resource utilisation and cost of care for women seeking treatment for urinary incontinence in an outpatient setting: Examples from three countries participating in the PURE study. *Maturitas* 2005;52(Suppl 2):S35–S47.

6. Nicolson P, Kopp Z, Chapple CR, Kelleher C, It's just the worry about not being able to control it! A qualitative study of living with overactive bladder. *Br J Health Psychol* 2008;13(Pt 2):343–359.

7. Vasvada S, Rackley R, Carmel, M, Urinary incontinence. 2015. emedicine.medscape.com/article/452289-overview#showall (accessed September 2016).

8. Parsons M, Cardozo L, *Female Urinary Incontinence in Practice.* The Royal Society of Medicine Press. 2004.

9. Sarris I, Bewley S, Agnihotri, S, The pelvic floor and continence. In Gardiner M (editor), *Training in Obstetrics and Gynaecology: The Essential Curriculum.* Oxford University Press. 2009:380–390.

10. Avery K, Donovan J, Peters T, Shaw C, Gotoh M, Abrams P, ICIQ: a brief and robust measure for evaluating the symptoms and impact of urinary incontinence. *Neurourol Urodynam* 2004; 23(4):322–330. ICIQ modules can be requested through the ICIQ website: www.iciq.net (accessed September 2016), and are free for clinical and academic use.

11. Abrams P, Avery K, Gardener N, Donovan J, The international consultation on incontinence modular questionnaire: www.iciq.net. *J Urol* 2006; 175:1063–1066.

12. Donovan J, Peters T, Abrams P, *et al.* Scoring the short form ICSmale SF questionnaire. *J Urol* 2000; 164(6):1948–1955.

13. Donovan J, Abrams P, Peters T, *et al.* The ICS-'BPH' study: the psychometric validity and reliability of the ICSmale questionnaire. *BJU* 1996;77:554–562.

14. Herbison G, Dean N, Weighted vaginal cones for urinary incontinence. Cochrane Database Syst Rev 2013;(7): CD002114.

15. Norton PA, Zinner NR, Yalcin I, Bump RC. Duloxetine versus placebo in the treatment of stress urinary incontinence. *Am J Obstet Gynecol* 2002;187(1): 40–48.

16. Wood S, Botulinum Toxin (BOTOX A) in the treatment of refractory detrusor overactivity. Patient information leaflet, Norfolk and Norwich University Hospitals. 2013. www.nnuh.nhs.uk/viewdoc.asp?ID=1190&t=Leaflet (accessed September 2016).

17. Robinson R, Cardozo L. Urinary incontinence. In Edmonds DK (editor), *Dewhurst's Textbook of Obstetrics and Gynaecology, 8th edn*. Wiley-Blackwell. 2011:635–691.

Chapter 21

Managing Cystitis in Primary Care

Tim Sayer

Key Points

- All symptomatic women need culture of their urine and where patients have repeated negative cultures the laboratory should be asked to look for atypical organisms.
- Women with repeated negative cultures also need testing for sexually transmitted infections (i.e. chlamydia).
- Prophylactic low-dose antibiotics in women with recurrent cystitis are still used, but alternative treatments are improving.
- Bladder instillations help significant numbers of women with interstitial cystitis to avoid antibiotics.
- Surgery has a minor role in treatment, but severe cases of interstitial cystitis need MDT review and referral to a tertiary referral centre.

Definition

Cystitis is inflammation of the bladder. Usually this refers to the mucosa, but may in some circumstances involve the muscular level. Commonly the lay press refers to cystitis as urinary tract infection but infective elements are not always present.

Cystitis like all bladder problems causes significant problems with a patient's quality of life. Bladder dysfunction is often seen as socially unacceptable and the problems of interstitial cystitis often affect relationships and work.

Case Scenario

Andrea is a 45-year-old woman who works in the local benefits office. She attends surgery and asks for a sick note. She is feeling stressed about her work as she is having a performance review. The main problem is that she has to go to the toilet regularly and finds this very painful when she goes. She sometimes has to leave a meeting, which is embarrassing for her and means that she struggles to keep up when taking the minutes of the meeting.

You note that she has attended frequently, including the out-of-hours service with symptoms suggestive of urinary tract infections (UTIs), and on each occasion was given a course of antibiotics.

The result of the last MSSU, sent two years ago, demonstrated no growth of organisms, but she has been given at least 10 courses of antibiotics since then.

Urinary Tract Infection

The classical symptoms of a urinary tract infection involve urinary urgency, frequency, dysuria and lower abdominal pain. Simple urinary tract infections in women who are premenopausal require a mid-stream sample of urine (MSSU) and appropriate simple antibiotic treatment. Recurrent urinary tract infections are defined as those that occur more than twice in a six-month period or three times in a 12-month period. Postmenopausal women are commonly afflicted.

There is often no apparent underlying cause for the infection, but poor fluid intake and constipation will add to the risk, as does bladder instrumentation or having been a hospital inpatient. In some women sexual activity is the provoking factor. Postmenopausal women are more at risk if they also present with vaginal mucosal changes associated with lowered circulating oestrogen levels. This results in a dry atrophic mucosa and maybe associated dyspareunia.

Women's Health in Primary Care, edited by Anne Connolly and Amanda Britton. Published by Cambridge University Press
© Cambridge University Press 2017

The risk of stones, pyelonephritis or bladder tumour should always be considered in women with recurrent bacterial cystitis and the investigations are simple, namely renal ultrasound and local anaesthetic flexible cystoscopy.

Recurrent Bacterial UTI

Where no aetiological factors can be found it is assumed that the urothelium is damaged and susceptible to bacterial infection. Very often prophylactic low-dose antibiotic treatment is used. Trimethoprim 200 mg nocte for three to six months is commonly prescribed. Nitrofurantoin has until recently been used, but with the long-term concerns it is being prescribed less often. In the postmenopausal group vaginal oestrogen in either cream, pessary or ring form often means that oral hormone replacement therapy can be avoided. If sexual activity is the precipitating factor then postcoital voiding and/or antibiotic prophylaxis may help. General measures for all groups of patients involve good hygiene, good fluid intake and avoidance of caffeine. Cranberry supplements have also been shown to be helpful.

Non-Infective Cystitis

It is recognized that infective cystitis is a troublesome problem for many women, but non-infective cystitis can be even more difficult to manage. Both patients and doctors are often frustrated by presentations of classical symptoms of cystitis, a negative urine culture and increasingly frequent requests for antibiotics which only give temporary relief. Some authorities do believe that there is an infective cause, but that traditional urine culture fails to identify this. Very often the laboratory report states that the level of pyuria is not sufficient to allow for culture. It is always worth asking for culture to specifically identify atypical organisms in women with recurrent abacterial cystitis.

Case Scenario

Andrea's MSSU is reported as negative. On enquiry you establish that she is having regular periods, but admits to being very anxious as she is avoiding having sex, because of her regular episodes of pelvic discomfort and urinary frequency and fears for her continence.

The history does not give any other suggestive cause for her symptoms, a repeat MSSU is used to exclude atypical organisms and STIs are excluded. She is relieved when you suggest referring her on to secondary care to exclude other causes.

Non-infective cystitis seems to affect all age groups and often there are no specific trigger factors.

Although not life-threatening, recurrent abacterial cystitis affects the quality of life of these women. Problems include absence from work, poor sexual function, lack of sleep and poor social interaction.

Cause of Non-Infective Cystitis

Most women will have idiopathic abacterial cystitis. Rare causes include:

- Bladder tumours
- Drugs, particularly those to treat bladder cancer
- Ketamine abuse
- Radiation treatment to the pelvis
- Radical surgery, often for malignancies.

It is thought that an insult to the mucosa of the bladder causes damage to the GAG (glycosaminoglycan) layer. This layer of mucosal chemicals protects the bladder from infection, but once damaged becomes inflamed. A decrease in the GAG layer means that new non-antibiotic treatments have a rationale.

Painful bladder, infective or non-infective cystitis, when chronic, is a debilitating disorder causing severe distress to patients and affecting their quality of life.

Interstital Cystitis/Painful Bladder Syndrome

Interstitial cystitis (IC) is a condition that results in bladder pain and pelvic pain. Symptoms vary from mild discomfort to severe pain. Urgency and the need to urinate frequently to reduce the pain are common and the symptoms are often worse around the time of menstruation. Sexual intercourse will often aggravate the situation.

Most clinicians believe that IC is a group of disorders and usually it is only diagnosed when all other physical problems have been eliminated.

The bladder becomes inflamed, leading to a stiff, low-compliant organ. Urodynamic tests show a reduced capacity and high pressure at capacity. Cystoscopy reveals postdistension pin point bleeding. The classical description is of Hunner's ulcers, where the urothelium appears to be ulcerated.

IC is most common in women, who account for 90% of the cases.

The aetiology is still poorly understood, but no infective cause has been found, hence antibiotics have a poor success rate. The association of IC with polymyalgia might imply an inflammatory cause. Commonly IC does not run in families.

Diagnosis is based on history of pain when the bladder is full and on the cystoscopic appearances. Biopsy is helpful to confirm chronic inflammatory changes and to see if there is a raised mast cell count. This will also exclude bladder neoplasm.

Treatment of Interstitial Cystitis

Treatment remains difficult as there is no cure nor is there a means to identify which patient will respond to which therapy. Many patients do improve after cystoscopic cystodistension, but the symptoms often recur at varying times. The risk with this treatment is bladder perforation as the bladder, as well as being stiffer, is also more brittle. Should perforation occur, simple catheterization for 10 days will allow time for healing to occur.

Oral medications range from the simple anti-inflammatory medications such as ibuprofen for pain relief. Tricyclic antidepressants such as amitriptyline may also help, especially at night. Pentosan polysulfate sodium (Elmiron) was first licensed in 1996, but sadly only helps in a third of patients. Liver and platelet function need to be observed during this treatment, but there do not appear to be any known drug interactions. Elmiron should be discontinued before surgery due to its effect on platelets.

Diet has been widely thought to be important in patients with IC. High-acid foods, alcohol, caffeine citrus drinks and chocolate may all aggravate the symptoms in patients to varying degrees. Smoking does affect the bladder and certainly predisposes to an increase in the risk of bladder cancer.

Physiotherapy and bladder retraining may help some patients along with some of the anticholinergic drugs.

The mainstay of treatment has been the use of intravesical instillation. Initially this was with dimethyl sulfoxide. This unpleasant treatment caused pain to the bladder during instillation, caused the patient to temporarily smell and could potentially

affect the refractoriness of the eye. Thankfully this treatment is now rarely used.

Newer bladder instillations aim to heal the GAG layer as this is said to be deficient in IC patients. Such instillations use hyaluronic acid and/or chondroitin sulfate in varying proportions. There is significant evidence that Cystistat improves outcomes in 80% of patients. These instillations are classed as a medical device, allergic reactions are rare and instillation regimes simple. Patients attend weekly for a month and then monthly for a further two to four treatments depending on their response. Subsequently some may need instillation two to three times a year.

Case Scenario

Andrea was seen in secondary care and diagnosed as having IC, and the bladder distension done at cystoscopy significantly improved her symptoms. She was given dietary advice and links to The Interstitial Cystitis Association, as there is the possibility symptoms could recur. Her life, her job and her relationship all improved as a result of this intervention.

Many patients need concurrent psychological help with their treatments, as do all patients with chronic pelvic pain.

There is increasing evidence that Botox injections to the bladder do help with the pain. A standard dose of 200 IU can be injected under local or general anaesthesia, but patients must be warned that 20% may need to self-catheterize postoperation and that the effects of Botox seem to wear off in nine to twelve months.

Once medical treatments have been exhausted, surgery is a last resort. Some patients do find repeated cystodistenion of benefit, but this requires repeated anaesthetics and the time interval between treatments seems to decrease with time. Many surgeons are hesitant to operate as cure rates for pain are not good and some patients seem to switch to other debilitating symptoms.

Cystoscopic cauterization of bladder ulcers has been used, as has laser treatment. Inflammatory bladder can be resected and the bladder augmented with a piece of bowel, namely a Clam cystoplasty. Patients may suffer postoperatively with mucus in the urine, may need to self-catheterize and are at increased risk of bladder cancer due to the effect of urine on bowel mucosa. Such procedures are only performed in tertiary centres. Despite surgical intervention, some patients continue with intractable bladder pain and may need cystectomy with the formation of a urostomy.

As in all treatments for chronic pain, 'phantom' pain can occur.

Patients with IC need support from family and friends. Help is available through The Interstitial Cystitis Association and other support groups. There is no contraindication to pregnancy and no direct evidence that IC predisposes to cancer.

Anecdotal Cases

All doctors remember their good and bad outcome cases. In the younger sexually active patient, bladder instillations certainly help to reduce the incidence of postcoital cystitis, but not in those patients with urethritis. Miss X was significantly improved with dietary advice in reducing coffee and cola, but still had some episodes of postcoital cystitis, especially around menstruation. She benefitted from postcoital trimethoprim at this time.

Postmenopausal women benefit significantly from vaginal oestrogen and bladder instillation. Mrs Y, a 60-year-old patient, had an excellent response to vaginal oestrogen pessaries and a course of iAluril. She stopped her vaginal oestrogen and her cystitis returned after three months. She was concerned regarding the risk of breast or uterine cancer if using long-term oestrogen, but was reassured that this is not significant when using local vaginal preparations. She continues to use vaginal oestrogen once or twice weekly and remains well.

Not all women do well. Mrs Z, a 42-year-old patient, had a two-year history of recurrent abacterial cystitis, frequency and bladder pain. Urodynamics showed a poorly compliant bladder with reduced functional capacity of 230 mL and bladder biopsy confirmed chronic inflammation with a raised mast cell count. Antibiotics have never helped; she has an excellent diet, never drinks alcohol and two courses of bladder instillations have failed. Botox failed and repeat cystoscopy and cystodistention showed a bladder with numerous bleeding pin point areas (Figure 21.1) and the procedure has been minimally successful. Her symptoms now dominate her life with pain and frequency every 40 minutes. She is contemplating alternative surgery to make life bearable.

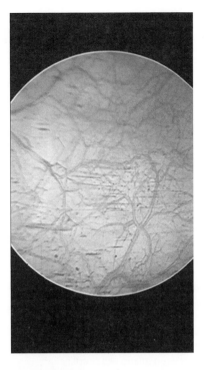

Figure 21.1 Pin point bleeding of the bladder seen during cystoscopy. (For the colour version, please refer to the plate section.)

Conclusion

Women often present with symptoms of cystitis to primary care. In those presenting with recurrent problems, a careful history to exclude other causes should be considered and lifestyle addressed. A negative MSSU should prompt different management, including looking for the possibility of atypical organisms, also of referring to secondary care for investigation that may result in a diagnosis by exclusion of interstitial cystitis. Bladder instillation and, in refractory cases, surgery may help some of these women. Managing some of the disabling symptoms and their psychological effect on a woman's wellbeing and quality of life needs understanding and additional support should be offered.

Further Reading

The Cystitis and Overactive Bowel Foundation. www.cobfoundation.org/ (accessed September 2016).

TevaUK Leaflet entitled MIMS Shared Care Management – Moderate-to-severe chronic cystitis. Issued August 2015. UK/CYS/15/0003.

Bladder and Bowel Foundation. www.bladderandbowelfoundation.org/ (accessed September 2016).

Chapter 22

The Management of Ovarian Cysts in Primary Care

Sally Louden

Key Points

- Almost all ovarian cysts in premenopausal women are benign.
- A transvaginal scan is far superior to a transabdominal scan.
- Care with the nomenclature used with patients helps to manage anxiety.
- The CA 125 assay is of little value in premenopausal women, but should be used in all postmenopausal women.
- Risk assessment tools are more useful in postmenopausal women and will simplify management.
- In premenopausal women:
  · A simple cyst, measuring less than 50 mm in diameter, requires no follow-up.
  · A larger simple cyst (50–70 mm) requires annual follow-up, and those greater than 70 mm are more likely to cause problems and should be referred.
- In postmenopausal women, where the risk of a malignancy is greater:
  · Simple cysts less than 50 mm in diameter and a normal CA 125 should be rescanned in three months.
  · Persistent simple cysts should be reassessed with a scan and a CA 125 every four months for one year.
  · Any woman with concerning features on ultrasound or a raised CA 125 should be referred.
- A widespread screening programme is not thought to be cost effective.
- The combined contraceptive pill is of uncertain benefit in the prevention of ovarian cysts in premenopausal women.
- Research is ongoing into new tumour markers.

Case Scenario: Alice

Alice, aged 47, attends the morning surgery. She is distressed. She presented with right iliac fossa pain one month ago, and some irregularities of her periods. She takes the progesterone-only pill as contraception. An ultrasound scan was requested, and this was performed yesterday. The report of the abdominal scan has not yet arrived, but on accessing the online report, it would appear that she has a right-sided loculated thin-walled simple ovarian cyst measuring 48 mm in its maximal diameter. The septum is thin. Her endometrial thickness is 10 mm and appropriate for the time in her menstrual cycle. Her aunt had ovarian cancer at the age of 72 and she wants to know what is going to happen next.

Definition

An ovarian cyst is a fluid-containing structure arising from the ovary measuring more than 30 mm in diameter. An ovarian follicle is an integral part of the ovary and should not exceed 30 mm in diameter.

Introduction

Ovarian cysts are extremely common, and up to 10% of women will have an operation during their life for investigation of an ovarian mass [1,2]. The majority of ovarian cysts are incidental findings on ultrasound scans performed for non-specific reasons such as irregular or heavy menstrual bleeding, pain or bloating. Of healthy postmenopausal women, 21% may have an ovarian cyst [3].

The risk of malignancy in a unilocular ovarian cyst in a premenopausal woman is low at 0.1% [1], but the finding of solid and cystic elements on the ultrasound

Women's Health in Primary Care, edited by Anne Connolly and Amanda Britton. Published by Cambridge University Press
© Cambridge University Press 2017

scan increases the risk of malignancy up to 17%. The risk of malignancy increases with cyst size, patient age and menopausal status.

The 2011 NICE guidelines [4] suggest that non-specific symptoms, such as persistent abdominal distension, satiety, bloating, pain, difficulty eating and urinary symptoms occurring regularly, particularly in the postmenopausal woman, should raise the index of suspicion. Further investigations are warranted, with the recommendation that a vaginal examination is undertaken, and then the appropriateness of a serum CA 125 and transvaginal ultrasound considered. Particular care should be taken in menopausal women with a family or personal history of ovarian or breast malignancies.

> **Case Scenario: Alice**
>
> Alice is aged 47. We do not know if she is still menstruating. Let us assume that she is. If her ovarian cyst is simple she has approximately a 1:1000 risk of malignancy.

Physiology of the Menstrual Cycle

During the first half, or follicular phase, of the menstrual cycle, follicle-stimulating hormone (FSH) is released to stimulate follicular growth, of both the endometrium and the ovaries. One of the ovarian follicles grows, and by about day seven, a dominant follicle will be established, usually in just one ovary. This follicle continues to grow, but any other stimulated follicles start to degenerate. The developing follicle produces oestrogen and this has several effects. Firstly, it encourages the thickening of the endometrium, but secondly, at a certain level, the oestrogen also has a negative effect on the FSH production, ensuring that only one follicle matures. Thirdly, the rising oestrogen triggers the release of luteinizing hormone (LH) from the pituitary gland over a 24-hour period (the LH surge), which is the stimulus for the follicle to release the ovum. The release of the ovum, or ovulation, generally occurs 36 hours after the LH surge.

The second half, or proliferative phase, of the menstrual cycle, sees the remains of the dominant follicle (or corpus luteum as it is now called) producing oestrogen. This is driven by the LH. If fertilization has not occurred, then the corpus luteum regresses, and levels of both hormones fall. The falling progesterone level is associated with the shedding of the endometrium, and menstruation begins.

Physiology of Ovarian Cysts

With the complex relationships between FSH, LH, oestrogen and progesterone, and the production of a dominant follicle with every menstrual cycle, it is not difficult to understand why, in some women, ovulation and the subsequent disintegration of the corpus luteum does not occur. Several dominant follicles may appear without one single follicle dominating. Why some premenopausal women appear to be regular cyst formers, and why it occurs at all in postmenopausal women, remains a mystery. There is no doubt, however, that the use of the correct terminology can alleviate anxiety. Women generally consider a 'cyst' to be pathological but a 'follicle' to be physiological, so care with the nomenclature at the outset of the diagnosis can pave the way for less stressful management. In gynaecological terms, a 'follicle' is anything up to 30 mm in diameter, but 'cyst' is anything larger than this.

> **Case Scenario: Alice**
>
> So what do we do with Alice? She wants to know if she has cancer.

Assessment of Patients with Ovarian Cysts

Initially, a thorough history should be taken, and particular attention should be paid to her risk factors, protective factors, her menopausal status and her symptoms.

Risk factors include personal or family history of breast, uterine, colonic or ovarian cancer, including the hereditary cancer syndromes (BRCA gene mutation or Lynch syndrome).

Protective factors include a previous pregnancy and breastfeeding, which confer a 50% reduction in risk. It is thought that current use of the combined oral contraceptive pill also confers protection, but use of HRT can increase the risk [5].

Symptoms of concern include persistent abdominal bloating, feeling full and/or loss of appetite, pelvic or abdominal pain and increased urinary urgency and/or frequency, particularly if they occur more than 12 times each month. Other worrying symptoms would be unexplained weight loss, fatigue or changes in bowel habit. It is rare for women to develop irritable bowel syndrome over the age of 50, so symptoms suggestive of this should trigger the exclusion of ovarian pathology. These are, of course, very common symptoms in primary care, making it easy to overlook the diagnosis of ovarian malignancy.

Clinical examination should include an assessment for a pelvic or abdominal mass, ascites, abdominal pain and lymphadenopathy.

The Vaginal Examination

If a cyst has already been diagnosed on ultrasound scan, then a pelvic examination will not offer much additional information. An assessment of mass tenderness, mobility, nodularity and the presence or absence of ascites or lymphadenopathy may aid the diagnosis. The vaginal examination is known to have really poor sensitivity in the detection of ovarian masses (between 15 and 51%), and one study suggested that junior doctors were better at picking up pathology than more experienced doctors [6].

What Sort of Scan is Best?

It is now widely accepted that a transvaginal ultrasound scan is considered the gold standard and is preferable to an abdominal ultrasound scan, because the better resolution gives much clearer images. This is particularly true for women with a high BMI, simply because the TV transducer starts imaging much closer to the pelvic organs, with less chance of artefactual deterioration of the scanned images. Women may be initially concerned at the appearance of the TV probe, which can look quite intimidating, but anecdotal evidence would suggest that women prefer the TV scan to the discomfort associated with the pressure being applied to the abdomen in the presence of a full bladder. The TV probe has a scanning depth of 5–10 cm whereas the abdominal transducer has a scanning depth of 10–15 cm. Certainly the TV scan is essential when looking for small pelvic changes, such as a tiny intrauterine gestation sac, or a possible ectopic pregnancy. However, the abdominal transducer may be preferred in some groups of women:

- Those who have never experienced sexual intercourse
- Those with such a large pelvic mass that 10 cm is an inadequate scanning depth to visualize the mass fully
- Those with an axial uterus (as opposed to anteverted or retroverted), which can be more difficult to visualize with the TV probe, particularly in the larger woman.

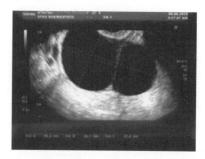

Figure 22.1 Bilocular ovarian cyst on TV scan.

The use of colour doppler has not really helped scanning diagnostic accuracy, but may help in the more detailed assessment of a complex mass, and is favoured by some specialists. Unless the cyst is really large (greater than 10 cm in diameter), the use of CT or MRI scanning often adds little to the diagnostic process, but may help in the assessment of complex lesions, lymphandenopathy or metastases.

How Does a Clinician Assess an Ovarian Cyst on Scanning?

The system most widely used in the assessment of ovarian cysts is that of 'pattern recognition' of specific ultrasound findings [7,8]. Pattern recognition assesses the appearance of the cyst on ultrasound, and classifies the findings into benign (B-rules) and malignant (M-rules). The sonographer essentially considers the:

- Size
- Wall thickness
- Whether it is unilocular or multilocular
- The thickness of the division between the locules
- The presence or absence of solid components
- The presence of acoustic shadowing
- The presence of ascites
- Bilateral lesions
- Blood flow.

This allows the clinician to assign an objective numerical score to the ultrasound report. A small, thin-walled unilocular cyst with no solid components would be described as being simple and of low concern. Unsurprisingly, the expertise of the sonographer is extremely important in this assessment.

Clinical Scenario: Alice

Alice will be best assessed with a transvaginal scan undertaken by an experienced sonographer. The scan she had done was an abdominal scan, with consequent images, and it may be that she needs to be re-referred for a second TV scan, because in Alice's case the cyst is not truly 'simple'.

Which Are the Best Serum Markers to Use, and How Are They Interpreted?

The serum CA 125 glycoprotein antigen serum marker is currently considered the best serum marker available. However, it can be affected by many conditions seen in the premenopausal woman, such as menstruation, fibroids, adenomyosis, endometriosis and pelvic infection, and to avoid unnecessary confusion, should ideally be taken when the woman is not menstruating. It is raised in only 50% of early epithelial carcinomas. A raised result should be treated with caution, and considered only in addition to the ultrasonographic findings. It does not need to be assayed in all premenopausal women [1], and indeed, some [8] consider it useless in these women.

The RCOG therefore states that:

- A serum CA 125 is not necessary when a clear ultrasonographic diagnosis of a simple ovarian cyst has been made.
- If a serum CA 125 is slightly raised, but less than 200 u/mL, further investigations may be necessary to exclude/treat the common differential diagnoses.
- When a CA 125 level is raised, serial monitoring (after four to six weeks) may be helpful, as rapidly rising levels are more likely to be associated with malignancy.
- If a CA 125 level is greater than 200 u/mL, discussion should take place with a gynaecological oncologist for further evaluation.

Lactate dehydrogenase (LDH), aFP and hCG should also be measured in all women under the age of 40 years with a complex ovarian mass, because of the possibility of germ-cell tumours. Human epididymis protein4 (HE4) is a tumour marker currently undergoing evaluation, and may be superior to CA 125.

The Risk of Malignancy Index

The risk of malignancy index is a risk assessment tool, used by hospital gynaecologists, first developed in 1991 by Sassone [9]. Used in the assessment of complex cysts, it is most useful in postmenopausal women. The RCOG suggests that it should only be employed if ovarian carcinoma is suspected in a premenopausal woman, but used every time for a postmenopausal woman. Sassone [9] suggested:

$$RMI = U \times M \times CA125$$

where U = ultrasound score, M = 3 for all postmenopausal women, but M = 1 for premenopausal women multiplied by the absolute value of the CA 125. Postmenopausal status was considered to be the absence of periods for 12 months, or women over 50 years of age who have had a hysterectomy. Anything above 250 was deemed to be at high risk of malignancy. This index, set at this level, has a sensitivity of 70% and a specificity of 90% [10].

- RMI <25, the risk of cancer is <3%
- RMI >25, but <250, risk of cancer 20%
- RMI >250, risk of cancer 75%.

Many other models have been produced in an attempt to improve upon the RMI, but the original 1991 model remains the best and most widely used.

Ovarian Cysts in Premenopausal Women

The chance of sinister pathology in premenopausal women is very low. The overall incidence of a symptomatic ovarian cyst in a premenopausal woman being malignant is approximately 1:1000, increasing to 3:1000 by the age of 50. Differentiation between benign and malignant ovarian masses in the premenopausal women can be difficult, as the CA 125 serum marker is not very helpful. The markers, AFP, hCG, and LDH [11] may be of use with a complex cyst.

A functional or simple ovarian cyst is a thin-walled cyst without any internal structures seen on the ultrasound scan, and measuring less than 50 mm in their maximum diameter. The Society of Radiologists in Ultrasound concluded that asymptomatic simple cysts 30–50 mm in diameter do not require further imaging or follow-up as these usually resolve over two to three menstrual cycles [12]. Test of resolution is not required. A cyst greater than 50 mm is more likely to incur an ovarian accident, including torsion, rupture or haemorrhage.

Clinical Scenario: Alice

Alice has some concerning features on her ultrasound scan. The cyst is described as being loculated, 40 mm in diameter, thin-walled and the septum between the locules is described as being thin. As her cyst is loculated, she requires a serum CA 125 performing. However, assuming she is premenopausal, her RMI will remain low.

Management of Ovarian Cysts in Premenopausal Women

The RCOG states that:

- As the majority of women with small (less than 50 mm diameter) simple ovarian cysts are likely to be physiological, and will almost always resolve within three menstrual cycles, these women do not require follow-up and can be managed conservatively.
- Those with slightly larger simple unilocular ovarian cysts (50–70 mm in diameter) should have annual ultrasound follow-up.
- Those with symptomatic or larger simple cysts (>70 mm) should be considered for further imaging or surgical intervention.

Alice's thin-walled 48 mm ovarian cyst with two locules and a family history of ovarian carcinoma may cause continuing concern. With this ultrasound appearance, however, her CA 125 and RMI will almost certainly be low. However, her family history may persuade you to rescan her in three to four months time, specifically requesting a transvaginal scan, for reassurance for both her and yourself.

Asymptomatic cysts that persist or increase in size are unlikely to be functional, and may warrant surgical management. Mature cystic teratomas (dermoid cysts) will grow over time, increasing the risk of pain and ovarian accidents. These cysts have a characteristic ultrasound appearance and would not be described as 'simple', so the guidelines would suggest CA 125 and referral. An evidence-based consensus regarding the upper limit of size that would indicate surgical management does not exist, but most studies would suggest an arbitrary maximum diameter of 50–60 mm.

Clinical Scenario: Alice

Alice accepts that you have considered her clinical condition and ultrasound findings carefully and you have agreed with her that as her CA 125 is low, in view of her family history, she should be rescanned in three to four months.

However, after 10 weeks, Alice re-presents to you with right iliac fossa pain of sudden onset six hours previously. She has been vomiting with the pain. Her bowels remain normal. She assures you that she has continued to take the contraceptive pill on a regular basis with no missed pills. Clinical examination reveals that she is apyrexial, her pulse is 85 b/min, she has significant abdominal pain, but no guarding or rebound. Her bowel sounds are normal. A pregnancy test is negative and her urine is clear on dipping.

What Can Go Wrong with Ovarian Cysts?

Rupture

Women who present acutely with lower abdominal pain, and a collapsed cyst on USS with free fluid in the pouch of Douglas, may have a ruptured ovarian cyst. An ectopic pregnancy needs to be excluded by ensuring a pregnancy test is negative. Uncomplicated cyst ruptures can be managed at home with analgesia and advice, as symptoms usually resolve within 24–72 hours. However, some patients develop a haemoperitoneum, and management in a hospital may be required. Occasionally, a laparoscopy may be indicated.

Torsion

If an ovary twists partially or completely on its pedicle of supporting ligaments, it may cut off its blood supply. The patient might present with sudden onset lower abdominal pain, vomiting and possibly a palpable, tender adnexal mass. The diagnosis is usually made clinically, but a USS will contribute to the diagnosis, and could show a reduced ovarian blood flow on Doppler and sometimes the presence of free fluid in the pouch of Douglas. Benign cysts greater than 50 mm, and particularly dermoid cysts, are at the greatest risk of torsion.

Laparoscopy is usually required to de-tort and conserve the ovary, but oophorectomy may take place if the ovary is not viable.

Pregnant Women with Ovarian Cysts

Women are scanned more frequently in pregnancy and incidental ovarian cysts are commonly found; 50% resolve spontaneously during the pregnancy. These may be related to a persistent corpus luteum of early pregnancy. With expectant management, the reported rate of complications is <2% [13]. A cyst seen on an eight-week dating scan will be reviewed regularly at routine antenatal scans. Intervention will be required if there is a suspicion of malignancy, if there is a complication, such as torsion, or if the size is so large that it is likely to cause obstetric problems. The best time to intervene is after the first trimester, when the miscarriage rate decreases. The risk of cancer in a pregnant woman is less than 1% [14].

The Treatment and Prevention of Ovarian Cysts in Premenopausal Women

A small Cochrane review concluded that the combined oral contraceptive probably did not prevent the formation of new cysts [15] or the resolution of existing cysts.

If intervention is required, the consensus is that it should be performed laparoscopically as it is safer, aesthetically more pleasing and more cost effective. However, with a large mass, with solid components and a possible risk of malignancy, a laparotomy may be considered more appropriate. The aspiration of ovarian cysts, either vaginally or laparoscopically, is associated with high recurrence rates.

Clinical Scenario: Alice

Alice is admitted acutely under the gynaecologists and is rescanned later that day. Her ovarian cyst has gone, but she has some free fluid in the pouch of Douglas. Her symptoms settle quickly with analgesia and with the reassurance that her scan is normal she is soon discharged from hospital.

Ovarian Cysts in Postmenopausal Women

Ovarian cysts are less common in postmenopausal women, but many are still found as incidental findings with the increasing use of ultrasound. Up to 21% may have abnormal morphology [2]. The RCOG states that as the risk of malignancy is greater in ovarian cysts in postmenopausal women, a TV ultrasound and a CA 125 assay should be performed in all of these women. However, the risk of malignancy in a simple, unilateral, unilocular cyst less than 50 mm in diameter is still less than 1% [16]. A CA 125 of more than 30 u/mL has a

sensitivity of 81% and specificity of 75% for the diagnosis of ovarian cancer in older women. The transvaginal ultrasound, in experienced hands, achieves a sensitivity of 89% and specificity of 73%. This result should be used in conjunction with the ultrasound findings and menopausal status. Other markers, such as the CEA and cancer antigen 19.9, are of uncertain clinical significance.

Management of Ovarian Cysts in Postmenopausal Women

The RCOG states that:

- Simple unilateral, unilocular ovarian cysts of less than 50 mm with a normal CA 125 can be managed conservatively; 50% of these will resolve spontaneously within three months.
- Cysts of 20–50 mm should be rescanned every four months [16,17] for one year, with repeat CA 125 assays every four months for one year [2].
- Women with concerning features on ultrasound or raised CA 125 should be referred to the gynaecological oncologist.
- Any woman who does not meet the criteria for conservative management should be offered surgical management. An oophorectomy is recommended rather than a cystectomy, if a malignancy is suspected, as this allows complete removal of the cyst and the avoidance of any spillage into the peritoneal cavity. Bilateral oophorectomy may be appropriate, as the contralateral ovary could be affected either now or in the future.

Screening The Population For Ovarian Cancer

For the general population routine screening does not have adequate sensitivity or specificity to be used as a mass screening test, but is useful on an individual basis. Screening with the transvaginal ultrasound has a high false positive rate, as it is difficult to differentiate between malignant and benign masses. The serum CA 125 is affected by benign conditions and is not always raised. Women with a strong family history of ovarian or breast malignancies should have genetic counselling. Those who carry the BRCA1 mutation have a lifetime risk of ovarian cancer of 60%, and BRCA2 in the region of 40% [18].

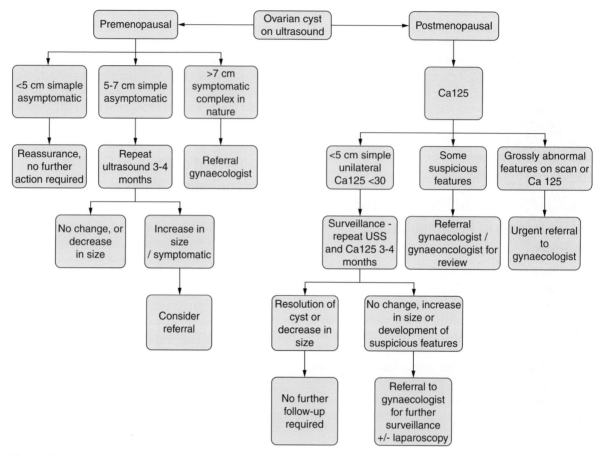

Figure 22.2 Management of ovarian cysts.

The Approach to Managing Ovarian Cysts in General Practice

Conclusion

The discovery of an ovarian cyst can cause a great deal of anxiety for both patients and doctors. Appropriate risk assessment using the available tools in the correct hands will simplify their management and reduce concern. Using the correct nomenclature early in the diagnosis is important. Much more care needs to be taken with the postmenopausal woman, but a screening programme is not, as yet, thought to be cost effective.

References

1. Royal College of Obstetricians and Gynaecologists. Management of suspected ovarian masses in premenopausal women. Green-Top Guideline. No 62. RCOG 2011.

2. Royal College of Obstetricians and Gynaecologists. Ovarian cysts in postmenopausal women. Green-Top Guideline No 34. RCOG 2003.

3. Menon U, Gentry-Maharaj A, *et al.* Sensitivity and specificity of multimodal and ultrasound screening for ovarian cancer, and stage distribution of detected cancers: results of the prevalence screen of the UK Collaborative Trial of Ovarian Screening (UKCTOCS). *Lancet Oncol* 2009;10(4):327–340.

4. NICE. Clinical guidance on ovarian carcinoma guidelines. CG 122. 2011.

5. Kmeitowicz Z. Short term use of HRT increases the risk of ovarian carcinoma. *BMJ* 2015;350:840.

6. Padilla L, Radosevich D, Milad M. Accuracy of the pelvic examination in detecting adnexal masses. *Obstet&Gynecol* 2000;96(4):593–598.

7. Timmermann D, Valentin L, Bourne TH, *et al.* Terms, definitions and measurements to describe the sonographic features of adnexal tumors: a consensus opinion from the International Ovarian Tumour

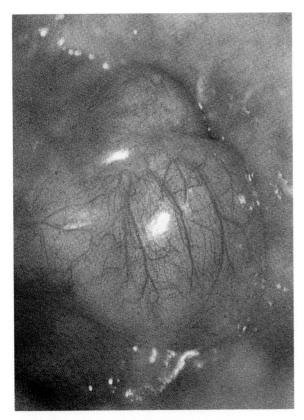

Figure 7.2 Colposcopic appearance of nabothian follicles with characteristic branching pattern of vessels overlying mucous-filled cysts. (A black and white version of this figure will appear in some formats.)

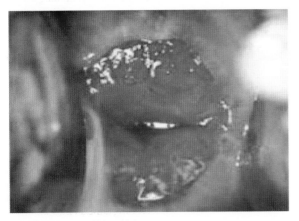

Figure 7.3 Ectropion. (A black and white version of this figure will appear in some formats.)

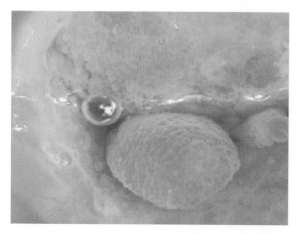

Figure 7.4 Cervical polyp. (A black and white version of this figure will appear in some formats.)

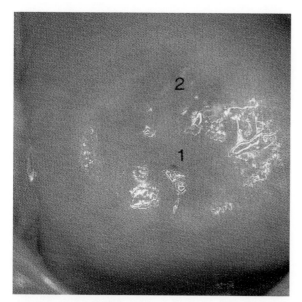

Figure 7.6 Stenosed cervix (1: cervical os; 2: transformation zone). (A black and white version of this figure will appear in some formats.)

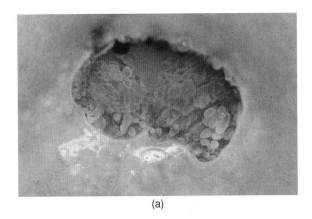

(a)

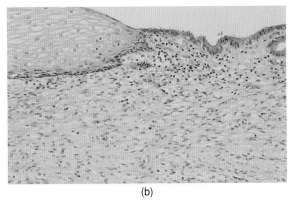

(b)

Figure 7.9 *Colposcopy.* (a) Colposcopic appearance of the external OS showing the SCJ. (b) Histology slide showing SCJ. (A black and white version of this figure will appear in some formats.)

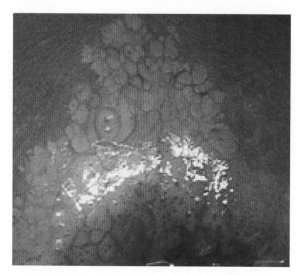

Figure 7.10 Colposcopic image showing mosaicism and punctation. (A black and white version of this figure will appear in some formats.)

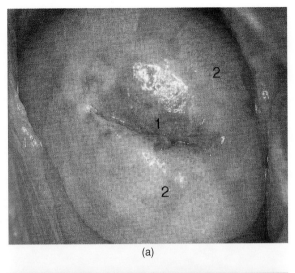

(a)

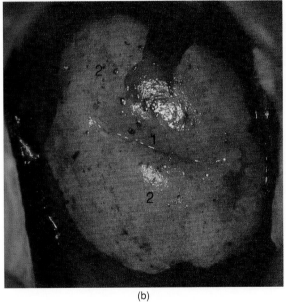

(b)

Figure 7.11 Effect of iodine on abnormal squamous tissue. (a) Before application of Shillers iodine (1: s–c junction; 2: aceto-white staining suggestive of CIN). (b) After application (1: s–c junction; 2: iodine – negative staining suggestive of CIN). (A black and white version of this figure will appear in some formats.)

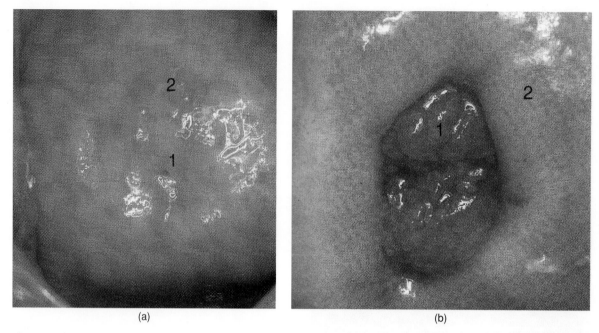

(a)   (b)

Figure 7.14 Common appearances post-LLETZ: (a) stenosis (1: cervical os; 2: transformation zone), (b) rosetting (1: columnar epithelium; 2: squamous epithelium). (A black and white version of this figure will appear in some formats.)

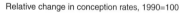

Relative change in conception rates, 1990=100

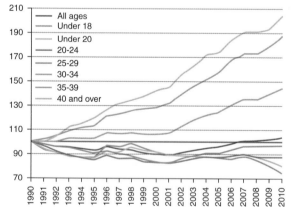

Figure 9.1 Average age of women giving birth to their first child, 1990–2010. (A black and white version of this figure will appear in some formats.)

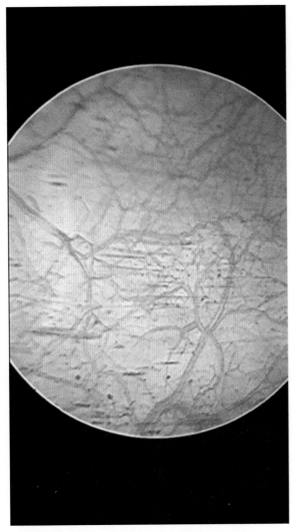

Figure 21.1 Pin point bleeding of the bladder seen during cystoscopy. (A black and white version of this figure will appear in some formats.)

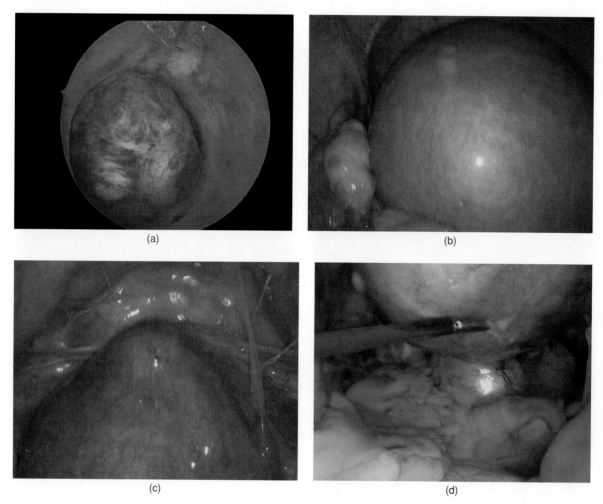

Figure 28.1 (a) Submucosal fibroid. (b) An enlarged uterus due to a large intramural fibroid. (c) Anterior wall subserosal fibroid. (d) Posterior wall pedunculated fibroid. (A black and white version of this figure will appear in some formats.)

Analysis (IOTA) Group. *Ultrasound Obstet Gynecol* 2000;16:500–505.

8. Timmermann D, Testa AC, Bourne T, *et al*. Simple ultrasound based rules for the diagnosis of ovarian cancer. *Ultrasound Obstet Gynecol* 2008;31: 681–690.

9. Sassone AM, Timor-Tritsch IE, Artner A, Westhoff C, Warren WB. Transvaginal sonographic characterization of ovarian disease: evaluation of a new scoring system to predict ovarian malignancy. *Obstet Gynecol* 1991;78:70–76.

10. Davies AP, Jacobs I, Woolas R, Fish A, Oram D, The adnexal mass: benign or malignant? Evaluation of a risk of malignancy index. *Br J Obstet Gynaecol* 1993;100:927–931.

11. American College of Obstetrics and Gynecology. Management of adnexal masses. *ACOG Bulletin* 2007;110:1.

12. Levine D, Brown DL, Andreotti RF, *et al*. Management of asymptomatic ovarian and other adnexal cysts imaged at US: Society of Radiologists in Ultrasound Consensus Conference Statement. *Radiology* 2010;256:943–954.

13. Zanetta G, Mariani E, Lissoni A, *et al*. A prospective study of the role of ultrasound in the management of adnexal masses in pregnancy. *BJOG* 2003;110:578.

14. Leiserowitz GS, Xing G, Cress R, *et al*. Adnexal masses in pregnancy: how often are they malignant? *Gynecol Oncol* 2006;101:315.

15. Grimes DA, Jones LB, Lopez LM, Schulz KF, Oral contraceptives for functional ovarian cysts. *Cochrane Database Syst Rev* 2009;(2):CD006134.

16. Bailey CL, Ueland FR, Land GL, *et al*. The malignant potential of small cystic ovarian tumors in women over 50 years of age. *Gynecol Oncol* 1998;69:3–7.

17. Aubert JM, Rombaut C, Argacha P, *et al*. Simple adnexal cysts in postmenopausal women: conservative management. *Maturitas* 1998;30:51–54.

18. National Health and Medical Research Council. Clinical practice guidelines for the management of women with epithelial ovarian cancer. CP98. NHMRC 2004.

23

Managing Menopause in Primary Care

Sarah Gray

Key Points

- Consider the possibility that loss of ovarian function could contribute to the patient presentation – listen to the patient.
- There are only limited instances where an FSH measurement can be helpful – menopause is generally a clinical diagnosis.
- Women vary greatly in the symptoms they experience – many may be satisfied with an explanation and reassurance.
- Lifestyle optimization should be discussed with all women.
- Intervention should be discussed if the woman's life is being adversely affected by menopause-related symptoms.
- Involve the patient such that she can make an informed decision.
- Hormone treatment can be considered for prevention and treatment of osteoporosis, even if symptoms are not intrusive.
- Tailor a hormone treatment regimen to the individual profile, review at three months after any change and at least annually.
- For women with premature ovarian insufficiency replace until the typical age of menopause (about 51). Beyond this use the lowest dose that is effective for as long as the benefits outweigh the risks and she wishes to continue.

Surveys of women and their health care providers have shown both groups to be confused regarding the diagnosis and management of menopause.

This chapter will:

- Revise the physiological changes at the end of the reproductive phase.

- Improve clinical confidence in the diagnosis of menopause and identification of associated symptoms.
- Outline the management options to be discussed in the primary care setting.
- Indicate how to develop an individualized management plan.
- Provide suggestions regarding further care and options for modification.

Background

The term 'menopause' is derived from the Greek language and refers to the very last menstrual bleed that a woman experiences. It is a retrospective diagnosis identified when no bleeding has occurred during a further year. This can be obscured if the bleeding response is suppressed by intrauterine or systemic hormone treatments or surgery. Symptoms relating to the reduction in hormone production can begin years before, at or after the last bleed and a significant minority of women will have none.

Physiology

This last bleed generally represents the cessation of cyclical ovarian activity. Women are born with their full complement of oocytes and these are progressively lost throughout reproductive life through programmed cell death (apoptosis). Each cycle involves recruitment and stimulation of one or more oocytes which produce oestrogen as they develop. Oestrogen levels peak at ovulation and then fall away, this becoming more marked with age. It is common for women in

Women's Health in Primary Care, edited by Anne Connolly and Amanda Britton. Published by Cambridge University Press
© Cambridge University Press 2017

their 40s to describe oestrogen deficiency symptoms at the end of their cycles and during the early menstrual phase that then resolve.

The first change that is usually noticed at the beginning of menopause transition is a shortening of the menstrual cycle. This is attributed to the increasing oocyte resistance to stimulation, higher levels of follicle-stimulating hormone (FSH) and more rapid progression when response occurs. Fertility services will check FSH early in the cycle as a marker of diminishing ovarian reserve. It cannot be used to predict when menopause might occur. Persistently raised levels suggest persistent lack of response and are consistent with, but not diagnostic of, the postmenopausal state. One measurement is not enough, repeat at least once after four to six weeks.

Progressively, oocyte resistance increases and if ovulation fails the woman will experience a longer than usual cycle length and miss a period. She may or may not experience symptoms in the gap which resolve with the next period. It is impossible to predict an individual women's experience other than to say that anything could happen.

In the phase of menstrual chaos it is important to remain alert for potential endometrial disease. Women who are obese, diabetic or have previous polycystic ovarian syndrome may be more at risk. Bleeding which is postcoital, persistent or more than a year after the last period should be investigated.

Early loss of ovarian function can occur spontaneously and if under the age of 30 significant genetic/chromosomal causes should be considered.

Age at menopause can be affected by family history, nutrition, smoking, medication (particularly chemotherapy), radiation, infection, surgery and many other factors. It is particularly important to identify premature ovarian insufficiency in order to avoid degenerative sequelae – particularly osteoporosis, but also coronary artery disease and loss of cognition. The term premature ovarian insufficiency has replaced ovarian failure as sometimes function will return.

In women, the circulating androgen level is much less than in men but is functionally important. Approximately half is derived from the ovarian stroma. Therefore surgical removal, radiotherapy, significant vascular disruption or infection affecting the ovaries can compromise androgens as well as oestrogen and some of the women affected will have symptoms as a result.

Symptoms

Typical symptoms result from sensitivity to the reduction in hormone production. This sensitivity will vary between women and is an explanation for the difference in experience. Oestrogen is pervasive, with receptors in many tissues and the potential spectrum of deficiency symptoms is broad. The reduction in progesterone produced may be seen as positive if this resolves a previous premenstrual syndrome. Androgen lack should only be considered after correction of oestrogen deficiency.

Consider the following groups of deficiency symptoms.

Centrally modulated effects of oestrogen – due to its effect on the central nervous system

- *Flushes and sweats* – these are due to over-reactivity of heat-losing mechanisms and are thought to result from a loss of temperature homeostasis (the thermoregulatory centre is located in the hypothalamus). Women will say that they feel as if their thermostat has 'packed up' and this appears to be close to the truth. After extreme sweating some women will feel cold and shiver as the response swings in the opposite direction.

  These vasomotor symptoms are the most generally recognized menopause-associated complaint, but are not universally experienced. They tend to resolve with time but this varies greatly. The typical experience is three to five years but some women continue to flush through their 60s and into their 70s with a few continuing beyond that. In trials of intervention, flush frequency and severity is used as the primary marker of efficacy.

- Sleep disturbance – Though night time sweating can disturb sleep, it is now recognized that sleep disturbance, waking for no apparent reason, is a separate phenomenon which can persist beyond the resolution of flushing. For some women this can be quite disabling.

- Mood change – A proportion of women will experience mood change. This can manifest as low mood, heightened anxiety, loss of confidence and emotional lability with a tendency to cry. Some describe themselves as irritable. Many of these women have had similar problems earlier in their lives with postnatal depression or premenstrual syndrome.

Some women who previously experienced premenstrual mood change will paradoxically feel better after menopause if intolerance of progesterone had been their main problem rather than lack of oestrogen.

- Concentration and memory problems – These are very difficult to tease out as being menopausal, as life stresses, sleeping difficulties and age-related changes will all have an effect. Word-finding difficulty is commonly recognized and may be linked as there are many oestrogen receptors in the centre for verbal memory. Difficulty concentrating and making decisions are often described by women after early surgical menopause and abrupt loss of ovarian function. There is some research linking this to an increased risk of dementia in later life.

Musculoskeletal Effects of Oestrogen

Oestrogen has many roles in the metabolism of collagen, cartilage and bone. It is well established that bone resorption increases as oestrogen is depleted. Early menopause is a significant risk for subsequent osteoporosis and fracture. Bone loss does not cause symptoms until fracture occurs. Some women do experience quite separately, otherwise unexplained aches and pains which resolve with oestrogen replacement.

Urogenital Effects of Oestrogen

Oestrogen exerts a trophic influence on the tissues of the vagina and lower urinary tract. With depletion comes progressive atrophic change that results in thinning, loss of elasticity and vaginal dryness, which affects almost 50% of women by three years after the last period. There may be itching (often misinterpreted as fungal infection), soreness and difficulty with intercourse, tight clothes or even walking. Urinary symptoms include urgency, frequency, nocturia, cystitis and an increased likelihood of infection. Surveys have shown these symptoms to be under-reported. It is important to determine if and how much of a problem they are as this factor will significantly affect management decisions.

Testosterone-Deficiency Symptoms

Women who have had a significant ovarian insult, are adequately replaced with oestrogen and continue to have problems with myalgia, lethargy and loss of sexual interest that is otherwise unexplained may have an associated testosterone deficiency.

Clinical Pathway (Figure 23.1)

Presentation

A proportion of women will present directly, identify that their problem is menopause and ask to discuss. This has reduced since the Women's Health Initiative (WHI) study first published in 2002 and the Million Women Study (MWS) in 2003. The findings of both studies were reported in a manner which created misunderstanding and fear which has persisted. In the clinical setting menopause is more often presented indirectly. You may have to explore the presentation, integrate the information provided and then arrive at this conclusion.

Consider the following general practice scenario.

Case Scenario

Linda is 52. She does not come to the surgery often and there is nothing of particular note in her medical summary. She is concerned as she has always been very calm and organized but recently has become irritable and struggles to cope with previously minor challenges. This is a problem as she teaches at a local secondary school and the youngsters exploit any perceived weakness. She feels that this is worse because she is not sleeping and asks for some sleeping tablets.

Do not simply take this at face value and assume that it is a mental health issue. The simplest way to begin to unravel the problem is to ask about her periods.

She tells you that her last period was six months ago and the previous one was three months before that.

This is enough information to indicate that she is perimenopausal. It allows you to explore further. As flushing and sweating are the most common problems, ask about these.

She gets very hot at night and so wet that she has to get out and change her nightclothes most nights, she is then cold and shivery so gets back in and often finds it difficult to get back to sleep. She has a few daytime flushes, but manages by wearing layers of clothes and takes her cardigan on and off.

You now know that she is missing periods and she is troubled by the most typical of menopausal symptoms. At this point you can make a clinical

---

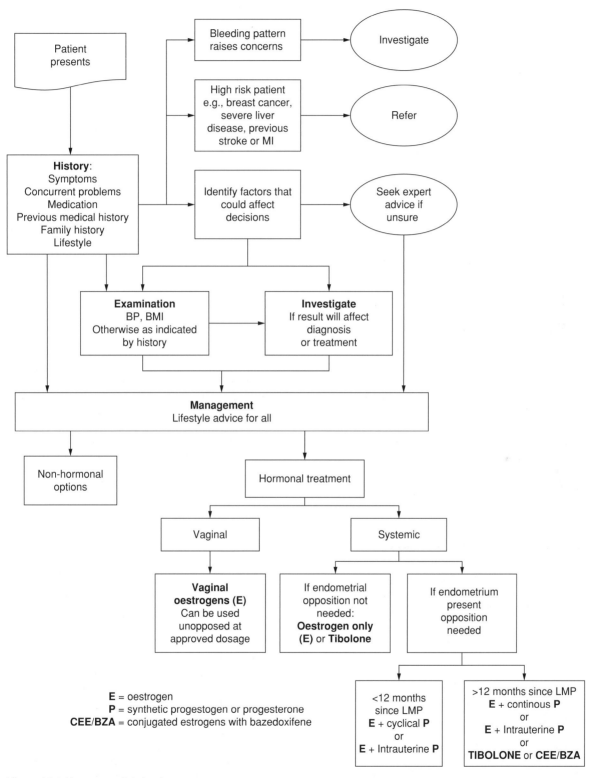

Figure 23.1 Menopause clinical pathway.

diagnosis, she does not need any further biochemical tests.

Linda has come to discuss her sleeping difficulties so return to that issue and ask if her problem is going to sleep or staying asleep. If she is waking, ask if she can tell why and is it because of the sweating.

She tells you that going to sleep is not the problem, but that she wakes three or four times in the night starting at 01:30. Sometimes it is because she is hot but mostly she wakes up and then sweats. It can be difficult to get back to sleep and that is why she is so tired.

Linda is grateful that you have listened and taken some interest. You can reflect that you think that her hormones may have a role in this and would like to ask some more questions. If you have built sufficient rapport and use appropriate language (but not the vernacular) it will not be difficult to ask about the next most common issues of menopause – urogenital atrophy and sexual function.

Linda tells you that she does have some vaginal dryness and it is uncomfortable to have sex, but she is really not interested and would rather go to bed with a cup of hot milk and a good book to help her to get to sleep. This is causing some tension at home which is not helped by her lack of patience and tendency to snap at her husband.

From the above it can be seen that being alert to the issue and asking a few carefully chosen questions can unravel the problem quite simply. You can appreciate that there are many aspects of her life that are currently more difficult and coping is a problem. The next stage is to explain why it is happening and outline her options. Reassure her that resignation from work does not need to be considered. You have no information so far that raises any concerns or requires any physical examination or investigation.

There are a variety of NHS and other organizations providing accredited information and support and the patient can be signposted to these. In most primary care settings consultation time is limited. It will be helpful for the patient to read about and consider her options and then return if she wishes to discuss how they might apply to her. Many women will not be so affected as Linda above and will be satisfied to understand why their symptoms are happening and reassured that there is no more sinister explanation. Others may choose not to pursue a medical route.

Managing Menopausal Symptoms

Menopause is a biological marker and an ideal opportunity to take stock of health issues and consider cardiovascular, bone and cancer risk profiles. Where there are concerns, the relevant risk assessment tools (QRisk2, FRAX or Qfracture, etc.) can be used to inform your discussion.

Whether or not the concept of hormone treatment is accepted, all women should benefit from lifestyle advice. This should include increasing exercise, stopping smoking, reduction in weight, moderation in caffeine and alcohol consumption. These changes will optimize ongoing health and may mitigate symptoms (though evidence for the latter can be conflicting).

Women may choose to manage their difficulties with techniques such as mindfulness, CBT, acupuncture or relaxation therapy though there is no established evidence that they specifically help individual symptoms.

There is some evidence that isoflavones (botanicals with some oestrogenic properties) and black cohosh may relieve flushing in the short term, but their safety profile is unclear and longer-term trials have not shown benefit. They are not available on prescription in the UK. Should they wish to try these women should be advised to choose a quality accredited standardized brand.

Research has shown that other therapeutic options can address some, but not all of the symptoms of menopause:

- Serotonin reuptake inhibitors (SSRIs) and serotonin and norepinephrine reuptake inhibitors (SNRIs) can ease the symptoms of flushing at lower dosage ranges. They are not as effective as oestrogen and may exacerbate flushing at high dose. The side-effect profile includes loss of sexual interest and anorgasmia, and this should be taken into consideration. They are not licensed in the UK for this indication and are not recommended as a first-line option.
- Gabapentin has been shown to reduce flushing at moderate dose, but is not licensed and not recommended first-line.
- Vaginal moisturizers and lubricants can help vaginal dryness and sexual difficulty and can be recommended. Some are available on prescription in the UK.

The content, efficacy and safety of compounded hormones (promoted as 'bioidentical') are unknown and they are not recommended.

Most menopausal symptoms are attributable to oestrogen deficiency. Many systematic reviews have confirmed that hormone therapy remains the most effective and holistic therapeutic option where symptoms have sufficient impact to require intervention. It should be considered for women with early loss of ovarian function for bone protection.

Women should be provided with up-to-date and evidence-based information regarding what is known and what is not known, to allow them to form an opinion about whether this is a course of action they wish to try. Guidance published by the National Institute for Health and Care Excellence (NICE NG23 November 2015) can be used as a reference.

Choosing an HRT Regimen

Determine

- Where is she in the menopause transition?
- What symptoms does she complain of?
- What is her main problem?
- What are her concerns?
- What is her risk profile? – consider
  - Lifestyle
  - Gynaecological factors
  - Cardiovascular factors
  - Breast factors
  - Musculoskeletal factors
  - Metabolic factors
  - Mental health

Consider the example of Linda given earlier. When she returns it is possible to determine very quickly the following:

Decision-Making

- Consider if vaginal (local) oestrogen alone may be adequate.
- If a systemic regimen is needed:
  - Choose an oestrogen, route of administration and dose
  - Add progestin if endometrial tissue is present to suppress proliferation
    - Cyclical for predictable bleeding
    - Continuous once postmenopausal.

For Linda we have no information that would point to an indication for a bespoke combination and a ready-formulated first-line cyclical combination would be reasonable. She has had a period within the last year so is not postmenopausal and would potentially bleed if prescribed a continuous preparation. This could lead to unnecessary anxiety and investigation. Two distinct advantages of a cyclical regimen are that any bleeding should be predictable and that assessment of response to the two different hormones involved is facilitated.

Consider starting at the lower end of the effective dose range (e.g. 2 mg oral oestradiol for young women and 1 mg for those at typical menopausal age), and allow three months before reassessment and potential increase.

Choosing Components (Figures 23.2 and 23.3)

Prescribers are advised to develop a simple and logical list of familiar preparations which allow:

- Change in oestrogen dose
- Progression from cyclical to continuous to low dose with the same combination of hormones

Information	Relevance
Para 2 some postnatal depression	She has previously had a hormone-related effect on mood – and to have a mood effect at menopause would not be unusual
Previously used condoms, but husband had a vasectomy 10 years ago Periods never a problem before No bleeding between periods now	Contraception is not needed (guidance is to allow a year after the last period in women over 50) No gynaecology issues No information about previous hormone intolerance
No personal or family history of breast problems	No raised background risks or anxieties
Mother has had a recent hip fracture age 81 and has thoracic kyphosis	Parental history of hip fracture approximately doubles risk and there is a concern to avoid this. Consider using a risk calculator
BP 132/80 – never smoked – BMI 26.5–not diabetic – 10 units alcohol/week	In primary care these are usually recorded, but check that information is up to date to provide a current cardiovascular risk profile This would not represent a higher risk
No other medication	No interaction to be considered

Types		Comment
Oral oestrogens		Familiar Easy to take Inexpensive *But:* Potential to interact via first-pass effects in the liver and affect: • Thrombotic pathways • Concomitant medication • Other hormone treatment via SHBG induction • Gall bladder physiology Potential for direct gastrointestinal side effects
Conjugated equine oestrogens (CEE)		Mixture of oestrogens derived from the urine of pregnant mares. Products used for > 60 years and in many of the trials
Oestradiol valerate (E2Val)		Oestradiol that is esterified to allow absorption rather than digestion
17β-Oestradiol (E2)		Oestradiol that is micronized to allow absorption rather than digestion (1 mg~1.2 mg E2Val)
Non-oral oestrogens		Minimize hepatic and gut effects, limit drug interaction and preferred in higher cardiovascular risk women
Gel	17β-oestradiol (E2) – 0.06% pump provides 0.75 mg/dose 0.1% sachets provide 0.5 mg or 1 mg options	Applied to clean dry skin of upper arm or thigh daily Early peak in serum levels then trough from reservoir in fat tissue
Patch	All 17β-oestradiol (E2)	Applied to clean dry skin below the waist and changed weekly or twice weekly Some differences in adhesive and dose ranges between brands, but all use matrix technology providing reasonably consistent release
Implant	17β-oestradiol (E2) in oily crystalline matrix 25 mg 50 mg	Implanted into fat tissue No licensed product in the UK; may be available in specialist clinic
Vaginal ring	17β-oestradiol (E2) 7.5 mcg/day	Retained for 12 weeks and then replaced Only currently available product releases very low dose and is licensed for atrophic vaginitis – not effective for systemic symptoms – opposition not needed
Vaginal tablets	17β-oestradiol (E2) 10 mcg	Used daily initially then twice a week (licensed) – more frequent use out of license but consistent with previous 25 mcg product Very low dose – licensed for atrophic vaginitis – not effective for systemic symptoms – opposition not needed
Vaginal cream	Oestriol 0.1% – delivers 1 mg/dose 0.01% – delivers 500 mcg/dose	Used daily initially then twice a week Very low dose – licensed for atrophic vaginitis – not effective for systemic symptoms – opposition not needed
Progestogens		Required to prevent hyperplasia and malignant change in endometrial tissue
Testosterone derivatives	Norethisterone	Available in form of progesterone-only contraceptive pills and as a component of many oral proprietary regimens in both continuous and cyclical forms Can be absorbed through skin and used in some combination patches
	Levonorgestrel and norgestrel	Available in form of progesterone-only pills and as a component of limited number of oral proprietary regimens Can be absorbed through skin and used in some combination patches Delivery via an intrauterine system highly effective with limited systemic impact
Progesterone derivatives	Dydrogesterone	Available in one range of fixed dose oral combinations
	Progesterone	Available as: • Micronized oral capsules (licensed) • Micronized vaginal capsules (unlicensed) • Pessaries/suppositories (unlicensed)
	Medroxyprogesterone acetate	Available as oral tablets and as a component of limited number of oral proprietary regimens

(Cont.)

Types		Comment
Mineralocorticoid derivative	Drospirenone	Available in one fixed dose continuous combination
Selective oestrogen receptor modulator (SERM)	CEE/Bazedoxifene	New continuous combination using a 3rd generation SERM to oppose the endometrial effects of 0.45 mgs combined equine estrogen
Testosterone		For relief of androgen deficiency symptoms, particularly low libido
Gel	1% testosterone tubes or sachets	Not licensed for women but may be used fractionated into tiny doses – specialist practice initiated
	2% testosterone pump	Not licensed for women and bolus dose too high for most women
Implants	100 mg in oily crystalline matrix	Only used in specialist practice – dose too high for most women
Gonadomimetic	Tibolone 25 mg tablets	Steroidal pro-drug metabolized to active metabolites with oestrogenic, androgenic and progestogenic activity. Limited breast and endometrial activity, not prothrombotic Consider for postmenopausal women with low libido

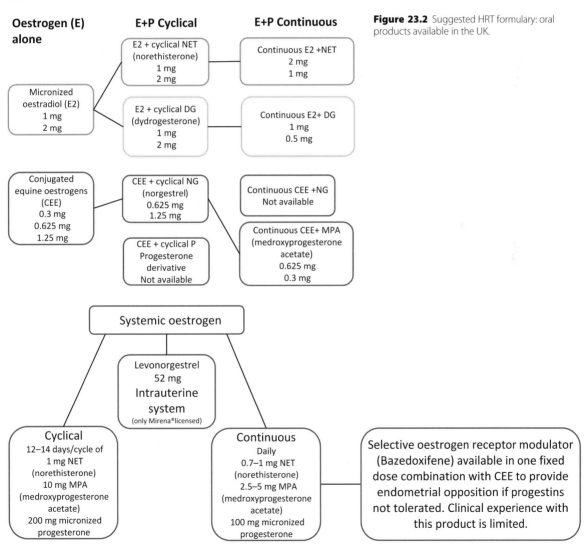

Figure 23.2 Suggested HRT formulary: oral products available in the UK.

Figure 23.3 Bespoke regimens: progestogenic opposition options.

- Change in progestogen if intolerance is an issue
- Change in delivery if oral route is an issue.

Linda could very reasonably be prescribed three cycles of a low-dose cyclical oral combination containing oestradiol 1 mg with norethisterone 1 mg for 12 days. There are no clues or risks that would suggest this to be unsuitable. It is important to ensure that the relevant risk and benefit advice is explained and that she should expect it to take six to eight weeks to achieve full benefit. Advise her to monitor when she bleeds and if any unexpected change occurs note where in the pack she is.

Counselling

Vaginal Products

Vaginal oestrogen products are highly effective for urogenital atrophy and can be used alone or in conjunction with systemic therapy.

Vaginal oestrogen products used in accordance with manufacturer's advice have not been shown to affect systemic risks due to the very low dose used. However, patient information leaflets are required to include all cautions for systemic oestrogen without making this distinction.

Seek expert advice regarding use of all hormone containing products in women with breast cancer. This includes the low-dose vaginal oestrogen products, though their use may not be precluded.

Vaginal moisturizers and lubricants can be used by all women, including those with breast cancer and women already using oestrogen-containing products.

Cardiovascular Risk

This is most easy to explain in three parts. It is important to evaluate the background risk of the woman in each area in order to overlay any effect of hormone therapy.

- *Coronary artery disease*: For women starting HRT up to 10 years after typical menopause there is little or no increase in the risk of coronary artery disease and younger women may be offered protection. There is no increased risk of death. If existing risks are managed this does not exclude the choice to use HRT.
- *Stroke*: Oral oestrogen may have a small effect to increase stroke risk, but this is not significant for up to 10 years after typical menopause. Most

women at this age have a low baseline risk. Standard doses of non-oral oestrogens have not shown an increase and are preferred if the patient has a higher risk profile.

- *Venous thromboembolism*: Oral oestrogens have been shown to increase risks of deep vein thrombosis (DVT) and pulmonary embolism (PE). Standard doses of non-oral oestrogens have not shown this effect and are preferred if the patient has a higher risk profile.

Breast Disease

Benign breast disease may remain uncomfortable if taking HRT, but this is not a risk for malignant transformation.

HRT is believed to act as a growth promoter of pre-existing breast cancer and its effect is lost after stopping. Oestrogen alone is associated with little or no increase in breast cancer diagnosis. Oestrogen with progesterone is associated with an increase in diagnosis after about five years of exposure. The size of this effect is small and of similar magnitude to that associated with regular alcohol consumption or having a BMI of 30.

HRT is not associated with a higher chance of dying from breast cancer.

Musculoskeletal Problems

The risk of fracture is reduced while taking HRT. This effect increases with time. While some effect is lost after stopping, a difference can persist for many years. There is some evidence that HRT may improve muscle mass and strength.

Diabetes

HRT does not adversely affect blood sugar control or increase the risk of a diagnosis of Type II diabetes.

Dementia

We do not know enough about the effects of HRT on dementia to be able to advise.

Review and Modification

Encourage your patient to return before the end of three months for review. Consider:

- Relief of original symptoms
- Onset of new symptoms (and when this is)
- Bleeding
- Any change in risk profile.

To return to Linda: after 11 weeks she says that:

- *Sleeping has improved, but is better in the first two weeks of the pack.*
- *She is generally not as good and the tearfulness returns when the pills change colour.*
- *Bleeding is fine: starting two to three days into the new pack and much like it was before.*
- *Really grateful and agrees that she is better, but thinks that more is possible and would like further improvement.*

In this case you can make two deductions

1. That the low oestrogen dose is not enough and the standard 2 mg dose is needed.
2. That the progestogen is counteracting the benefit of the oestrogen on mood. This tends to be a class effect so change class.

Looking back to Figure 23.2, you see there is a ready-made combination with the same oestrogen, but at a higher dose and an alternative progestogen. Linda is prescribed oestradiol 2 mg with 10 mg dydrogesterone in the second phase.

Three months further on Linda comes back in with a big smile and says '*thank you so much – you have given me my life back*'. This is one of the few areas in medicine where you really can make a difference. It is, however, important to be realistic and reading a good book at bedtime may persist if there are other relationship issues.

Problem-Solving Suggestions

- Persistence/reappearance of flushing
  - Increase oestrogen
  - Consider change to non-oral regime
- Breast tenderness
  - Often settles in four to six weeks
  - Reduce oestrogen and increase very slowly
  - Try a non-oral oestrogen
  - Change progestogen class or consider LNG-IUS
  - Consider tibolone
- Premenstrual syndrome
  - Change class of progestogen
  - Change route of progestogen – consider LNG-IUS
  - Increase oestrogen
- Bleeding too early in cyclical regime
  - Increase progestogen dose
  - Change progestogen class

- Investigate if previously bled to schedule
- Bleeding after starting a continuous combined regime
  - Allow three to six months to settle initially
  - Reduce oestrogen
  - Increase progestogen
  - Consider IUS
  - Try Tibolone
  - Revert to cyclical regime
- Unscheduled bleeding with any regime
  - May reflect endogenous hormone release, but should be investigated if previously settled for the last six months – it may be a sign of structural or histological abnormality.

Stopping

There is little evidence regarding the best way to stop HRT and most experts reduce gradually. If symptoms return then these have not been deferred merely masked and it may be that an informed decision is made to continue for longer at the lowest effective dose. In the longer term it makes no difference whether stopped gradually or abruptly.

Further Reading

NICE. Menopause: Diagnosis and management. NG23 www.nice.org.uk/guidance/NG23 (accessed September 2016).

Boardman H, Hartley L, Eisinga A, *et al*. Hormone therapy for preventing cardiovascular disease in post-menopausal women. *Cochrane Database Syst Rev* 2015;(3):CD002229.

FSRH Clinical Effectiveness Unit. Contraception for women aged over 40 years (July 2010). www.fsrh.org/pdfs/ContraceptionOver40July10.pdf (accessed September 2016).

Qfracture: 10 year fracture risk. www.qfracture.org (accessed September 2016).

FRAX: 10 year fracture risk and guide to intervention (UK). www.shef.ac.uk/FRAX/tool.aspx?country=1 (accessed September 2016).

Qrisk: cardiovascular risk calculator. www.qrisk.org/ (accessed September 2016).

The International Menopause Society provides the international consensus and has a range of educational materials – some generally available. www.imsociety.org (accessed September 2016).

The British Menopause Society. www.thebms.org.uk/ (accessed September 2016).

Menopause matters provides information and support to women and health care professionals. www.menopausematters.co.uk/ (accessed September 2016).

Vulval Dermatoses in Primary Care

Susan Towers and Kate London

Key Points

- It is important to proactively ask about vulval symptoms in a woman with a generalized skin condition such as eczema or psoriasis as she may be too embarrassed to complain about the problems she is experiencing.
- The principles of management of a vulval skin problem are the same as many skin conditions; with irritant avoidance, repair of skin function and reduction of inflammation.
- Emollients require regular use so decanting some into a small, easy to carry pot is useful for frequent application.
- Using small amounts of high potency steroid are important to reduce inflammation and the consequences of persistent vulval scratching.
- Women find different emollient and steroid preparations more acceptable and may need support and understanding to find the most appropriate for them to use.
- Women with vulval problems are often embarrassed and feel stigmatized. They may experience significant emotional distress, which requires careful assessment and possible referral for psychological support.
- Signposting women to useful web resources may help them understand the importance of self-management and improve compliance with their treatment regimen.
- Women with lichen planus need to be aware of the small increased risk of developing vulval intraepithelial neoplasia. This may present as an unresolving vulval lump, ulceration or change in skin appearance and requires an early medical review.

Introduction

Vulval skin conditions may not be revealed by patients to health professionals due to a number of factors, including:

- Embarrassment
- Not knowing who to talk to
- Physical pain
- Fear of being stigmatized
- Previous misdiagnoses or treatment failure.

The British Association of Dermatology (BAD) Vulval Health Survey 2015 revealed that one in five women had experienced thoughts of self-harm as a result of their vulval condition [1].

Comments recorded include:

'*I feel broken, hopeless and often at times less of a woman*'
'*disgusted with my own body*'
'*like a freak*'
'*going out was difficult and I couldn't talk to anyone about my symptoms in detail*'.

However, treatment of some of the most common vulval conditions, though not curative, can make a significant difference to quality of life and alleviate the significant emotional distress experienced by these women.

History-Taking

A good history is paramount in making a correct diagnosis and in effective management. Stopping the patient from doing some things can be just as important to a successful outcome as active treatment.

Women's Health in Primary Care, edited by Anne Connolly and Amanda Britton. Published by Cambridge University Press
© Cambridge University Press 2017

Important points to cover include:

- Her symptoms: including any itching, burning, pain. Or she may have no symptoms, but a partner has noticed discolouration of the vulva.
- Which site is affected: including always asking about other sites, e.g. scalp, elbows, knees, nails and mouth.
- The duration of symptoms: which should also include her perception of cause of onset. This may be an important clue, e.g. a topical allergen, or an important misconception, e.g. food allergy, not being clean, excessive washing after a 'one night stand'.
- Any aggravating and relieving factors: previous treatment success or failure.
- Does she have any urinary and bowel symptoms: in particular incontinence and measures to cope with those issues, e.g. use of pads, deodorizers.
- Has she or any of her family members had any history of skin problems.
- Does she have any other medical problems, e.g. diabetes, auto-immune conditions or thyroid disease.
- What are her washing habits/grooming: use of soap, sponges, hair removal, douches, liners and pads, clothing.
- Does she have any hobbies which might aggravate a vulval problem: wearing tight lycra for exercising, cycling, horse riding.

Examination

As the vulva is modified skin it is important to check the whole skin surface, including the oral mucosa, as particular sites may provide significant clues to help diagnose the problem.

The scalp, elbows and knees may reveal typical rough scaly plaques and the natal cleft and axilla may show flexural disease, which is red, shiny and well demarcated. These findings may confirm a diagnosis of psoriasis.

Nail changes can be present and suggestive of eczema, psoriasis or lichen planus.

Examination of the skin of the wrists, sacrum and ankles may reveal the shiny flat topped purplish papules of lichen planus. Additional findings

may include eroded areas on the buccal mucosa (lacy appearance) or gingivitis.

Vulval examination may demonstrate findings including:

- Erythema which may be:
  - Diffuse or well demarcated
  - Dusky or bright red
  - Flexural creases may be spared or affected
- Lichenification which is suggestive of chronic scratching from irritation
- Specific patches or generalized pigmentation or depigmentation

On parting the labia majora you may see:

- Depigmentation suggesting vitiligo or pallor suggestive of lichen sclerosus.

Or architectural change such as:

- Loss of the labia minora, fusion of the clitoral hood or midline fusion, which may be secondary to disease or female genital mutilation (FGM)
- Scarring secondary to ulceration or trauma
- The introitus may show changes of redness or erosion
- The perianal skin must also be examined for skin changes by turning the woman into the left lateral examination position.

Following this careful history and examination a diagnosis should be made if possible and may be due to:

- Lichen sclerosus
- Lichen planus
- Eczema; consider atopic, irritant, seborrhoeic
- Psoriasis
- Intertrigo.

Management

In medicine it is unusual for 'always' and 'never' to apply; however, in the management of vulval conditions these may be appropriate and include the following recommendations:

- *Always* stop irritants
- *Always* restore the skin barrier function
- Suppress inflammatory response where indicated.

Irritant Avoidance

Box 24.1 Irritants

Some of the most common irritants include:

- Washing with soap ± the sponge, loofah, flannel (cosmetic soaps and shower gels are all detergents – like washing up liquid!)
- Baby wipes
- Cosmetic bath additives
- Excessive frequency/duration of washing
- Vigorous drying
- Topical anti-itching remedies

Patients think what they are using to wash with and how they are doing it are normal. It is important to be very specific in understanding the washing/hygiene procedures for that particular patient in detail.

'What exactly do you use to wash with?'

'How long do you bath/shower/wash for?'

'How often do you shower or bath and how hot is the water?'

'Then what do you do?'

Avoidance of tight-fitting clothes of synthetic material should also be avoided if possible, e.g. tight layers of Lycra, thongs, etc.

Restoring Barrier Function

Having identified the potential causes of loss of the skin's barrier function, the patient needs a new regime to restore it.

Emollients are important to restore the barrier function of the skin by improving the water-resistant lipid lamellae encasing the corneocytes (bricks). The corneocytes are held together by corneodesmosomes (cement), which are dependent on a balance of proteases to remain intact.

This important barrier function can be destroyed by environmental factors, such as soap and other detergents, which enhance protease activity. This causes the corneodesmosomes to break and inhibits lipid lamellae synthesis and subsequent 'brick' shrinkage. In this way there is increased water loss from the skin allowing for increased ingress of irritants and allergens producing a vicious cycle of skin barrier breakdown.

An emollient should be used as a soap substitute. The woman needs to be advised that this will not foam up as it is not a detergent. Nor will this leave the skin feeling 'squeaky clean' because it is leaving the natural barrier of the skin intact; but the skin will still be clean.

Clear instructions should be given on how to use emollients as a soap substitute. A 50p size amount of emollient should be placed in the palm of the hand and applied to the vulva as she would with a soap and then rinsed off. The water used should not be too hot or too cold. After bathing she should "pat" the vulva dry with a soft towel and apply emollient again directly to the area which should then be left. Emollients can be used liberally (in contrast to topical steroid) and should be applied several times a day, possibly also putting some on the toilet paper before wiping.

The choice of emollient will be the one that the patient prefers, however Diprobase cream is commonly recommended as this is tolerated well by most women. Further advice about choosing an emollient can be found in Box 24.2.

Tip: Recommend a prepaid prescription to your patient. Ideally several small quantities of different emollients can then be issued for the patient to choose from.

The use of the emollient as above is essential for the management of vulval disease. Bath additives or shower gels such as balneum, oilatum, etc. can be used in addition, but not instead of the above.

An important exception to the 'emollient rule' is that aqueous cream has never been licensed to leave on as a moisturizer, as it contains sodium lauryl sulfate which can have a detrimental effect on the skin pH and may aggravate the condition.

Box 24.2 Choosing an Emollient

Things to consider in choosing an emollient:

- Creams work better than emollients as soap substitutes and are often more acceptable to patients.
- Emollients work in different ways, some are occlusive (prevent water loss from the skin) and others draw water up into the stratum corneum and some do both.
- Creams need preservatives which can themselves be irritant, ointments less so.
- You can refer to the 'emollient ladder' [2] to assist in your choice of emollient with a patient.

Box 24.3 Emollient Choices

- Greasy
  - Hydromol ointment
  - Epaderm ointment
  - Diprobase ointment
  - Cetraben ointment
- Rich cream
  - Unguentum M
  - Doublebase gel
  - Dermamist spray
  - Doublebase dayleve gel
  - Neutrogena dermatological cream
- Creamy
  - Diprobase cream
  - Cetraben cream
  - Oilatum cream
  - E45 cream
  - Aveeno cream
  - Dermol 500 cream
- Urea-containing creams
  - Aquadrate
  - Calmurid
  - Eucerin
  - Balneum Plus
  - E45 Itch Relief
- Light
  - Aveeno lotion
  - Keri lotion
  - Dermol 500 lotion
  - Eucerin lotion (urea containing)

Suppress Inflammation (Disease Control)

The next issue for management is to suppress any inflammatory process. This is likely to require the use of a topical steroid preparation regularly or intermittently, depending on the condition.

Steroid and emollient application should be separated by about 30 minutes to avoid 'dilution'. Patients are very keen to know whether to use their emollient or steroid first. Dermatologists disagree on which should be used first however *the* most important point is that *both* are used, never steroid alone.

Cream or ointment formulations of most steroids are available and the steroid ladder (Box 24.4) can clarify the preparations in order of potency. The potency required will depend on the condition and the patient. An ointment rather than a cream is a preferred option as this contains fewer preservatives and stabilizers and is therefore less likely to cause a contact allergy.

The Finger Tip Unit (FTU) is a helpful guide to the quantity of topical steroid to use. One FTU is the length of cream squeezed from a tube which spreads from the distal fold on the index finger to the tip and is about 0.5 g. One FTU can treat an area equivalent to the area of both palms.

Who to Refer

Referral is important for:

- Those with unusual presentations: 'It just doesn't look right'

Box 24.4 An Example of a Steroid Ladder

Potency	Active ingredient	Trade name
Very potent	Clobetasol propionate 0.05%	Dermovate
	Diflucortolone valerate 0.3%	Nerisone Forte
Potent	Betamethasone (as valerate) 0.1%	Betnovate
	Mometasone furoate 0.1%	Elocon
	Fluocinolone acetonide 0.025%	Synalar
	Hydrocortisone butyrate 0.1%	Locoid
	Diflucortolone valerate 0.1%	Nerisone
	Betamethasone (as dipropionate) 0.05% with salicylic acid 3%	Diprosalic
Moderate potency	Clobetasone butyrate 0.05%	Eumovate
	Betamethasone (as valerate) 0.025%	Betnovate RD
	Fluocinolone acetonide 0.00625%	Synalar 1 in 4
Mild potency	Hydrocortisone 1%	Hydrocortisone 1%
	Hydrocortisone 1% + clotrimazole 1%	Canesten HC
	Hydrocortisone 1% + miconazole nitrate 2%	Daktacort
	Hydrocortisone 0.5% + nystatin 100,000 u/gm + chlorhexidine 1%	Nystaform HC

- Those failing to respond to treatment, having checked compliance with treatment
- Diagnostic uncertainty
- Persistent lesions, e.g. thickened white areas, ulceration.

Putting the Theory Into Practice with Our Cases

Case Scenario 1

Hayley aged 27 comes to surgery angry and upset because of her psoriasis. She feels she gets 'fobbed off' with different creams which don't work and she hasn't been clear for at least seven years. Your careful history-taking and empathetic approach reveal that Hayley has plaque psoriasis affecting her elbows and knees, but she also has genital psoriasis, which is particularly embarrassing for her with her partner.

Hayley is unlikely to admit that she has genital psoriasis unless specifically asked. Women experience a lot of very negative feelings about themselves which make it hard for them to be open about genital problems and we must ask specifically at times.

Genital psoriasis is thought to affect between 3 and 7% [2] of patients with psoriasis, however the true prevalence is unknown.

Hayley hasn't been using any treatment in the genital area as she is 'frightened' and does not know what ointments she can use for this problem. In fact she isn't too bothered by the elbows and knees, but the genital psoriasis is causing her difficulty with sex because she is embarrassed and the condoms are making her sore. She is also finding the itching embarrassing if she needs to scratch when she is in a public setting.

Confirming the diagnosis is not difficult in this case. Hayley has classic changes of psoriasis on the other typical sites and the redness in the vulva is well demarcated and shiny, as expected. The vagina is not involved and the labial structures look normal. Examining the natal cleft you see the typical splits seen in genital psoriasis. Unlike other affected body sites, the genital area and flexures are not generally scaly due to the hydrating effect of the skin folds.

Hayley is currently washing with water alone. She uses Dovobet on her elbows and knees, but nothing else in the genital area.

Management

Hayley should be advised to use an emollient, e.g. Diprobase, and instructed how to use this as a soap substitute as well as a 'leave on' emollient, explaining why this is important.

For management of the inflammation from psoriasis a moderately potent topical steroid ointment should be applied once daily in the morning. Eumovate is suitable or one of the vitamin D analogues such as Curatoderm or Silkis at night.

Dovonex and Dovobet are not suitable for genital psoriasis due to the irritant effect of Dovonex and the potency of the topical steroid.

Using condoms may have aggravated the psoriasis due to a Koebner effect from trauma, therefore advice about use of a suitable lubricant may be helpful. It is important to also advise Hayley that condoms are not ideal for her as topical preparations have the potential to affect the integrity of the condom if they are oil-based and have been applied just before sex.

Case Scenario 2

Rita, a 58-year-old lady, comes in to morning surgery. She doesn't want to take up too much of your time as she can see you are as busy as usual, but she has thrush again and would like some more Canesten HC cream, which seemed to help last time.

Looking through her records you see she has had a diagnosis of 'thrush' made on three occasions in the past eight months, but you cannot see any details of examination findings.

Taking a history from Rita you find that she does not have a discharge and Canesten HC eases the symptoms a little while she is using it, but the vulval irritation returns when she finished the course of treatment. She is very careful about keeping clean, but has stopped using soap as it seemed to make the 'thrush' worse. Her last period was about eight years ago and she did not have much trouble with menopausal symptoms.

Rita is embarrassed about being examined, but this is essential as the problem is recurring and the examination findings will help determine the diagnosis and organize correct management.

Vaginal candidiasis is uncommon in post-menopausal women, though studies have shown that of the third who still suffer, those patients may have a more vigorous and resistant form of the condition [3].

On examination you find changes consistent with lichen sclerosus. The vulva appears red and there is shrinkage of the labia minora bilaterally and some pallor consistent with lichen sclerosus.

Management

It is important to review anything that may be irritating the problem that Rita has by making sure that she is not using any soaps or detergents that could be reducing her skin barrier function.

It is also important that she understands that her problem is not due to 'thrush' but due to the changes that you have found.

Rita should be advised about 'soap avoidance' and commenced on a regime to restore the skin barrier function by using an emollient as a soap substitute and as a 'leave on' emollient.

Lichen sclerosus requires a very potent topical steroid such as Dermovate (clobetasol 0.5%) or Nerisone Forte. She needs to use this on a daily basis for up to four weeks until itching is controlled, followed by a weaning down period, e.g. alternate day use followed by maintenance of possibly once or twice a week. She should use the FTU as a guide to the amount of steroid cream needed.

A review appointment should be made for two to three weeks after treatment is started to assess the response and compliance with treatment. It is important to advise that it is essential to control the itching she has to prevent the inflammatory process from damaging the vulval structures.

There is also a small increased risk of developing vulval intraepithelial neoplasia (VIN) with lichen sclerosis. Compliance with treatment may be improved if she is made aware that she has a 5% risk of developing vulval carcinoma, which is reduced if the lichen sclerosus is well controlled. Rita should be warned that if she notices any changes to the vulval skin which do not resolve, such as white patches, lumps or ulceration, she needs a medical review. Otherwise yearly examination by a doctor is advised.

Case Scenario 3

Mary is aged 74. She walks awkwardly into your clinic room and sits down carefully. She is clearly in discomfort and on questioning informs you that for the past four months she has been very sore 'down there' and occasionally has to scratch. Any embarrassment is overcome by the fact that this soreness is 'unbearable'. She has tried Canesten, Sudocrem and Vagisil, all to no avail.

Mary's previous medical history reveals IHD and Bowen's disease of the lower leg.

She is washing with water alone now and cannot bear any intimate contact with her husband due to the soreness of her vulva.

She agrees to examination reluctantly as she knows this will be painful. Examination reveals a well-defined, red, angry erosion which extends into the vagina and appears to have caused some resorption of the right labia minora. The findings are consistent with those of lichen planus. She had no other signs on her body, however a check of the oral mucosa is necessary as oral lichen planus is present in 30–70% of those with lichen planus elsewhere.

The treatment for lichen planus follows the same lines as for lichen sclerosus, with irritant avoidance, emollient use and potent steroids.

Conclusion

Vulval conditions cause embarrassment, debilitating physical symptoms and emotional upset to women. In the majority of cases relatively simple irritant avoidance and restoration of barrier function will make life much more comfortable. It is important that women can feel able to talk about their bodies without fear of stigma.

Examination of women who complain of vulval symptoms is important, particularly if the problem is recurrent. Women who have a chronic skin disease, such as psoriasis and eczema, may not report the symptoms unless specifically asked and if they admit to or present with vulval problems, examination is essential.

The principles of irritant avoidance and restoration of barrier function are applicable across a wide range of vulval conditions, similar to the advice necessary to improve other skin conditions routinely managed in primary care.

The British Society for the Study of Vulval Disease (BSSVD; www.bssvd.org) is an excellent resource for professionals and patients wanting to know more about vulval conditions. The BSSVD in addition to the British Association of Dermatologists (http://www.bad.org.uk), have excellent patient information leaflets relating to vulval skin disease, including helpful self-management advice.

Images of vulval skin disorders can be found on the BSSVD website or in Danderm Atlas of Dermatology, Dermnet or Google Scholar.

References

1. British Association of Dermatologists. BAD Vulval Health Survey. 2015.

2. Wang G, Li C, Gao T, Liu Y, Clinical analysis of 48 cases of inverse psoriasis: a hospital-based study. *Eur J Dermatol* 2005;15:176–178.

3. Ventolini G, Baggish MS, Post-menopausal recurrent vaginal candidiasis: effect of hysterectomy on response to treatment, type of colonization and recurrence rates post-treatment. *Maturitas* 2005;51(3): 294–298.

Chapter 25

Management of the Patient with Pelvic Organ Prolapse in Primary Care

Christian Phillips and Charlotte Hutchings

Key Points

- A prolapse is a protrusion of any pelvic organ or structure beyond its normal anatomical position. These are graded first, second and third degree, depending on their severity.
- Damage to the major supports of the vagina (endopelvic fascia, ligaments and levator ani) leads to prolapse.
- Childbirth is the major risk factor for development of prolapse.
- Patients with prolapse present with a variety of symptoms depending on the compartment affected.
- Patient should only be referred for treatment for prolapse if their symptoms are bothersome. Asymptomatic prolapse can be left alone.
- Patients with anterior compartment prolapse often have urinary symptoms and should be questioned for this.
- Patients with posterior compartment prolapse often have concomitant bowel symptoms and need to be questioned for this.
- Diagnosis is made on clinical examination, usually with the patient in a left lateral position with a Sims speculum.
- Surgery is the mainstay of treatment, but should only be considered after all risk factors have been treated and the patient's family has been completed.
- Women opting for conservative management with a ring pessary can be managed successfully in primary care with regular review.

Introduction

Prolapse is a common condition that presents regularly in primary care. Many women with a prolapse will be asymptomatic and can be reassured and provided with general advice about risk avoidance and pelvic floor exercises. However, those with symptoms need a methodical history and examination to help determine the type and stage of their prolapse in order to determine the management options available to them.

Case Scenario

Andrea is a 33-year-old woman who attends your general practice clinic to discuss her problems with prolapse. This was noted by the practice nurse when the woman came for a cervical smear. She works as a health care worker in a nursing home, smokes 20 cigarettes a day and has a body mass index of 36. She has had two vaginal deliveries in the past with children aged five years and seven years. She had one forceps delivery with an episiotomy and one normal vaginal delivery when she sustained a second-degree tear which was sutured by the midwife. She is divorced, but has recently had a new partner with whom she co-habits. Andrea is worried and concerned about her prolapse and wants your advice about having something done about it. She has heard that her friend has had a 'sling procedure' and she was wondering whether she should have the same.

What are the Structives that Support the Pelvic Organs?

Let us first consider the mechanisms of support for the pelvic organs. The pelvic organs comprise of:

- In the anterior compartment – urethra and bladder
- In the apical compartment – uterus and vaginal vault

Women's Health in Primary Care, edited by Anne Connolly and Amanda Britton. Published by Cambridge University Press
© Cambridge University Press 2017

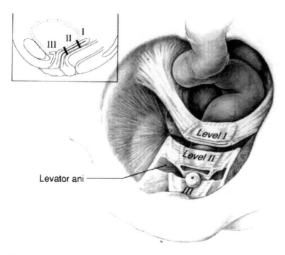

Figure 25.1 Levels of support for pelvic organs.

- In the posterior compartment – small bowel, peritoneum and rectum.

The pelvic organs are supported by three mechanisms of support [1].
- The endopelvic fascia with its condensations forming the uterosacral and cardinal ligaments
- The levator ani with its intact nerve supply
- The posterior angulation of the vagina when the woman is standing.

Fascia

The endopelvic fascia is formed of connective tissue with occasional smooth muscle and these envelope the pelvic organs. They form condensations of fascia inserted to the top of the vagina (paracolpium) and cervix/uterus (parametrium). These form the uterosacral ligaments posteriorly, the transverse (cardinal) ligaments laterally and the thin pubocervical ligaments anteriorly.

DeLancey describes three levels of pelvic organ support (Figure 25.1). The condensations of fascia that insert into the cervix and upper vagina are the 'Level 1' supports. Tears or avulsion in the Level 1 support causes uterine prolapse or if the uterus is absent, vault prolapse. The vagina, with bladder anteriorly and rectum posteriorly, is, enclosed with connective tissue/endopelvic fascia. These form sheet-like structures to partition the vagina from the bladder and the rectum. These are the 'Level 2' supports. Tears in these structures can cause a cystocele or rectocele. The

'Level 3' supports form the sphincter complex and suburethral hammock anteriorly and the perineal body posteriorly [2].

Muscle

The levator ani muscles form a diaphragm for the pelvic organs to sit upon. Integrity between the connective tissue of the endopelvic fascia and its connections to the levator ani ensure that the pelvic organs are suspended within the pelvis. Denervation or direct injury to the muscle at the levator ani or avulsion of the endopelvic fascia/tears in the endopelvic fascia cause lack of continuity between the levator ani and the connective tissue and the pelvic organs. This will result in prolapse.

What are the Risk Factors that this Lady has for Pelvic Organ Prolapse?

The primary mechanism in the aetiology of pelvic organs prolapse is obstetric injury and childbirth [3]. This lady has had a forceps delivery and a spontaneous vaginal delivery. At both deliveries she sustained either an episiotomy or a tear. Parturition through the birth canal can cause injury both in the form of tears in the pelvic fascia, but also injury to the pudendal nerve which innervates the levator ani or direct injury to the levator muscles themselves and their attachments to the pelvic side-wall [4].

Andrea has had two children in the past, but it is noted from the history that she has started a new relationship and she may wish to have further children with her new partner yet. This needs to be taken into account when counselling her. Certainly any surgical correction (which will be discussed later) needs to be deferred until her family is complete. Furthermore, on counselling her about subsequent pregnancies there is sometimes the temptation to open the discussion about elective caesarean section with the aim of trying to prevent further obstetric injury and prolapse. There is however no evidence that caesarean section reduces the risk of a prolapse or urinary incontinence [5].

In this case, although she already has a degree of pelvic floor injury resulting in prolapse, a caesarean section will not prevent deterioration of this and on balance is likely to have a greater morbidity than a further vaginal delivery. The advice should therefore be to aim for a vaginal delivery unless there is an obstetric reason to plan otherwise and if the possibility of an elective caesarean section has been raised by another health care professional, any explanations to try and sway her from this are often questioned due to conflicting advice. The patient could receive conservative therapy for the prolapse until her family is complete and then surgical correction may be considered if she so wishes [5].

Other causes for the development of prolapse are those that predispose to prolonged or sustained periods of raised intra-abdominal pressure. In this case Andrea has a high body mass index, smokes, with a history of asthma, and in her occupation is lifting patients. She also may have chronic constipation. All these factors predispose her to having sustained periods of straining, which increases intra-abdominal pressure, forcing the pelvic organs down into the vagina. These would all need addressing before any form of treatment could be discussed.

Other risk factors for the development of prolapse include a genetic predisposition to collagen/connective tissue disorders [6]. The most severe forms of this would be Ehlers–Danlos syndrome. Ageing is the other major risk factor [7]. Atrophic tissues can be associated with prolapse. There is no evidence in the postmenopausal patient that HRT would reduce or reverse the development of a sustained prolapse. However, HRT (especially in the form of topical administration) can be useful as an adjunct to surgery or pessary usage. This will be discussed later.

What Should you Look for when Assessing this Patient?

History

As discussed previously, prolapse can affect all three compartments of the pelvis (anterior, apical and posterior). As such, prolapse from each compartment can cause symptoms from the organs that are present in each compartment. Anteriorly sits the urethra and bladder. Patients with cystocele and urethrocele can present with urinary symptoms, including concomitant stress incontinence, urinary frequency and nocturia, urinary urgency and poor voiding (in advanced prolapse). Posterior compartment involvement involves injury to the supporting structures of the rectum and small bowel. Patients can present with obstructive defecation and incomplete evacuation of the bowel requiring digitation and perineal splinting

and occasionally concomitant faecal urgency or faecal incontinence. Non-specific symptoms of prolapse include vaginal bulge, often worse at the end of the day or on straining, pelvic aching (which may extend down to both thighs), backache and dyspareunia. A careful detailed history is necessary to elicit which compartments may be affected before going on to clinical examination.

What Other Salient Features in this Woman's History Would You Want to Elicit?

The most important thing to ascertain from her is whether the prolapse does indeed 'bother her' in day-to-day life. In other words, does it affect her quality of life? If the prolapse has been noted by the practice nurse and is an incidental finding and completely asymptomatic with little effect on her day-to-day living, the advice should always be to leave things well alone until it does become bothersome. Often reassurance that prolapse is not dangerous is all that is needed. Patients can sometimes be concerned that it may get worse in the future and would therefore like to have it corrected now while they are still young. The advice from the surgeon should always be only to undergo surgery when the prolapse becomes an issue, as age is seldom a cause not to operate.

Clinical Examination

It is first worth looking on clinical examination for risk factors of the development of prolapse including high body mass index, comorbidities such as COPD or asthma or any obvious trauma to the pelvis caused by obstetric injury in the form of episiotomy scars, etc. A bimanual abdomino-pelvic examination should be performed to exclude any pelvic masses and then the patient asked to lie in the left lithotomy position and the vagina inspected using a Sims speculum (Figure 25.2). This is inserted initially retracting the posterior vaginal wall to inspect the anterior compartment and the apex and then is slowly withdrawn back out through the introitus, to see if any ensuing enterocele or rectocele falls into the vagina behind the lip of the retracted speculum. Urinalysis should also be performed as routine to exclude haematuria and urinary tract infection.

Any obvious suspicious pelvic masses or haematuria should be referred to the appropriate rapid access clinic at the hospital and any urinary tract infection treated. Signs of atrophy should be noted and treated

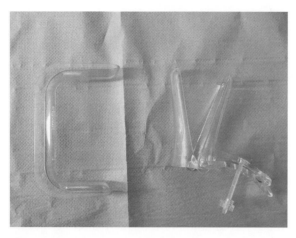

Figure 25.2 Sims and Cuscoes specula: Sims is used with the patient in the left lateral position, and used to inspect each compartment for prolapse.

with topical oestrogens if felt appropriate and symptomatic.

Classification of Pelvic Organ Prolapse

How do we classify a prolapse that is seen on examination?

As explained earlier, prolapses can be classified into the appropriate compartment:

- Anterior compartment – urethra, bladder
- Apical – uterus, vaginal vault (if uterus is absent)
- Posterior compartment – small bowel, rectum.

The prolapse derives its nomenclature from the affected organ (Table 25.1)

The prolapse can further be graded by severity. This can be done in two ways. Commonly clinicians in primary care and gynaecology use the Baden–Walker classification:

- Stage 1 – prolapse is deviated from its anatomical position, but has not reached the introitus.

Table 25.1 Classification of prolapse

Compartment	Structure	Prolapse
Anterior	Urethra	Urethrocoele
	Bladder	Cystocoele
Apex	Uterus	Uterine Prolapse
	Vault	Vault Prolapse
Posterior	Small Bowel	Enterocoele
	Omentum	Enterocoele
	Rectum	Rectocoele

- Stage 2 – the prolapse has deviated from its normal anatomical position and has extended down to the level of the introitus, but not beyond.
- Stage 3 – the prolapse has deviated from its normal anatomical position and has extended beyond the level of the vaginal introitus.

Clinicians in secondary care may sometimes refer to the PoPQ (pelvic organ prolapse quantification) grading. This involves taking nine measurements at certain points in the vagina and measuring how far these points have deviated from the level of the vaginal introitus [8].

Investigation

Very little in the way of investigation is needed for a patient with pelvic organ prolapse. Once abdomino-pelvic examination has excluded any pelvic masses and urine dipstick analysis is negative to exclude haematuria or urinary infection, investigations are dependent on the patient's symptoms and can be geared accordingly. If the patient has a retroverted uterus or is obese then pelvic masses can be difficult to feel on bimanual examination and a pelvic ultrasound scan may be necessary. Urodynamics are not necessary routinely unless surgery is being considered. Patients with concomitant bowel symptoms that are refractive to stool softeners may need referral to a coloproctologist or combined pelvic floor clinic (if available) for clinical assessment. Those with symptoms of obstructed defaecation may need proctography (conventional or MRI) to look for an intussusception, as well as rectocoele or enterocoele. If they have faecal urgency, anal or faecal incontinence, then endoanal ultrasound may be necessary to assess anal sphincter integrity. Anal manometry is occasionally indicated to assess sphincter function.

What are the Treatment Options for Prolapse?

Conservative Therapies

Conservative treatments are centred round reducing or preventing predisposing factors for the development or worsening of prolapse. These include weight loss in the obese patient, treatment of chronic asthma or COPD, or constipation. It is important to take a good, detailed history of the patient's bowel habit as often concomitant constipation and straining exist. Review of the patient's Bristol stool score can help to educate the patient on what a normal stool consistency should be [9]. The use of stool softeners such as Laxido, Fybogel or Movicol are all helpful in aiming to increase the water content of the stool and thus reducing its hardness. If obstructive defecation and incomplete emptying persists despite optimizing the patient's stool consistency, one may consider referral to a combined pelvic floor clinic, if available, where patients can be assessed with a proctogram or even MR proctography to rule out concomitant intussusception which may co-exist with the vaginal prolapse.

Although there is little evidence for the role of pelvic floor exercises to treat prolapse, a recent large randomized controlled multicentre study did demonstrate that physiotherapy may be helpful in the treatment of prolapse, especially in stage 1 and stage 2 [10,11]. Pessaries are also one of the most common forms of conservative therapy with a high (70–90%) level of patient satisfaction [12,13]. These are inserted into the vagina and require replacement every three to six months, depending on the type of pessaries used. Silicone ring pessaries can be changed every six months, whilst shelf pessaries have a greater chance of causing ulceration and incarceration, and need changing every three months. The size and shape necessary vary on type of prolapse and the patient's wishes. The use of pessaries can cause vaginal ulceration and infection, and therefore the vagina should be carefully inspected at the time of replacement or insertion. Topical oestrogens in the form of pessaries or creams may be beneficial in reducing the risk of vaginal ulceration. The main indications for pessary treatment are:

- Patient's wish for medical rather than surgical intervention.
- As a therapeutic test to ascertain whether correction of the prolapse will improve the patient's symptoms before considering surgery.
- The patient has not completed their family or is currently pregnant or in the early postpartum period/breastfeeding.
- The patient is medically unfit to undergo surgery.
- Symptomatic relief whilst waiting for surgery.

The commonest pessaries used in the past have been ring and shelf pessaries. There is now a greater variety such as the Gellhorn, cube pessaries and the hinged ring pessary, which the patient can take out and insert by themselves (Figure 25.3)

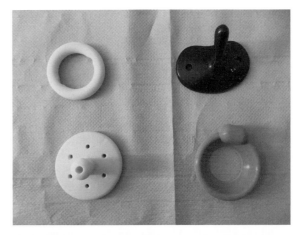

Figure 25.3 Common types of pessaries used in clinical practice.

Surgical Therapies

The aim of surgery is to restore normal anatomy, as well as normal function. There are a variety of vaginal and abdominal operations designed to correct prolapse. Although one would not expect a general practitioner to counsel a patient fully about the variety of surgical procedures, a knowledge of the surgery is essential to be able to counsel patients appropriately prior to referral and also to help manage any postoperative problems that may occur, but may not necessitate admission or re-referral to secondary care.

Anterior Compartment Surgery

Anterior repair (colporrhaphy) is the most commonly performed surgical procedure. An anterior vaginal wall incision is made and the defect in the endopelvic fascia underlying the bladder is isolated and closed, usually with interrupted absorbable sutures. With the bladder position restored, any redundant vaginal epithelium is removed and closed. Anterior repair can sometimes be performed with concomitant surgery for stress incontinence, usually in the form of a sling procedure.

Posterior Compartment Surgery

Posterior colporrhaphy is the most commonly performed procedure for a rectocele. A similar incision is made to an anterior colporrhaphy and the fascial defect is closed, preventing the rectum herniating into the vagina. Once the anatomy of the rectum is restored, any redundant epithelium is excised and the incision closed.

Repair of an enterocele involves excision of the peritoneal sac containing the small bowel and then approximating the peritoneum and/or the uterosacral ligaments at the same time. This is often performed with concomitant posterior colporrhaphy.

Apical Compartment Prolapse

The commonest procedure for uterine prolapse is vaginal hysterectomy. This is one of the oldest major operations with the references dating back to Hypocrites in the fifth century BC. The operation involves incising the vaginal epithelium around the cervix and then entering the peritoneal cavity between the bladder and the uterus and the rectum and the uterus. The major blood vessels are then ligated and the uterus removed through the vagina. The vault is then closed and supported by sutures into the uterosacral-cardinal ligament complex.

Uterine-Preserving Surgery for Uterine Prolapse

The uterus can be preserved if the patient so wishes. Ideally, surgery should not be contemplated until the patient has completed their family; however, there have been case reports of successful pregnancies following uterine-preserving prolapse surgery. The uterus can be suspended to a variety of structures, including the anterior longitudinal ligament overlying the sacrum (by open or laparoscopic procedure) or to the sacrospinous ligament (by a vaginal procedure).

Manchester repair

This procedure is rarely performed any more. It involves accessing the uterus vaginally and performing an amputation of the cervix and then using the uterosacral and cardinal ligament complex to support the uterus. This has gone out of vogue due to problems with cervical stenosis or cervical incompetence and risk of miscarriage.

Le Fort's colpocleisis

This operation is used in very frail patients who are unfit for major surgery. It involves partial closure of the vagina by suturing the anterior and posterior vaginal walls together, thus preventing the uterus from falling through the vaginal opening.

Vault Prolapse

After a hysterectomy, failure of support to the vaginal vault can occur in a proportion of patients. In this situation the vault needs to be attached back within the pelvis either to the anterior longitudinal ligament that overlies the sacrum (open/laparoscopic sacrocolpopexy) or to the sacrospinous ligament (vaginal sacrospinous fixation).

Vaginal Mesh Procedures

After the relative success of synthetic vaginal slings in treating stress urinary incontinence, (see relevant chapter) vaginal mesh has been used to treat vaginal wall and uterine prolapse. The mesh is inserted via a variety of techniques, often using a specially designed introducer device. A range of different meshes can be introduced and attached to a variety of anatomical points within the pelvis to support the uterus, bladder and rectum. The use of these has declined significantly since a report by the FDA in 2009 recommended caution in their usage due to risks of mesh erosion and dyspareunia [14]. NICE guidance recommends patients should be counselled about the possible short- and long-term risks of synthetic mesh and cases where vaginal mesh is used, should be followed up for service evaluation purposes [15]. Although reducing in popularity, a few centres still may utilize these devices, provided they have suitable clinical governance arrangements.

Conclusion

Prolapse is a common condition that presents regularly in primary care. Treatment is only necessary if the patient has symptoms from their prolapse. Asymptomatic prolapse requires reassurance alone. Pessaries and physiotherapy can be maintained in the community if the patient wishes. Although the mainstay of treatment is surgery, referral for surgery should only be considered if the patient is symptomatic, has completed their family and wishes surgical intervention.

References

1. Bonney, V, The principles that should underlie all operations for prolapse. *BJOG* 1934; 41(5):669–683.

2. DeLancey, J, Anatomy and biomechanics of genital prolapse. *Clin Obstet Gynecol* 1993; 36(4):897–909.

3. MacLennan AH, Taylor AW, Wilson DH, Wilson D, The prevalence of pelvic floor disorders and their relationship to gender, age, parity and mode of delivery. *BJOG* 2000; 107(12):1460–1470.

4. Mant J, Painter R, Vessey M, Epidemiology of genital prolapse: Observations from the Oxford Family

Planning Association Study. *Br J Obstet Gynaecol* 1997; 104(5):579–585.

5. Dietz HP, Simpson JM, Levator trauma is associated with pelvic organ prolapse. *BJOG* 2008; 115(8):979–984.

6. Malfouz I, Asali F, Phillips C, The management of urogynaecological problems in pregnancy and early postpartum. *Obstet Gynaecol* 2012; 14(3): 154–158.

7. Phillips CH, Anthony F, Benyon C, Monga AK, Collagen metabolism in the uterosacral ligaments and vaginal skin of women with uterine prolapse. *BJOG* 2006; 113(1):39–46.

8. Persu C, Chapple CR, Cauni V, Gutue S, Geavlete P, Pelvic Organ Prolapse Quantification System (POP–Q): A new era in pelvic prolapse staging. *J Med Life* 2011; 4(1):75.

9. McCallum I, Ong S, Mercer-Jones M, Chronic constipation in adults. *BMJ* 2009; 338:b831.

10. Hagen S, Stark D, Maher C, Adams E, Conservative management of pelvic organ prolapse in women. *Cochrane Database Syst Rev* 2004;(2):CD003882.

11. Hagen S, Stark D, Glazener C, *et al.* A multicentre randomised controlled trial of a pelvic floor muscle training intervention for women with pelvic organ prolapse. *41st Annual Meeting of the International Continence Society, 29 August–2 September 2011*, Abstract 000129.

12. Lamers BH, Broekman BM, Milani AL, Pessary treatment for pelvic organ prolapse and health-related quality of life: a review. *Int Urogynecol J* 2011; 22:637–644.

13. Bugge C, Adams EJ, Gopinath D, Reid F, Pessaries (mechanical devices) for pelvic organ prolapse in women. *Cochrane Database Syst Rev* 2013; (2):CD004010.

14. US Food and Drug Administration. FDA Safety Communication: UPDATE on Serious Complications Associated with Transvaginal Placement of Surgical Mesh for Pelvic Organ Prolapse. 2011. www.fda.gov/MedicalDevices/Safety/AlertsandNotices/ucm262435.htm (accessed September 2016).

15. NICE. Surgical repair of vaginal wall prolapse using mesh. www.nice.org.uk/guidance/ipg267 (accessed September 2016).

Chapter 26

Ovarian Cancer: Improving Outcomes
A Primary Care Perspective

Ken S. Metcalf

Key Points

- 90% of ovarian cancers are from the epithelium.
- Ovarian cancer presents late – only 30% are diagnosed in an early stage when the prognosis is better.
- There is no screening process with an acceptable risk/benefit profile.
- The presenting symptom with the greatest positive predictive value (PPV) is abdominal distension – the ppv is over 5% if this is associated with appetite loss.
- CA 125, examination and USS are important in the assessment of suspected ovarian cancer, as is calculating the Risk of Malignancy Index. Advances in USS assessment are likely to be of greater importance in the immediate future.
- CA 125 over 200 in a premenopausal and over 65 in a postmenopausal woman would give a high RMI and a high level of suspicion and alone act as a red flag.
- The commonest hereditary syndrome is the breast ovarian cancer syndrome associated with BRCA 1 and 2. Lynch syndrome (hereditary nonpolyposis colorectal cancer) is another.
- Laparoscopic BSO is a safe and effective strategy for women identified as at increased personal risk.
- Use of the OCP confers considerable risk reduction for ovarian cancer.

The term ovarian cancer tends to represent the group of tumours arising from the ovarian surface epithelium (epithelial ovarian cancer, or EOC). EOC is numerically by far the commonest malignant tumour of the ovary and represents over 90% of all ovarian tumours.

One in 52 women will be diagnosed with ovarian cancer during their lifetime. Around 7000 women are diagnosed with ovarian cancer in the UK each year making it the fifth most common cancer and representing 4% of all new cancer cases in women. Amongst gynaecological cancers, ovarian cancer has the highest mortality, with over 4000 deaths per year, accounting for 6% of all cancer deaths in women [1].

Almost three-quarters of cases are diagnosed in women aged 55 and over, but 26% of cases occur in younger women.

Analysis of ovarian cancer mortality rates throughout the UK shows very little variation between health boundaries, and European age-standardized mortality rates do not differ significantly to those in the UK.

For patients where the stage was recorded at diagnosis, 57% were advanced disease (stage III or IV, indicating tumour spread beyond pelvis). The one-year relative survival rate for early-stage disease (stages I or II – tumours confined to pelvis) is excellent (88.6–98.1%) in comparison to late-stage disease (51.5–71.3%) [1,2] As such, a major goal in improving outcomes from this disease would be to stage shift diagnosis and increase the proportion of early-stage tumours detected.

Early Diagnosis

Currently, only 30% of patients are diagnosed with early-stage disease. Early symptom recognition and screening are two key areas where an effective outcome could lead to early-stage shift.

Symptoms

Symptoms associated with ovarian cancer are also common in non-malignant conditions and one

---

Women's Health in Primary Care, edited by Anne Connolly and Amanda Britton. Published by Cambridge University Press
© Cambridge University Press 2017

estimate suggested that as many as 95% of women attending primary care have a symptom potentially representing ovarian cancer [3]. Because of such confounding variables it is difficult to believe that this strategy could provide great advantage.

Hamilton et al. [4] looked at the positive predictive value (PPV) of symptoms for ovarian cancer, i.e. the chance that a woman with a symptom actually has ovarian cancer. This large case-control study involved a retrospective review of case records in 39 general practices to identify all (212) women aged >40 diagnosed with ovarian cancer in 2000–7. Their medical records were examined for a full year prior to diagnosis; 32% were stages I and II, 45% stage III and 23% stage IV. These cases were each matched with five controls. The PPV was calculated for seven key symptoms and was 2.5% for abdominal distension, 0.6% for loss of appetite, 0.5% for postmenopausal bleeding, 0.3% for abdominal pain, 0.2% for increased urinary frequency, 0.3% for abdominal bloating and 0.2% for rectal bleeding. Abdominal distension in combination with any other of the key symptoms increased the PPV, particularly with loss of appetite where the PPV was >5%.

The small PPVs identified in this study reflect the common nature of such symptoms overall and the low incidence of ovarian cancer, but it seems that persisting abdominal distension (in contrast to bloating, which is an intermittent symptom) should be a red flag symptom and lead to urgent further investigation. Whether early symptom recognition will lead to a stage shift diagnosis remains unproven, but it is noteworthy that in this study 34% of the early-stage cancers and 35% of late-stage cancers presented with abdominal distension within a year of diagnosis, in comparison to 0.6% of controls. One might hypothesize that a fraction of the late-stage disease patients may have progressed from an earlier stage during the course of the year.

NICE

In 2010, the NICE guideline [5] recommended that in women with suspicious symptoms for ovarian cancer, a clinical examination should be performed and a serum CA 125 measurement should be obtained. An elevation in CA 125 over 35 IU/mL or the presence of a pelvic mass should lead to a pelvic ultrasound assessment. For any woman who has normal CA 125 (less than 35 IU/mL), or CA 125 of 35 IU/mL or greater, but normal pelvic ultrasound, NICE recommended

careful assessment for other clinical causes of symptoms and investigation if appropriate, and if no cause apparent advise to return to GP if symptoms become more frequent and/or persistent.

Adopting the NICE guideline measures meant that many women were reassured on the basis of a normal CA 125 result. It has long been known that patients with early-stage ovarian cancers often have normal CA 125 levels [6]. More recent data from the United Kingdom Collaborative Trial of Ovarian Cancer Screening (UKTOCS) has shown serial CA 125 estimation to be important and that velocity change, even within the normal reference range, can confer high risk when interpreted using their risk of ovarian cancer algorithm (ROCA) [7]. These data indicate that a new paradigm will need to be defined to ensure maximum reassurance is provided.

Screening Tests

Employing a general population screening test to detect ovarian cancer at an early stage remains the subject of ongoing global research, but to date a successful screening strategy has not been found.

A major concern in screening is to establish a successful balance between sensitivity (the ability to detect the problem where present) and specificity (the ability to not detect a problem where absent) of the screening test. Sensitivity reflects the false negative rate and a high level of sensitivity will indicate a low false negative rate. Specificity reflects the false positive rate and a high level of specificity reflects a low false positive rate. An ideal test has very high sensitivity and specificity. In terms of cancer screening it is clearly important to have the highest sensitivity possible to ensure the tumour is detected and not missed by the test. A very high specificity will also reduce the likelihood of a false positive result. This is particularly important as the consequences of a positive result often include invasive tests or surgery, both of which have significant complication risks in terms of morbidity and even mortality.

Even with very good test performance (high specificity), the low background prevalence of ovarian cancer means that the number of unnecessary interventions can be unacceptable. Assuming the prevalence for ovarian cancer of 1:2500 women and a test specificity as high as 99.6% (i.e. 0.4 false positive cases in every 100 tests), there would be 10 false positives per case detected, an unacceptable ratio.

There is a wide range of commercially available biomarker blood tests for ovarian cancer. Whilst these are of significant value in secondary care triage for known pelvic pathology, none has demonstrated a high enough sensitivity and specificity to be recommended and at this time patients should be discouraged from using commercially available screening kits.

Current screening strategies are most focused on combinations of transvaginal ultrasound scanning and CA 125 testing. Two large studies have looked at this, but in different ways.

The PLCO multicenter American trial [8] looked at annual screening with ultrasound and CA 125. It failed to show any reduction in mortality and in those women with false positive results, 15% sustained a major complication from the subsequent surgical intervention.

In 2001, the UKTOCS trial commenced and recruited more than 200,000 women aged between 50 and 64 who were randomly assigned to one of three groups – control, annual ultrasound or annual CA 125 test. In the latter group, instead of relying on the absolute value of the CA 125 level, the result was utilized as part of the ROCA test (see earlier). Early published data showed an increase in the number of ovarian cancers diagnosed at an early stage, but the latest published results have not shown any confirmed impact on overall mortality from this trial in either screening arm [9]. The early results suggest that approximately 15 ovarian cancer deaths could be prevented for every 10,000 women who attend for screening that involves annual blood tests for between 7 and 11 years, but longer-term follow-up is required to confirm this. In the UKTOCS study, for every three women having surgery for presumed ovarian cancer (based on their blood test), two of them turned out not to have cancer. This represents a lot of unnecessary surgery for the screened population. Notwithstanding the undoubted psychological effects of false positive results, major complications occurred in 3% of women having surgery. It is still unclear whether the risk:benefit ratio is in favour of screening in this fashion.

Results Assessment and Secondary Care Referral Patterns

Where investigations indicate an abnormality, correct interpretation is vital in both counselling the patient and also determining the most appropriate route for secondary care referral. In many cases the results will indicate a greater likelihood of benign abnormality. In such cases expectant management may be appropriate or referral on a non-urgent pathway for a general gynaecological opinion and management. For others at greater risk, urgent referral to a specialist gynaecological oncology multidisciplinary team is essential, as there is strong data to indicate better outcomes for women with gynaecological malignancies, particularly ovarian cancer, where treatment is undertaken in specialized centres [10].

In a postmenopausal woman, an abnormal CA 125 level or the presence of a pelvic mass on ultrasound should lead to urgent referral for a secondary care opinion, usually as a cancer two-week wait referral. This approach is also appropriate for the premenopausal patient where CA 125 level is greater than 200 IU/mL or the ultrasound report indicates suspicion of malignancy. For other premenopausal cases where the CA 125 level is not normal but <200 IU/mL and where the ultrasound report indicates a cystic adnexal mass with minimal complexity, there may be a dilemma faced by the referring clinician in terms of the urgency and/or best place for secondary care referral. In such circumstances it may be helpful to consider the calculation made by secondary care specialists for overall risk of malignancy, the Risk of Malignancy Index (RMI) [11]. This simple calculation is easily made.

The RMI assessment involves calculating the product of the formula:

$$\text{Age score} \times \text{CA 125 score} \times \text{Ultrasound score}$$

Commonly, an RMI calculation of >200 would be taken as conferring a significant enough risk of malignancy to merit urgent and specialist referral. The age score relates to menopausal status (score 1 for premenopausal, 3 for postmenopausal). The CA 125 score is the absolute level of CA 125 in IU/mL. The ultrasound score is either 1 or 3, where 3 would be an ultrasound report indicating more than one of five possible features on scan (multilocularity, bilaterality, presence of solid components within cyst, presence of pelvic fluid/ascites, presence of possible abdominal implants).

It is noteworthy that a CA 125 level of 200 in a premenopausal patient or 65 in a postmenopausal patient will result in a high risk RMI calculation even where the ultrasound findings are not particularly suspicious (i.e. score 1). It is useful to keep these two CA 125 levels in mind as red flags.

Advances in ultrasound technology and operator-dependent skills are leading to much greater accuracy with risk prediction using ultrasound alone. The International Ovarian Tumour Analysis (IOTA) Study algorithms show a better sensitivity and specificity for cancer prediction than RMI in both pre- and postmenopausal women [12]. The ultrasound variables which IOTA has shown to be required are within the capacity of non-expert ultrasonographers and will undoubtedly soon become represented widely in mainstream ultrasound reporting. This will much more easily facilitate ideal choice of referral stream from primary care level, leading to the most appropriate level of triage and choice of surgical specialist at secondary and tertiary care level.

Identifying High-Risk Women

The recognition of women at significantly increased risk of developing ovarian cancer and referral for preventative surgery is an important component in any strategy to improve ovarian cancer outcomes.

The strongest known risk factor is a family history of the disease, which is present in 10–15% of women with ovarian cancer. Women with a single family member affected with ovarian cancer have a 4–5% lifetime risk (general population risk 1.4%). With two affected relatives the risk is 7%. In some circumstances a definite hereditary ovarian cancer syndrome can be identified and such women have a lifetime risk as high as 50%.

The commonest hereditary syndrome is the breast ovarian cancer syndrome accounting for over 90% of hereditary ovarian cancers. This syndrome is associated with mutations in the BRCA1 or 2 genes and confers high risk for both ovarian and breast cancer. Risk-reducing strategies therefore have to take account of both ovarian and breast cancer. BRCA1 mutations increase risk significantly for both cancers from age 35, so it is important that risk-reducing measures are implemented early for both. For BRCA2 mutations, breast cancer risk is significantly increased from age 35, whereas ovarian cancer risk appears to only be significantly increased from age 45. This leaves the opportunity to delay ovarian cancer risk-reducing measures for BRCA2 cases if desired.

Lynch syndrome, also known as hereditary non-polyposis colorectal cancer (HNPCC), is the other common hereditary ovarian cancer syndrome. This syndrome is associated with mutation of the MLH1, MSH2, MSH6 and PMS2 genes. Affected patients have high risk to develop colon, endometrial and ovarian cancers, so risk-reduction strategies must consider all sites.

Where a patient is identified as having a family history of ovarian, breast, colon or endometrial cancer it will be helpful to refer for a formal genetics consultation. In many circumstances this will be initially conducted by genetic counsellors and where high risk is suspected, more formal genetic testing pursued and a more accurate risk stratification calculation.

Risk-Reducing Surgery

Even in high-risk women who have a known familial or genetic increased risk for ovarian cancer, annual screening has no impact on mortality. Further study is underway to establish if more frequent screening intervals might confer greater advantage. Until such time risk-reducing surgery remains the only way to reduce mortality from ovarian/fallopian tube cancers for these women [13].

Bilateral salpingo-oophorectomy (BSO) in women who carry the BRCA1 or BRCA2 mutations will very considerably reduce the lifetime risk for ovarian, tubal or peritoneal cancers, although not eliminate it completely (residual risk approximately 0.1%). BSO in these women reduces their breast cancer risk by 50% also [14]. Compared to women who do not undergo risk-reducing BSO, undergoing surgery is associated with a lower all-cause mortality (10% vs 3%), breast-cancer-specific mortality (6% vs 2%) and ovarian-cancer-specific mortality (3% vs 0.4%) [15].

For the vast majority of cases surgery will be laparoscopic. This approach is associated with little morbidity and BSO is usually performed as day case surgery. In practice, most women are concerned about timing of surgery, whether to have a concurrent hysterectomy and the hormonal implications of the intervention.

In BRCA1 carriers the risk for both breast and ovarian cancer starts to rise significantly from age 35 and general consensus would be that risk-reducing surgery to both breasts and ovaries should be considered after this age, as soon as childbearing is complete. For BRCA2 carriers, whilst increased breast cancer risk still occurs early, as for BRCA1, the ovarian cancer increased risk occurs later (significantly from age 50). These women may choose to delay risk-reducing BSO, but they would not then get the benefit of breast cancer risk reduction from earlier BSO.

A minimum surgical intervention for risk reduction is BSO in isolation. The fallopian tubes should be removed in addition to the ovaries as it is highly likely that some apparent ovarian cancers arise in the fallopian tubes [16]. In some circumstances there are convincing concurrent gynaecological indications for total hysterectomy also. The presence of a significant increase in endometrial cancer risk with Lynch syndrome (HNPCC) is a compelling indication, but women on tamoxifen therapy also may choose to eliminate the small associated increased endometrial cancer risk with concomitant hysterectomy. Concerns raised in relation to the increased risk of breast cancer in combined HRT users compared with oestrogen-only users [17] is a strong stimulus for many women choosing hysterectomy as part of their risk-reducing surgery as subsequent HRT may then be oestrogen-only-based and safer.

The inclusion of hysterectomy as part of the surgical strategy obviously increases the scale of the surgical intervention and potential risk in comparison to BSO alone, but many women will be suitable candidates for a total laparoscopic approach (TLH), which has clear benefits in terms of perioperative morbidity and time to recovery.

For those women having risk-reducing surgery with a preceding history of breast cancer, oestrogen replacement therapy would be inadvisable as some data suggests an increase in recurrence risk. Nevertheless, where intractable menopausal symptoms arise, decision-making will need to be individualized. For others, available data suggests that HRT may be given to women up to the age of 50 with no loss of benefit in terms of breast cancer risk reduction [18]. This guidance appears to be reasonable for BRCA1 carriers also, where only 3.9% of breast cancers are oestrogen-receptor positive. A slightly greater anxiety may be required for BRCA2 carriers where incident breast cancers are more often oestrogen-receptor positive [19].

Non-Surgical Risk-Reduction Strategies

Screening may be offered to women who decline risk-reducing surgery. In this setting a six-month screening interval should be considered. This should start from age 35 (or 5 years earlier than the youngest age of ovarian cancer diagnosis in the family).

It has long been known that use of the oral contraceptive pill (OCP) is associated with a significant reduction in risk of ovarian cancer. This effect increases with duration of use. The odds ratio for ovarian cancer incidence in ever-users compared to never-users is 0.73. With more than 10 years OCP use, lifetime incidence of ovarian cancer is reduced by 50% [20].

In BRCA mutation carriers, OCP use has a significantly protective effect for ovarian cancer (odds ratio 0.58) and whereas the association with breast cancer showed a suggestion of increased risk, this was non-significant [21].

Summary

EOC remains a major health problem with poor overall outcomes. Strategies for early diagnosis have so far proven disappointing and shown negligible impact on overall mortality. However, continued recognition of the risk reduction conferred by OCP use and identification of those high-risk women who will benefit from risk-reducing surgery are clear goals from a primary care and public health perspective.

References

1. www.cancerresearchuk.org/health-professional/cancerstatistics/statistics-by-cancer-type/ovarian-cancer/mortality (accessed January 2016).

2. McPhail S, Johnson S, Greenberg D et al. Stage diagnosis and early mortality from cancer in England. Br J Cancer 2015;112:S108–S115.

3. Goff B, Mandel L, Melancon C, Muntz H, Frequency of symptoms of ovarian cancer in women presenting to primary care clinics. JAMA 2004;291(22):2705–2712.

4. Hamilton W, Peters T, Bankhead C, Sharp D, Risk of ovarian cancer in women with symptoms in primary care: population based case-control study. BMJ 2009;339:b2998.

5. NICE. Ovarian cancer: the recognition and initial management. CG122. 2010. www.nice.org.uk/guidance/CG122 (accessed September 2016).

6. Zurawski J, Knapp R, Einhorn N et al. An initial analysis of preoperative serum CA125 levels in patients with early stage ovarian carcinoma. Gynecol Oncol 1988;30:7–14.

7. Menon U, Ryan A, Kalsi J et al. Risk algorithm using serial biomarker measurements doubles the number of screen detected cancers compared with single

threshold rule in the United Kingdom Collaborative trial of Ovarian Cancer Screening. *J Clin Oncol* 2015;33:2062–2071.

8. Buys S, Partridge E, Black A *et al*. Effect of screening on ovarian cancer mortality: The Prostate, Lung, Colorectal and Ovarian (PLCO) Cancer Screening Randomized Controlled Trial. *JAMA* 2011;305 (22):2295–2303.

9. Jacobs I, Menon U, Ryan A *et al*. Ovarian cancer screening and mortality in the UK Collaborative Trial of Ovarian Cancer Screening (UKCTOCS): A randomized controlled trial. *Lancet* 2016; 387(10022):945–956.

10. Woo Y, Kyrgiou M, Bryant A *et al*. Centralisation of services for gynaecological cancers: a Cochrane systematic review. *Gynecol Oncol* 2012;126:286–290.

11. Jacobs I, Oram D, Fairbanks J *et al*. A risk of malignancy index incorporating CA125, ultrasound and menopausal status for the accurate pre operative diagnosis of ovarian cancer. *Br J Obstet Gynaecol* 1990;97:922–929.

12. Kaijser J, Sayasneh A, Van Hoorde K *et al*. Presurgical diagnosis of adnexal tumours using mathematical models and scoring systems: a systematic review and meta analysis. *Hum Reprod Update* 2014;20:449–462.

13. Rosenthal A, Fraser L, Manchanda R *et al*. Results of annual screening in phase I of the United Kingdom familial ovarian cancer screening study highlight the need for strict adherence to screening schedule. *J Clin Oncol* 2013;31(1):49–57.

14. Rebbeck T, Lynch H, Neuhausen S *et al*. Prophylactic oophorectomy in carriers of BRCA1 or BRCA2 mutations. *N Engl J Med* 2002;346:1616–1622.

15. Domchek S, Friebel T Singer C *et al*. Association of risk reducing surgery in BRCA1 or BRCA2 mutation carriers with cancer risk and mortality. *JAMA* 2010;304(9):967–975.

16. Nik N, Vang R, Shih IeM *et al*. Origin and pathogenesis of pelvic (ovarian, tubal and peritoneal) serous carcinoma. *Ann Rev Pathol* 2014;9:27–45.

17. Kuhl H, Schneider H. Progesterone: Promoter or inhibitor of breast cancer. *Climacteric* 2013;16(suppl 1):54–68.

18. Scottish Intercollegiate Guidelines Network. Sign 135: Management of epithelial ovarian cancer. 2013. www.sign.ac.uk (accessed September 2016).

19. Foulkes W, Metcalfe K, Sun P *et al*. Estrogen receptor status in BRCA1 and BRCA2 related breast cancer: the influence of age, grade and histological type. *Clin Cancer Res* 2004;10(6):2029–2034.

20. Havrilesky L, Moorman P, Lowery W *et al*. Oral contraceptive pills as primary prevention for ovarian cancer: a systematic review and meta-analysis. *Obstet Gynecol* 2013;122(1):139–147.

21. Moorman P, Havrilesky L, Gierisch J *et al*. Oral contraceptives and risk of ovarian cancer and breast cancer among high-risk women: a systematic review and meta-analysis. *J Clin Oncol* 2013;31(33):4188–4198.

Chapter 27

The Management of Endometrial Hyperplasia and Carcinoma in Primary Care

Dileep Wijeratne and Sian Jones

Key Points

- The natural history of endometrial cancer is a progression through various stages of endometrial hyperplasia offering opportunities for treatments if the problem is identified at an early stage, before progression to cancer.
- Endometrial cancer is the commonest gynaecological malignancy in the UK and the incidence is increasing alongside the current obesity epidemic.
- The majority of cases of endometrial hyperplasia and cancer result from unopposed oestrogenic stimulation of endometrial growth. Risk factors include obesity, increasing age, anovulatory conditions such as PCOS and women with a uterus using oestrogen-only HRT.
- Postmenopausal bleeding (PMB) is the commonest presentation of endometrial malignancy. Women presenting with PMB require cervical examination, to exclude a cervical cause, and referral using the urgent two-week suspected cancer pathway.
- In younger women presenting with menstrual dysfunction a risk stratification is required to determine who can be managed in primary care and which women require early investigations.
- Measurement of endometrial thickness using ultrasound scanning, preferably by the transvaginal route, is usually the first-line investigation to exclude endometrial malignancy. In postmenopausal women endometrial thickening provides a reliable recommendation for further endometrial assessment.
- The management of endometrial hyperplasia without atypia is usually by medical means using intrauterine progestogen alongside management of any treatable cause, i.e weight reduction. Oral progestogens are considered as second-line treatment.
- Monitoring of women with endometrial hyperplasia without atypia is important to ensure disease regression. This will be recommended or managed by secondary care.
- Hysterectomy is the first-line treatment for women with endometrial hyperplasia with atypia, provided they are considered to be fit for major surgery.
- The majority of women with endometrial cancer are diagnosed at stage 1 disease which with early surgical treatment has five-year survival rates of at least 96%.

Introduction

Endometrial cancer is the commonest gynaecological malignancy in the UK with more than 8000 cases diagnosed every year [1]. The natural history of endometrial cancer is that of a progression through various stages of endometrial hyperplasia, which if left untreated, can progress to cancer. The incidence of endometrial hyperplasia is at least three times higher than that of endometrial cancer [2]. Early detection of endometrial hyperplasia therefore offers an opportunity for intervention and treatment before progression to endometrial cancer occurs.

The incidence of both endometrial cancer and endometrial hyperplasia has been steadily rising over the past 20 years, mainly due to increasing levels of obesity. In spite of this, mortality from endometrial cancer has not increased. This is due, in large part, to the presence of clear guidelines, robust referral pathways and well co-ordinated care for women presenting with symptoms such as postmenopausal bleeding. Accordingly, around 75% of cases of endometrial cancer are diagnosed at stage I disease, for which early treatment confers a five-year survival rate of at least 96% [1].

In the coming years, an increasing number of younger women will present to primary care with symptoms of menstrual dysfunction in the context of risk factors for endometrial hyperplasia and cancer. Risk stratification of these women, followed by prompt referral for appropriate investigations and treatment will be key in ensuring that deaths from endometrial cancer remain low. In addition, primary care will have an increasingly prominent role in supervising the treatment of endometrial hyperplasia (especially in cases of medical/conservative management). In acknowledgement of this changing landscape, this chapter discusses in detail:

1. Risk factors common to endometrial hyperplasia and cancer
2. Classification of endometrial hyperplasia
3. The risk of progression of each hyperplasia subtype to endometrial cancer
4. Clinical presentation
5. Investigations
6. Management (conservative and surgical) and follow-up (with a focus on endometrial hyperplasia).

In addition, an illustrative case study is used to highlight some of the complexities in managing women with endometrial pathology.

Risk Factors for Endometrial Hyperplasia and Cancer

Both endometrial hyperplasia and endometrial cancer arise primarily in response to chronic oestrogenic stimulation of endometrial cell growth, unopposed by the suppressive effects of progesterone. Oestrogenic stimulation can be either intrinsic or extrinsic. Other factors such as genetic predisposition and immunosuppression can also play a role.

Obesity

- Androstenedione, produced by the theca interna cells of the ovary and the adrenal cortex, is

Table 27.1 Risk of atypical endometrial hyperplasia in relation to BMI [17].

BMI	Risk of atypical endometrial hyperplasia (odds ratio)
Normal BMI <24.9	1.0
Overweight BMI 24.9–29.9	2.3
Obese BMI 30–39.9	3.7
Morbidly obese BMI 40 and above	13.0

converted to oestrogen (oestrone) by aromatase enzymes present in adipose tissue. Increased levels of peripheral adiposity are therefore associated with elevated levels of oestrone, thus increasing the overall potential for oestrogenic stimulation of the endometrium [3].

- This is particularly relevant in situations where progesterone suppression is infrequent or absent, such as after the menopause or during episodes of amenorrhoea and anovulation seen in conditions such as polycystic ovarian syndrome.

Table 27.1 contains data from a case series of 446 women from the USA, illustrating the risk of developing atypical endometrial hyperplasia in relation to BMI. In this series, morbid obesity conferred a 13-fold increase in the risk of developing atypical hyperplasia.

Other Forms of Endogenous Oestrogenic Stimulation

- Anovulatory menstrual cycles, whereby there is a significant reduction in the usual progestogenic suppression of the endometrium in the second half of the menstrual cycle, are more common at the extremes of reproductive life. Early menarche (at or before the age of 11) and late menopause (after the age of 55) are therefore relative risk factors for endometrial hyperplasia and cancer.
- Nulliparity confers a two- to threefold risk of developing endometrial cancer. There may be an association between the nulliparity and anovulatory menstrual cycles.

Exogenous Oestrogens

- *Oestrogen-only HRT* in women with an intact uterus (i.e. who have not undergone hysterectomy) has been shown to increase the risk of endometrial hyperplasia at all doses and is therefore not recommended [4].

- *Tamoxifen* is a selective oestrogen receptor modulator which has different effects depending on the site of action. In breast tissue, tamoxifen has an anti-oestrogenic effect, hence its use in the treatment of breast cancer. Tamoxifen has a pro-oestrogenic effect on the endometrium, increasing the risk of hyperplasia and carcinoma. This increase is not thought to be of significance in premenopausal women. The American College of Obstetricians and Gynaecologists suggests that postmenopausal women using tamoxifen should be 'closely monitored', but concludes, in keeping with the evidence, that there is no role currently for monitoring of asymptomatic women either by ultrasound or endometrial biopsy [5].

Oestrogen-Secreting Tumours

The prevalence of endometrial hyperplasia in women with *granulosa cell tumours* of the ovary has been estimated at up to 40% [6].

Genetic Risks

- *Lynch syndrome or HNPCC* (hereditary non-polyposis colorectal cancer, a DNA mismatch repair mutation) confers a lifetime risk of developing endometrial cancer of up to 50%. Although there is no clear evidence to guide practice, women with Lynch syndrome are frequently offered surveillance, usually after the age of 35, in the form of annual endometrial biopsy [6].
- *Cowden syndrome* is a rare autosomal dominant disorder characterized by multiple harmatomatous growths and an increased risk of certain cancers. Women with Cowden syndrome have a lifetime risk of endometrial cancer of up to 19% [6].

Immunosuppression

Evidence from small case series involving renal graft recipients suggest that immunosuppressed individuals with abnormal uterine bleeding have up to a twofold increase in the incidence of endometrial hyperplasia at biopsy [7].

Classification of Endometrial Hyperplasia

In 2014 the WHO proposed a simple revised classification which divides endometrial hyperplasia into two groups:

- Hyperplasia without atypia
- Atypical hyperplasia.

This new classification is based on the observation that from a clinical perspective, it is the presence or absence of nuclear atypia that is most significant with regards to risk of progression to endometrial cancer [8].

The Risk of Progression From Endometrial Hyperplasia to Endometrial Cancer

There a paucity of high-quality data to help provide detailed and nuanced risk stratification with regards to the likelihood of endometrial hyperplasia progressing to cancer. However, the association between the presence of nuclear atypia and a significant risk of developing endometrial cancer is well established. The most useful general risk data come from a retrospective case series of 170 patients. In the study, hysterectomy specimens were examined from women who had previously undergone endometrial sampling for abnormal menstrual bleeding. The time between endometrial sampling and hysterectomy ranged between 1 and 27 years (13 on average). The risk of progression to endometrial cancer based on the study's findings is shown in Table 27.2 alongside a brief description of the histological features of each hyperplasia subtype.

Practice point: importantly, women found to have atypical hyperplasia on histology are at significant risk of having a co-existent endometrial carcinoma. Some case series suggest that this risk may be as high as 37% [9].

Clinical Presentation

The commonest way that women with either endometrial cancer or hyperplasia present is with abnormal uterine bleeding. In some cases, such as with postmenopausal bleeding, the indication for referral and assessment is clear and straightforward. In other cases, the decision of when to refer for investigations can be more complex. In younger women presenting with abnormal bleeding, for example, the majority will be

Table 27.2 Risk of progression to endometrial cancer based on endometrial hyperplasia subtype [18]

Hyperplasia category	Histological features	Risk of progression to endometrial cancer
Simple hyperplasia (no atypia)	Mildly crowded glands. Mitoses may or may not be present	1%
Complex hyperplasia (no atypia)	Very crowded, disorganized glands (>50% gland-to-stromal ratio). Mitoses present	3%
Simple hyperplasia *with* atypia (rare)	Nuclear enlargement with either evenly dispersed or clumped chromatin	8%
Complex hyperplasia *with* atypia		29%

Once the progression to *endometrial cancer* has occurred (most commonly endometrial adenocarcinoma) the histological appearance becomes that of small, round, back-to-back glands without any intervening stroma. There will be varying degrees of nuclear atypia, depending on the level of differentiation of the malignant cells.

cases of benign menstrual dysfunction as only 6% of cases of endometrial cancer present in women aged 35–44 [10]. However, adopting a holistic approach to clinical assessment by taking into account the risk factors described above can help identify the small number of younger women who may be at risk of endometrial hyperplasia and cancer.

Occasionally, women may also present without abnormal bleeding. For example, postmenopausal women may be found incidentally to have an abnormally thickened endometrium on ultrasound/CT/MRI after investigations for other conditions. Endometrial cancer can also occasionally be detected when malignant cells are seen on cervical cytology in postmenopausal women (reported as glandular cells).

With regards to *abnormal uterine bleeding*, symptoms that should lead to a suspicion of endometrial hyperplasia and cancer depend on age and associated risk factors:

- *Postmenopausal women*: *Any type of bleeding*, including spotting, bleeding when wiping after passing urine and staining of underwear should prompt investigation. On average, 10% of women who present with PMB will be diagnosed with endometrial cancer. A further 5–15% will be diagnosed with endometrial hyperplasia [11].
- *Perimenopausal women (age 45–menopause)*: *Any abnormal bleeding* in this age group should prompt further investigation. 19% of cases of endometrial cancer occur in women aged 45–54 [11]. Abnormal bleeding includes:
  - *Heavy Menstrual Bleeding*: heavy and/or prolonged period loss, which is usually subjectively reported but may be supplemented by objective evidence such as microcytic anaemia.
  - *Polymenorrhea*: frequent periods with an interval between onset of bleeding episodes less than 21 days.
  - *Intermenstrual bleeding*.
  - *Oligomenorrhoea/Amenorrhoea*: an extended interval between episodes of bleeding may of course be a normal feature of the perimenopause. However, in women who are anovulatory (e.g. with PCOS) or have other risk factors such as severe obesity, endometrial pathology should be considered.
- *Younger than 45 years*: Abnormal uterine bleeding (as described above) that occurs in the context of significant risk factors or failed medical management should prompt further investigation.

Investigations

Hysteroscopy and Endometrial Biopsy

In women suspected of having endometrial hyperplasia or cancer, confirmation of the diagnosis requires histological examination of a specimen of endometrial tissue. Commonly, endometrial biopsy samples are obtained using miniature sampling devices (such as the Pipelle) in the context of an outpatient hysteroscopy service.

Outpatient vs Inpatient Hysteroscopy

Outpatient hysteroscopy can be undertaken using miniaturized hysteroscopes often without the need for anaesthesia or instrumentation of the cervix. The diagnostic accuracy for detecting endometrial hyperplasia and carcinoma is high. Outpatient hysteroscopy is well tolerated, requiring reduced time off work, reduced loss of income and reduced travel costs for women, in addition to substantially less cost per woman to the NHS [12].

For certain women, inpatient hysteroscopy under general anaesthesia is the preferred option. Such cases include: when outpatient hysteroscopy has failed – either due to patient discomfort or technical difficulties such as uterine position or cervical stenosis; when OP sampling has been insufficient for diagnosis; when the woman herself declines an OP procedure (for example due to vaginismus or anxiety).

Urgency of Referral

Women presenting with postmenopausal bleeding should be referred for investigation via urgent two-week suspected cancer pathways. Often, they will be sent to a one-stop service where they will receive a pelvic ultrasound (see below) with or without hysteroscopy and biopsy, combined with visual examination of the perineum and cervix. In perimenopausal women, the majority of referrals to hysteroscopy will be via routine pathways unless the referring clinician feels that the symptomatology or risk-factor profile warrants more urgent assessment. In light of the relatively low incidence of endometrial cancer in premenopausal women under the age of 45, it is unusual for women of this age group to be referred via suspected cancer pathways with regards to suspected endometrial pathology. However, as with older women, if there is a strong enough clinical suspicion based on risk factors (for example women with menstrual dysfunction and Lynch syndrome) then urgent referral pathways can be used.

Radiological Imaging

Ultrasound

Ultrasound of the pelvis (ideally transvaginal) is usually the first-line investigation for women with postmenopausal bleeding. This is because measurement of the endometrial thickness is useful for ruling out endometrial cancer. Evidence from systematic reviews suggests that when the endometrial thickness measurement is less than 4 mm, the probability of cancer is

less than 1% [13]. Women with an endometrial thickness greater than this can continue on to have a hysteroscopy and endometrial biopsy.

Ultrasound is less useful for risk stratification in premenopausal women as there is a significant overlap between normal endometrial thickness and that caused by endometrial pathology. The main use of ultrasound in premenopausal women is to rule out other structural anomalies such as fibroids or endometrial polyps which may be contributing to the menstrual dysfunction. However, guidance from the RCOG supports the use of endometrial thickness measurement in women with PCOS/anovulation and amenorrhoea. A combination of a thickened endometrium and/or cystic appearances would warrant referral for hysteroscopy and endometrial assessment.

CT and MRI

There is little evidence for the use of computerized tomography in the diagnosis of endometrial hyperplasia and cancer. When an incidentally thickened endometrium is detected on CT scans undertaken for other reasons, this is usually followed up by a pelvic ultrasound scan.

MRI is currently used in the staging of endometrial cancer to detect invasive disease. It may have the future potential to diagnose possible endometrial hyperplasia and to be used in women with atypical hyperplasia undergoing surveillance (see below) to detect malignant change. More evidence is needed, however, before these uses can be adopted as widespread practice [14].

Management and Follow-Up of Endometrial Hyperplasia and Early Endometrial Cancer

Endometrial Hyperplasia (Without Atypia)

The majority of cases of hyperplasia without atypia will regress back to normal endometrium during a period of observation. Data from cohort studies suggest spontaneous regression rates of around 74% at six months for (both simple and complex) hyperplasia without atypia. Observation alone, whilst addressing reversible risk factors such as HRT use and obesity, is therefore an acceptable treatment option [15].

Treatment with progestogens is associated with a higher rate of regression back to normal endometrium when compared with observation alone. Treatment is recommended either when women are symptomatic or if there is no regression after an initial period of observation (usually six months). Treatment may also be useful where risk factor modification may be difficult (such as in treating severe obesity) [14].

Risk Factor Modification

- *Obesity:* Tackling obesity is complex, but the usual principles of multidisciplinary management apply. There is evidence that the incidence of asymptomatic hyperplasia is reduced in severe obesity after bariatric surgery (surgery is not indicated for this reason alone).
- *HRT:* Women who present with abnormal bleeding and hyperplasia whilst on HRT should have a review of their need for ongoing HRT. Women who wish to continue and are taking sequential preparations should be switched to a continuous combined preparation. For women on continuous combined HRT preparations, a manipulation of the regimen to increase the proportion of progestogen may be enough to induce regression of the hyperplasia when atypia is not present. This is particularly important in postmenopausal women, as they will have no endogenous progesterone production. Women already taking an appropriate form of continuous combined HRT who develop hyperplasia should be advised to stop [14].
- *Tamoxifen:* Women who develop endometrial hyperplasia whilst taking tamoxifen will need a joint decision between oncology and gynaecology regarding ongoing management.

Progestogenic Suppression

Progestogens antagonize the stimulatory effects of oestrogens on the cells of the endometrium. The two modes of treatment which can reliably deliver high enough concentrations of progestogens to the endometrium are oral progestogens and the levonorgestrel-releasing intrauterine system (Mirena®).

Intrauterine (LNG-IUS) vs Oral Progestogens

- The LNG-IUS is recommended as the first-line treatment as it achieves the highest concentration of progestogen at the endometrium, resulting in higher rates of regression [14].
- Evidence is available from RCTs comparing LNG-IUS with continuous oral progestogens for the treatment of simple hyperplasia. After six months, regression rates for LNG-IUS varied between 88 and 100%. For continuous oral progestogens, regression rates varied between 56 and 95% [14].
- One RCT reported follow-up results at two years. For the oral progestogen group, the regression rate was 64%, for the LNG-IUS group the rate was 100%.
- For women with complex hyperplasia, a systematic review of uncontrolled observational studies found regression rates of 66% with oral progestogens and up to 92% with the LNG-IUS [16].
- The minimal systemic absorption of hormone via the LNG-IUS helps to produce a more favourable side effect profile, thus aiding compliance [14].
- In women of reproductive age, LNG-IUS also provides effective contraception.
- Some women will receive a diagnosis of endometrial hyperplasia after investigations for heavy menstrual bleeding for which LNG-IUS is also the recommended first-line treatment.

In light of the lower rates of disease regression and poorer compliance, oral progestogens are only recommended when the LNG-IUS is unacceptable to women or when its use is contraindicated (such as in women with suspected or confirmed pelvic infection or those undergoing investigations for cervical neoplasia).

Continuous oral progestogen regimens should be used, rather than cyclical schedules, which are known to be significantly less effective in inducing regression to normal endometrium.

The two continuous oral progestogen regimens with the strongest evidence base are:

- Norethisterone 10–15 mg/day
- Medroxyprogesterone 10–20 mg/day.

In women with endometrial hyperplasia without atypia, treatment with either the LNG-IUS or oral progestogens should continue for a minimum of 6 months [14].

Follow-Up for Women Undergoing Risk Factor Modification/Progestogenic Suppression

Endometrial surveillance in the form of a repeat endometrial biopsy should be undertaken at a minimum of six-monthly intervals. A shorter interval may be required in some women depending on the severity of risk factors (e.g. postmenopausal women undergoing HRT modifications may require repeat biopsies at three-monthly intervals) [14].

Generally, women can be discharged when they have had two consecutive six-monthly biopsies that show normal endometrium. However, women should be advised to report any symptom recurrence as this may represent the recurrent development of hyperplasia [14].

Women who have persistent, significant risk factors (such as severe obesity) are at higher risk of relapse and should be advised to have yearly surveillance, even when regression has been achieved [14].

Women who have the LNG-IUS inserted should be advised to continue treatment for the duration of its five-year lifespan unless they wish it to be removed for fertility purposes. Endometrial biopsies can be easily taken with the IUS *in situ*.

Surgical Treatment of Endometrial Hyperplasia Without Atypia

Hysterectomy is not offered as a first-line treatment in hyperplasia without atypia. The specific circumstances in which hysterectomy would be offered to women not wishing to preserve their fertility include:

- When progression to ATYPICAL hyperplasia occurs during follow-up.
- When the endometrium does not revert to normal after 12 months of treatment with progestogens.
- If there is a relapse of hyperplasia after completing progestogen treatment.
- If a woman has persistent, severe bleeding symptoms.
- If a woman declines to undergo endometrial surveillance or comply with medical treatment.

Endometrial ablation is not recommended in the treatment of endometrial hyperplasia because complete and permanent destruction of the endometrium cannot be guaranteed in every case. The adhesions that form after ablation may also render any further endometrial biopsies difficult or impossible [14].

Atypical Endometrial Hyperplasia

Hysterectomy

In women diagnosed with endometrial hyperplasia with atypia, the first-line treatment is total hysterectomy (removal of uterus and cervix) due to the high risk of co-existing malignancy or the high risk of progression to adenocarcinoma.

In postmenopausal women with atypical hyperplasia, the fallopian tubes and ovaries should also be removed at the time of hysterectomy as this will reduce the chance of ovarian malignancy in the future. For premenopausal women, the decision of whether or not to remove the ovaries will be individualized after discussion with a gynaecologist [17].

A randomized controlled trial has compared total laparoscopic hysterectomy vs open hysterectomy for women with atypical hyperplasia or grade I endometrial cancer. There were no differences in the rates of major complications between either approach and both allowed adequate visualization of the abdominal cavity to assess for further disease. Laparoscopic hysterectomy, however, was associated with a shorter hospital stay, less pain and faster resumption of daily activities [17].

Women Unsuitable for Surgery/Wishing Fertility Preservation

In premenopausal women found to have atypical hyperplasia who wish to preserve their fertility or in women who are unsuitable for surgery, progestogenic suppression with careful surveillance is the mainstay of treatment. As in the case of non-atypical hyperplasia, the treatment of choice is the LNG-IUS. Importantly, there is a paucity of clear evidence to guide treatment and follow-up in these cases.

Prior to commencing treatment with progestogens, women with atypical hyperplasia should be reviewed in a gynaecology/oncology multidisciplinary team meeting. Further investigations will likely be recommended, including MRI to rule out invasive endometrial cancer and measurement of CA 125 levels to help exclude ovarian cancer. An individualized plan for follow-up will usually be formulated with review intervals for repeat endometrial biopsies being set at three to six months until two negative biopsies are obtained. Thereafter, long-term follow-up is usually recommended, either every 6–12 months or until hysterectomy can be performed. At each follow-up a detailed history of bleeding symptoms and pelvic examination should also be undertaken.

In women wishing to conceive, at least one normal endometrial biopsy should be obtained before pregnancy is attempted. In these cases, the chance of a live birth is around 25% and assisted conception has been shown to be associated with more live births (30%) compared to natural conception (15%) and may also prevent relapse. An early referral for specialist fertility advice may therefore also be indicated.

Once fertility is no longer required, hysterectomy is recommended, due to the high risk of relapse and progression to endometrial cancer [14].

Endometrial Cancer

The treatment of endometrial cancer depends upon the stage at presentation and is planned and undertaken by multidisciplinary gynaecology/oncology services. It is worth noting that 75% of cases of endometrial cancer are diagnosed at stage I disease, for which early treatment in the form of total hysterectomy and bilateral salpingo-oophorectomy confers a five-year survival rate of at least 96% [1].

Conclusion

Diagnosis and management of endometrial hyperplasia is important both in terms of treating menstrual dysfunction and preventing endometrial cancer. The diagnosis of endometrial pathology can, however, be challenging, especially in younger women where there is a significant overlap in symptomatology with benign menstrual dysfunction. In this chapter we have highlighted how a holistic approach to history-taking and examination can help to identify those women who warrant further assessment and treatment. We have also discussed the need for careful follow-up for women undergoing treatment or observation and highlighted some of the complex multidisciplinary challenges that can arise, especially in

women of child-bearing age (see also case scenario below).

> **Case Scenario**
>
> Mrs B is a 39-year-old lady of South-East Asian (Bangladeshi) origin. She visits her GP requesting assistance due to an inability to conceive for approximately two years. She has one child, born by normal delivery five years ago. Prior to conception she had been prescribed a six-month course of clomiphene citrate for the purposes of ovulation induction. Until recently, her periods had been irregular with a cycle length varying between two and four months. In the past 12 months, however, her periods have become more frequent and heavy. She has occasionally had to take some time off work due to tiredness. Mrs B has a BMI of 33, an increase from her previously recorded value from five years ago, which was 28.

- *With regards to risk factors for endometrial pathology, what are the concerning features of this history?*
  Previous oligomenorrhoea and requiring ovulation induction for conception are suggestive of a diagnosis of polycystic ovarian syndrome. Taking into account the World Health Organisation's reclassification of BMI categories based on ethnicity, a BMI of 33 falls into the 'severe obesity' category for a lady of South East Asian origin. The history therefore combines a risk of excess oestrogenic stimulation secondary to obesity with episodes of absent progestogenic suppression secondary to anovulation. The new onset of heavier and more frequent menstruation may therefore represent the development of new endometrial pathology.

- *What would be the appropriate next steps in the investigation and management of this lady?*
  An important first step in this case would be careful counselling that the focus of care should shift, for the time being at least, away from fertility concerns towards the exclusion of endometrial pathology. The most important investigation would be hysteroscopy and endometrial biopsy. As the incidence of endometrial cancer is low in premenopausal women under the age of 45, fast track referral is not indicated. This lady could

therefore be referred as routine to a direct access outpatient hysteroscopy service if available, or for review by a gynaecologist.

Mrs B underwent outpatient hysteroscopy and endometrial biopsy. The biopsy results revealed endometrial hyperplasia with atypia.

- *What is the risk of progression to endometrial cancer and what are the options for management?*
Based upon the best available evidence, the risk of Hyperplasia with atypia progressing to endometrial cancer is up to 29%. There is also a significant risk (up to 37%) of co-existing carcinoma that was not detected at biopsy.

Mrs B's case is reviewed at a gynaecology oncology MDT meeting and the recommendation made for hysterectomy. Mrs B is emphatic, however, that she wishes to maintain her fertility. In association with the gynaecology oncology team, a plan is made for progestogenic suppression using a Mirena® coil, with repeat endometrial biopsies planned at three-monthly intervals.

- *Which other referrals might be helpful in this situation?*
Mrs B's major risk factor for developing hyperplasia is her obesity. She accepts referral for dietary support from a nutritionist. She declines referral for a specialist fertility consultation.

Unfortunately, at three and six months, there is no evidence of regression in Mrs B's atypical hyperplasia. Furthermore, Mrs B's BMI increases over this time to 34 and she states that worry over her risk of developing cancer is a significant contributory factor to this. After further discussion with her gynaecologist, she decides to opt for a hysterectomy. The procedure is uncomplicated and Mrs B makes a full recovery. Histopathological examination of the uterus confirms the diagnosis of endometrial hyperplasia with atypia.

References

1. Cancer Research UK. Uterine cancer statistics. www.cancerresearchuk.org/health-professional/cancer-statistics/statistics-by-cancer-type/uterine-cancer (accessed September 2016).
2. Reed SD, Newton KM, Clinton WL, et al. Incidence of endometrial hyperplasia. Am J Obstet Gynaecol 2009;200(678):e1–6.
3. Simpson ER, Role of aromatase in sex steroid action. J Molec Endocrinol 2000;25:149–156.
4. Furness S, Roberts H, Marjoribanks J, Lethaby A, Hormone therapy in postmenopausal women and risk of endometrial hyperplasia. Cochrane Database Syst Rev 2012;(8):CD000402.
5. American College of Obstetricians and Gynaecologists. Committee opinion: Tamoxifen and uterine cancer. 2014. www.acog.org/Resources-And-Publications/Committee-Opinions/Committee-on-Gynecologic-Practice/Tamoxifen-and-Uterine-Cancer (accessed September 2016).
6. Chen LM, Berek J, Endometrial cancer: clinical features and diagnosis. 2016 www.uptodate.com/contents/overview-of-endometrial-carcinoma (accessed September 2016).
7. Bobrowska K, Kaminski P, Cyganek A, et al. High rate of endometrial hyperplasia amongst renal transplanted women. Transplant Proc 2006;38:177–179.
8. Kruman RJ, Carcangiu ML, Herrington CS, Young RH (editors), WHO Classification of Tumours of Female Reproductive Organs, 4th edn. IARC, 2014.
9. Trimble CL, Kauderer J, Zaino R, et al. Concurrent endometrial carcinoma in women with a biopsy diagnosis of endometrial hyperplasia: A Gynecologic Oncology Group Study. Cancer 2006;106:812–819.
10. National Cancer Institute. SEER Stat Fact Sheets: Endometrial Cancer. 2013. seer.cancer.gov/statfacts/html/corp.html (accessed September 2016).
11. American College of Obstetricians and Gynecologists. ACOG practice bulletin: management of endometrial cancer. Obstet Gynaecol 2005;106(65):413.
12. RCOG/BSGE. Best practice in outpatient hysteroscopy. Green-Top Guidance Guideline No. 59. 2011. www.rcog.org.uk/globalassets/documents/guidelines/gtg59hysteroscopy.pdf (accessed September 2016).
13. Scottish Intercollegiate Guidelines Network (SIGN). Investigation of post-menopausal bleeding. SIGN publication no. 61. 2002. http://www.sign.ac.uk/guidelines/fulltext/61/ (accessed September 2016).
14. Royal College of Obstetricians & Gynaecologists. Management of Endometrial hyperplasia. Green-top guideline No.67, RCOG/BSGE joint Guideline, Feb 2016.
15. Terakawa N, Kigawa J, Taketani Y, et al. Endometrial Hyperplasia Study Group. The behaviour of

endometrial hyperplasia: a prospective study. *J Obstet Gynaecol Res* 1997;23:223–230.

16. Gallos ID, Shehmar M, Thangaratinam S, *et al*. Oral progestogens vs levonogestrel-releasing intrauterine system for endometrial hyperplasia: a systematic review and meta-analysis. *Am J Obstet Gynaecol* 2010;203(547):e1–e10.

17. Mourits MJ, Bijen CB, Arts HJ, *et al*. Safety of laparsocopy versus laparotomy in early stage

endometrial cancer: a randomised control trial. *Lancet Oncology* 2010;11:763–771.

18. Epplein M, Reed S, Voigt L, *et al*. Risk of complex and atypical endometrial hyperplasia in relation to anthropometric measures and reproductive history. *Am J Epidemiol* 2008;168(6):563–570.

19. Kruman RJ, Kaminski PF, Norris HJ. The behaviour of endometrial hyperplasia: A long-term study of 'untreated' hyperplasia in 170 patients. *Cancer* 1985;56:403–412.

Chapter 28

The Management of Fibroids in Primary Care

Elizabeth Burt and Ertan Saridogan

Key Points

- Uterine fibroids are common and a significant proportion is asymptomatic.
- Symptoms are usually related to abnormal menstruation, pressure or fertility.
- The aetiology of fibroids is unclear, but is likely to be related to sex steroids, genetics and stem cell biology.
- Submucosal fibroids tend to cause more symptoms compared to intramural and subserosal fibroids.
- Consider referral to secondary/tertiary care when the uterus is palpable abdominally, its length is longer than 12 cm on ultrasound or at hysteroscopy, when there are submucosal fibroids or when there are pressure or fertility symptoms.
- The main diagnostic tools are history, abdominal and pelvic examination, and pelvic ultrasound examination.
- Treatment should be tailored individually based on severity of symptoms, location/size of fibroids, fertility plans and acceptability of the options.
- Medical treatment options include levonorgestrel-releasing intrauterine system 52 mg (LNG- IUS) Mirena®, tranexamic acid, mefenamic acid, combined oral contraceptive pill, ulipristal acetate and gonadotrophin-releasing hormone analogues.
- Combined oral contraceptive pill, Mirena®, tranexamic acid and mefenamic acid can be started in the primary care setting.
- Non-medical options include hysteroscopic or abdominal (open or laparoscopic) myomectomy, uterine artery embolization and hysterectomy.

Case Scenario

Beatrice attends your GP practice. She is a 35-year-old nulliparous Afro-Caribbean lady. She has a long history of heavy periods, which are disrupting her daily life.

Introduction

Fibroids, also known as leiomyomas, are benign tumours of the uterine myometrium. They are extremely common, affecting up to 70–80% of women by the age of menopause [1]. Their high prevalence within the female population coupled with their related symptomatology renders them a source of significant morbidity, accounting for a large proportion of primary care consultations. Fibroids may cause a wide spectrum of clinical presentations with varying severity, making both their diagnosis and management a challenge.

Epidemiology

Fibroids mainly affect women in their reproductive years. With fibroids being rare prior to menarche and known to shrink in size after the menopause, it is thought that oestrogen and progesterone are the driving hormones responsible for fibroid stimulation and maintenance.

Fibroids are common in all ethnicities, however, the prevalence is higher in Afro-Caribbean women, with 60% of women having fibroids detected by the age of 35 increasing to 80% by the age of 49. In contrast, Caucasian women have an incidence of 40% at the age of 35 rising to 70% by the age of 49 [1]. This also highlights that the prevalence of fibroids increases progressively with age from puberty to menopause, with the peak age being the fifth decade. Afro-Caribbean women also have a distinctive natural history of fibroids, with fibroids occurring at an earlier age, being more numerous and clinically more apparent in comparison to their Caucasian counterparts.

Other risk factors increasing the susceptibility of uterine fibroids include environments with heightened and prolonged oestrogen and progesterone exposure. This would include early menarche, with later menarche appearing protective. In addition, increasing parity is also protective against fibroid development. Obesity, which is associated with a hyperoestrogenic state, due to increased adipose production of oestrogen, is associated with an increased risk of fibroids, as is polycystic ovary syndrome [2–4].

Histology and Aetiology

Fibroids are benign monoclonal tumours of the smooth muscle. The typical histological appearance is of spheres of myometrial cells nesting within increased amounts of extracellular matrix [4]. Alternative histological appearances may be apparent when fibroids undergo degeneration and this may occur when they outgrow their vascularity and undergo infarction and necrosis.

Fibroids range in size and can be solitary or occur in clusters. Most classically they occur within or around the uterine myometrium, but more rarely may be situated extra-uterine in the cervix, broad ligament or be peritoneal.

The aetiology of fibroids is still largely elusive, but is likely to be multifactorial. The growth of fibroids has been linked to sex steroids, genetics and stem cell biology.

Classification

Fibroids are classified according to their location within the myometrium. This in turn may be correlated to their clinical significance and their associated symptomatology, and is vital for the planning and recommendation of treatment strategies.

Submucosal

Submucosal fibroids (Figure 28.1a) are the least common of the fibroids, representing just 5%. Due to their position, these are most likely to cause the most

bothersome clinical symptoms, such as abnormal uterine bleeding (AUB) and fertility difficulties. Less frequently they may prolapse into the cervical canal or vagina.

These can be further subdivided depending on the degree of their projection within the endometrial cavity. Type 0 submucosal fibroids are polyp-like and are completely within the uterine cavity. Type 1 fibroids have less than 50% of the fibroid within the myometrium, whilst type 2 have more than 50% within the myometrium. This classification is particularly helpful when planning endoscopic surgical treatment.

Intramural

Intramural fibroids are located within the myometrium, and although they are the most common type of fibroids, they are less likely to manifest symptoms unless they are large (Figure 28.1b).

Subserosal

Subserosal fibroids are situated within the myometrium under the uterine serosa (Figure 28.1c). These are the least likely to cause symptoms. These tend to be related to pressure symptoms, but are only problematic if large.

Pedunculated

Pedunculated fibroids are connected to the uterus by a stalk and may cause pressure symptoms or cause acute pain as a result of torsion (Figure 28.1d).

Presentation

Fibroids produce a heterogeneous array of symptoms. The majority of women are asymptomatic, with an incidental diagnosis being made during ultrasound or surgery for other indications. Fibroids, however, may cause extreme symptoms, with significant impact on quality of life (Table 28.1). Symptoms attributable to fibroids may be related to their position within the endometrial cavity, their sheer size or from their effect on endometrial milieu and function. The symptoms can be grouped as menstrual disturbances, pressure symptoms and impact on fertility.

History

Specific questions in the *history* should include:

- Acute or chronic heavy menstrual bleeding (HMB)
- Intermenstrual or postcoital bleeding

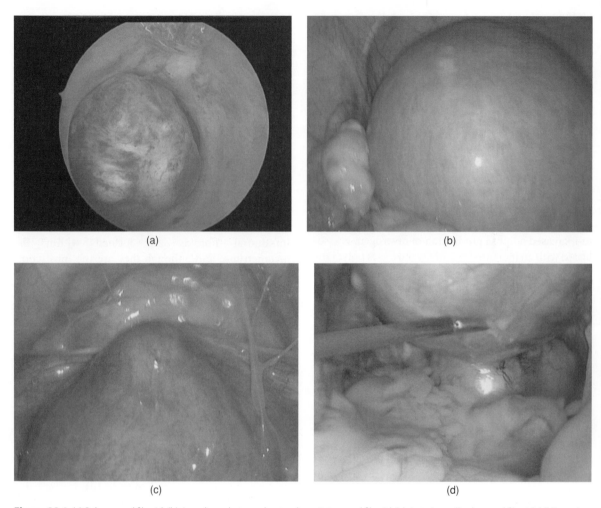

Figure 28.1 (a) Submucosal fibroid. (b) An enlarged uterus due to a large intramural fibroid. (c) Anterior wall subserosal fibroid. (d) Posterior wall pedunculated fibroid. (For the colour version, please refer to the plate section.)

- Dysmenorrhoea
- Urinary symptoms (frequency, nocturia, incontinence)
- Bowel symptoms (constipation, pressure on rectum)
- Palpable or visible abdominal mass
- Fertility desires

Table 28.1 Symptoms associated with fibroids

- 1. HMB
- 2. Urinary frequency, nocturia
- 3. Pelvic mass
- 4. Pain
- 5. Dyspareunia
- 6. Constipation
- 7. Subfertility

- Smear history
- Impact on quality of life.

Examination

An abdominal examination may reveal a palpable or even visible mass, which is often described as having a knobbly consistency. A bimanual vaginal examination may be necessary to further assess the size of the uterus, which is commonly documented in relation to the size of a gravid uterus.

HMB and Dysmenorrhoea

This is the most common presentation, with HMB affecting 64% of women with fibroids [5]. These symptoms are most commonly attributed to submucous fibroids, but may also be seen with larger intramural fibroids, or when the overall uterine size is very large.

Chronic heavy cyclical uterine bleeding may be as a result of the disruption of the endometrium or alternately, it has been postulated that fibroids have a direct effect on endometrial function, affecting both decidualization and haemostasis.

Sequale from heavy menstrual bleeding includes both anaemia and, in addition, may cause psychological implications if it affects and restricts a woman's day-to-day life.

A history of HMB may be obtained, but it is important to recognize that postcoital bleeding and intermenstrual bleeding are not classical features of fibroids and caution should be exercised [6]. Furthermore, the longevity of the HMB is an important factor. Acute menorrhagia starting over the age of 45 should prompt alarm bells and referral should be made for further endometrial assessment to rule out other conditions such as endometrial hyperplasia and cancer.

To exclude significant anaemia a full blood count (FBC) should be considered, especially if any signs (pallor) or symptoms of anaemia (tiredness, shortness of breath, dizziness) are disclosed.

Pelvic Mass

Due to the size of the fibroids women may present with the feeling of a pelvic or abdominal 'lump' that may have gradually increased in size over a number of years.

The growth of fibroids tends to be slow and the rare instance of leiomyosarcoma should be considered in a rapidly growing mass, although the vast majority of fast-growing fibroids are benign.

Pain and Pressure Symptoms

Large subserosal fibroids may result in many pressure symptoms secondary to their compression of adjacent pelvic structures. This includes:

- Lumbar and sacral nerve trunks resulting in chronic pelvic pain
- Bladder and ureters causing urinary symptoms (frequency and nocturia) and less frequently hydronephrosis
- Rectum leading to constipation
- Cervix producing dyspareunia
- Inferior vena cava and pelvic veins with subsequent vascular stasis leading to increased

susceptibility to the development of deep vein thrombosis.

Acute abdominal pain may be related to pedunculated subserosal fibroids. These may undergo torsion with subsequent infarction.

Subfertility

The majority of women with fibroids are fertile, but the relative risk of conception, implantation and successful ongoing pregnancy is lower in the presence of fibroids. Compounding the detrimental impact of fibroids on fertility further is their association with increased risk of miscarriage [7]. This is apparent in both spontaneous and assisted-conception pregnancies. It would seem intuitive that submucous fibroids which distort the cavity would be primarily responsibility for this effect, however it also appears that intramural fibroids reproduce this correlation, which may in part be related to their compression of the fallopian tubes, affecting gamete transfer or the effect on uterine blood flow. In contrast, subserosal fibroids are less likely to impact fertility outcomes, although with any type of large fibroids there may be significant distortion to the pelvic anatomy affecting the relationship between the fallopian tubes and ovaries, resulting in compromised ovum capture and gamete/embryo transport.

Sarcoma

Uterine sarcoma is a rare cancer and is frequently a histological diagnosis made posthysterectomy. More common in postmenopausal women, the majority are *de novo* lesions, and only 1:700 (0.14%) of presumed benign fibroids are indeed leiomyosarcomas [8]. As this is a rarity, diagnosis may pose a challenge and depends on excellent clinical acumen and a high index of suspicion in those women, especially postmenopausal, presenting with a pelvic mass, which had enlarged rapidly.

Obstetric

It is important to reiterate to women that the majority of those with fibroids experience an entirely normal pregnancy. Albeit, in pregnancy, fibroids tend to grow rapidly and may be associated with acute pain, malpresentation and postpartum haemorrhage, with complications occurring in 10–40% of women with fibroids [9]. It is thought that the size of the fibroids may be

Table 28.2 Alarm symptoms in gynaecological presentation

- Acute menorrhagia > 45 years
- Intermenstrual bleeding
- Postcoital bleeding
- New rapid growing pelvic mass
- Features of cancer – unexplained weight loss
- Pelvic mass (not fibroid)

Table 28.3 When to refer women with fibroids to secondary care

- Fibroids palpable abdominally
- Submucosal fibroids
- Alarm symptoms
- Medical management has failed
- Uterine length is greater than 12 cm on ultrasound or at hysteroscopy
- Pressure symptoms
- Fertility/obstetric problems

proportionally related to the chance of complications, however often women with very large fibroids have no difficulties.

With an increase in endogenous oestrogen, pregnancy is associated with promotion of fibroid growth. This may lead to degeneration causing acute pain during pregnancy. Malpresentation, especially breech, which is more common in the presence of fibroids, is in turn associated with an exponential risk of caesarean section. Abnormal uterine contractility has been implicated in the role of fibroids and postpartum haemorrhage.

See Tables 28.2 and 28.3.

> **Case Scenario**
>
> Beatrice has a very clear history of chronic HMB with no other worrying symptoms. On examination, a bulky uterus can be palpated just above the pubic symphysis, approximately 14-week pregnancy size.
> You organize a pelvic ultrasound and FBC.

Diagnosis

From a thorough history and examination, fibroids can be highly suspected and empirical medical treatment may be considered in primary care. An ultrasound should be arranged to confirm the diagnosis and plan further management and/or referral. Fibroid mapping is the detection and delineation of their classification, size and number.

Ultrasound

Ultrasound examination is the mainstay of diagnosis, with transvaginal ultrasound having a sensitivity of 100% and specificity of 94% for the detection of submucous fibroids; coupled with good patient acceptability, this is now the first-line investigation [10].

Fibroids classically appear as well-circumscribed hypoechoic lesions. Due to their histological makeup they have a typical 'whorled' appearance and acoustic shadowing is seen.

Subserous fibroids distort the external uterine contour, whilst submucous fibroids protrude into the endometrial cavity. In order to aid the diagnosis of submucous fibroids and their differentiation from an endometrial polyp, either three-dimensional ultrasound or saline infusion sonohysterography may be employed.

Sarcomatous changes are neither well described nor specific, therefore making their diagnosis problematic. Uterine sarcomas tend to be large (> 8 cm), have less defined demarcation, may exhibit foci of haemorrhage or necrosis and have amplified vascularity [8].

MRI

MRI is often not a prerequisite for fibroid diagnosis, the exception being when it is indicated prior to complex surgery or if fibroids are suspected in more rare locations. MRI is also advantageous to assess the suitability for and predict success of uterine artery embolization. For fibroid detection, MRI demonstrates a sensitivity of 88–93% and a specificity of 66–91% [11].

> **Case Scenario**
>
> Beatrice's transvaginal ultrasound demonstrated a 3 cm type 1 submucosal fibroid. The FBC was normal. Referral to secondary care is required due to the presence of a submucosal fibroid. In the interim, she would like to discuss possible treatment to alleviate her HMB.

Treatment Options

The majority of asymptomatic fibroids do not warrant treatment. Optimal treatment and patient satisfaction are dependent on tailored therapeutic strategies. Factors to enable this include:

- Symptoms
- Size and position of fibroids
- Age

- Patient wishes
- Fertility desires.

Surgery remains the only definitive curative treatment for fibroids; however, due to the inherent risks of surgery, this is not acceptable to many women and thankfully many other options exist to circumvent the immediate need for surgery.

Expectant Management

The natural history of fibroids is not well established, with the growth of fibroids being both variable and unpredictable. For women who have non-troublesome small, non-intracavitary fibroids, a conservative approach should be advocated [12].

Counselling women with regards to the conceivable future risks associated with their fibroids can be a clinical challenge. It has been found that the largest fibroid may have a 35% volume increase per year, but equally up to one-fifth of fibroids may become smaller [13]. Fibroid growth may be correlated to their initial size at presentation and their position. Higher growth rate is associated with fibroids measuring less than 20 mm and greater than 50 mm and those that are intramural [13].

Women who are approaching menopausal age may wish to delay treatment as with menopause fibroids shrink, with associated symptoms diminishing.

Medical Management

Medical management can be further categorized into symptom relief and that used as an adjunct prior to surgery.

Levonorgestrel-Releasing Intrauterine System (LNG-IUS) Mirena®

Marketed in the UK as Mirena®, the LNG-IUS is the preferred choice as first-line treatment for HMB in women who are not trying to get pregnant. It provides local release of progestogens, which, in turn suppresses endometrial growth. LNG-IUS may reduce the bleeding by 90%, and up to 20% of women may be amenorrhoeic after 12 months. In addition to being highly efficacious for HMB, it delivers reliable long-term contraception and it is licenced for up to five years' use.

LNG-IUS has specific beneficial effects on fibroid-related bleeding and a positive effect is witnessed on fibroid size reduction [14]. NICE recommend LNG-IUS only in the presence of fibroids less than 3 cm, but in clinical practice it is often used in the presence of bigger fibroids.

The main disadvantage of Mirena® cited by many women is the irregular bleeding, which may be troublesome for the first six months, and other progesterone-related side effects might be described. In the presence of submucous fibroids, fitting may be difficult or impossible and together with a large uterine cavity, expulsion may be more common, therefore LNG-IUS is less effective in women with large/multiple and submucosal fibroids.

Combined Oral Contraceptive Pill (COCP)

The COCP has been an established form of contraception for the last 50 years and, more recently, additional benefits have also come to light, making the COCP an attractive choice of treatment for a multitude of gynaecological conditions. Specifically, for use in HMB, the COCP reduces the production of gonadotrophins, inhibits folliculogenesis and, in turn, prevents endometrial proliferation. Once thought to be linked to fibroid growth, this fear has now been allayed and on the contrary, the COCP may be associated with a 17% reduction in growth [5]. Correspondingly the COCP delivers an overall 50% reduction in menstrual blood loss, including that attributable to fibroids [15].

Tranexamic Acid and NSAIDs

For women wishing to avoid hormonal/contraceptive preparations, the combination of mefenamic acid and tranexamic acid is often prescribed. Mefenamic acid is a non-steroidal anti-inflammatory drug (NSAID), which inhibits prostaglandin synthesis, and tranexamic acid is a plasminogen activator inhibitor, which acts as an antifibrinolytic agent.

Often a trial of three months is suggested, and mefenamic and tranexamic acid have been shown to reduce menstrual blood flow by 25% and 50%, respectively. Used solely at the time of menstruation, both are generally well tolerated. They may be used individually, in combination or in parallel to other treatment, such as LNG-IUS.

Selective Progesterone Receptor Modulators (SPRMs)

These are exogenous progesterone receptor peptides with a mixed agonist/antagonist ligand profile dependent on their target tissue. This allows a directed response, whilst concurrently minimizing side effects.

With fibroids being hormone sensitive, blockage of the progesterone receptor causes their shrinkage. Ulipristal acetate (UPA), trade name Esmya®, was initially licensed only for preoperative treatment; however, unlike gonadotrophin-releasing hormone analogues (GnRHa), which have limited long-term use, intermittent UPA may provide a long-term pharmacological option, which offers good patient tolerability. UPA is now licensed for long-term intermittent medical treatment of fibroids.

UPA has been shown to reduce both menorrhagia, with improvement seen in 98% of women and amenorrhoea occurring in up to 90%, and a reduction in fibroid size by 72% after four treatment courses. Unlike GnRHa, UPA causes a longer sustained effect on fibroid size, even six months post a three-month course of treatment [16,17].

UPA has minimal adverse effects, however concerns were initially raised with regards to sustained use of UPA and its prolonged effect on the endometrium. UPA may induce changes mimicking endometrial hyperplasia. This has been coined progesterone-associated endometrial changes (PAEC) and clinicians need to be aware of this to avoid both misdiagnosis and patient anxiety.

UPA may be given in a daily oral dose of 5 mg and can be used for three months preoperatively or used in a repeated intermittent dose regime (up to four courses have been studied). In both scenarios, UPA should be started with menstruation. With retreatment UPA should recommence after a two menses break.

Surgical Pretreatment

To facilitate surgical management, concurrent medical treatment may be clinically warranted in the preoperative planning period. The intended benefits are reduction in bleeding, optimization of haemoglobin, to permit a less invasive surgical route and to overall lessen surgical morbidity risk.

GnRHa

GnRHa are synthetic molecules which block the GnRH receptor at the level of the pituitary, thereby modifying the release of FSH and LH. Initially causing an elevated level of release there is subsequent down-regulation and hypogonadotrophism. This simulates a temporary menopausal state. Deprived of the stimulatory effect of oestradiol and progesterone, amenorrhoea occurs and fibroid regression is observed, which can be in the order of 50% volume reduction.

The side effect profile of GnRHa is comparable to an artificial menopause with hot flushes, vaginal dryness, mood swings and bone density loss. This, therefore, restricts its continuing usage and currently can only be used for six months. An alternative to prevent these side effects is to use concomitant add-back therapy; however, this combination is less efficacious in the context of fibroid volume reduction and does not fully mitigate the side effects. The side effects, except osteoporosis with more than six months' usage, are transitory complaints and fully reversible on cessation of the medication; equally fibroids tend to regrow posttreatment within approximately three months.

Summary of Medical Options

See Table 28.4.

Case Scenario

After full discussion, Beatrice was not keen on hormonal preparations and decided to try the combination of tranexamic acid and mefenamic acid. This has reduced her bleeding to a more manageable level. She is subsequently seen in secondary care and counselled regarding further treatment options.

Uterine Artery Embolization (UAE)

Uterine artery embolization (UAE) is a minimally invasive, surgery-sparing, commonplace technique. This is a percutaneous procedure performed by interventional radiologists. A catheter is inserted into the femoral artery and, using x-ray, the uterine arteries are injected with an embolic agent. This in turn induces avascular necrosis within the fibroids.

Patient satisfaction postprocedure is high, with an associated 40–70% reduction in fibroid volume and 80–90% of patients having significant symptom relief after one year [18]. Results are comparable to both hysterectomy and myomectomy, but in favour of UAE, this is associated with shorter hospital stay and is overall more cost effective [19–21].

Although UAE is considered both safe and efficacious, women should be fully aware of the fact that fibroid shrinkage is not permanent and up to one-third of women may require further treatment [22].

Table 28.4 Medical management of fibroids

Pharmacological agent	Mechanism of action	Reduction in menorrhagia	Reduction in fibroid growth	Side effects
LNG –IUS Mirena®	Prevents endometrial proliferation	90%	Reduction in uterine volume	• Irregular bleeding • Expulsion • Progesterone effects • Ovarian cysts
Tranexamic acid	Antifibrinolytic	50%		• Gastrointestinal effects
Mefenamic acid	Inhibits prostaglandin synthesis	25%		• Gastrointestinal effects
COCP	Inhibits folliculogenesis, ovulation and induces endometrial atrophy	50%	17%	• Thromboembolic events • Break through bleeding • Progesterone effects
GnRHa	Down regulation at pituitary levels reducing gonadotrophin release	Amenorrhoeic during treatment	50%	• Menopausal symptoms • Bone demineralization
Ulipristal acetate	Selective progesterone receptor modulation	98% improvement 90% amenorrhoea	72%	• PAEC • Headache and breast tenderness

In addition, although complications of UAE are rare, they include premature ovarian failure (1%), which is more common in those over the age of 45, postembolization syndrome and the need for urgent hysterectomy.

Desire for pregnancy was once considered a relative contraindication as UAE was thought to affect endometrial blood flow, which in turn may affect implantation and placentation, nevertheless successful pregnancies have been reported after UAE. Although data are minimal, the consensus is that UAE is associated with an increased rate of miscarriage compared to untreated fibroids and myomectomy (35% vs 17% vs 23%). Caesarean section delivery and postpartum haemorrhage are also higher post-UAE. Reassuringly other pregnancy outcomes, namely intrauterine growth restriction, malpresentation and preterm delivery are not amplified after UAE [23]. Due to potential impact on fertility and pregnancy outcomes, many clinicians do not offer UAE as a first-line treatment for fibroids in women planning to become pregnant in the future.

Surgical Management

Surgical intervention may be indicated in a variety of circumstances:

- Failure of medical treatment
- Large fibroids
- Pressure symptoms
- Intracavitary fibroids
- Patient wishes.

Hysterectomy is obviously contraindicated in those wishing to conceive and therefore other uterus-preserving surgical options exist.

Myomectomy

Myomectomy, which is the surgical removal of fibroids with preservation of the normal myometrium, can be further classified depending on the surgical route employed. Preoperative treatment with GnRHa or UPA may be recommended.

Transcervical Resection of Fibroids (TCRF)

Submucous fibroids, which are predominately intracavitary, i.e. type 0, type 1 and some type 2, are amenable to resection via the vaginal route with hysteroscopy. Subject to the size of the fibroids, this may be carried out under general or local anaesthesia. This is a relatively short procedure and well tolerated with a reduction in bleeding in 90% of patients [11]. Potential complications include haemorrhage, infection, uterine perforation, irrigation fluid overload and intrauterine adhesions.

Pertinent to fertility, the elimination of submucosal fibroids appears to enhance conception and reduce miscarriage rates [7].

Open/Laparoscopy Myomectomy

Abdominal myomectomy can be either open (laparotomy) or via laparoscopy. With the advent of morcellation, even large fibroids can be treated laparoscopically with the associated benefits of minimal access surgery.

Hysterectomy

This is the only option that conveys symptom relief with no possibility of fibroid recurrence. Hysterectomy may be completed through the abdominal, vaginal or laparoscopic route, a decision that will depend on the preoperative size and location of the fibroids and experience of the surgeon.

Hysterectomy is only an option for women who have completed their family with no desire for further fertility and may not be suitable for women who have significant surgical risks.

Case Scenario

After further consultation in secondary care, given Beatrice's principal complaint of HMB in the presence of an intracavitary fibroid, a TCRF was advised. This was performed as a day case with excellent postoperative recovery.

References

1. Baird D, Dunson D, Hill M, Cousins D, Schectman JM, High cumulative incidence of uterine leiomyoma in black and white women: ultrasound evidence. *Am J Obstet Gynecol* 2003;188(1):100–107.

2. Valez Edwards D, Baird D, Hartmann K, Association of age at menarche with increasing number of fibroids in a cohort of women who underwent standardized ultrasound assessment. *Am J Epidemiol* 2013;178(3):426–433.

3. Baird D, Dunson D, Why is parity protective for uterine fibroids? *Epidemiology* 2003;14(2):247–250.

4. Chabbert-Buffet N, Esber N, Bouchard P, Fibroid growth and medical options for treatment. *Fertil Steril* 2014;102(3):630–639.

5. Moroni R, Vieira C, Ferriani R, Candido-dos-Reis F, Brito L, Pharmacological treatment of uterine fibroids. *Ann Med Health Sci Res* 2014;4(Suppl 3):S185–S192.

6. National Institute for Health and Care Excellence Heavy menstrual bleeding: Assessment and management. NICE clinical guideline 44. www.guidance.nice.org.uk/cg44 (accessed September 2016).

7. Pritts E, Parker W, Olive D, Fibroids and infertility: an updated systematic review of the evidence. *Fertil Steril.* 2009; 91(4):1215–1223.

8. Brölmann H, Tanos V, Grimbizis G, *et al.* Options on fibroid morcellation: a literature review. *Gynecol Surg* 2015;12(1):3–15.

9. Guo X, Segars J, The impact and management of fibroids for fertility: an evidence-based approach. *Obstet Gynecol Clin North Am* 2012;39(4):521–533.

10. Uterine fibroids. *BMJ Best Practice.* http://bestpractice.bmj.com/best-practice/monograph/567.html.

11. Khan A, Shehmar M, Gupta J, Uterine fibroids: current perspectives. *Int J Women's Health* 2014;29;6:95–114.

12. National Institute for Health and Care Excellence. Fibroids. Clinical Knowledge Summaries. 2013. cks.nice.org.uk/fibroids (accessed September 2016).

13. Mavrelos D, Ben-Nagi J, Holland T, *et al.* The natural history of fibroids. *Ultrasound Obstet Gynecol* 2010;35(2):238–242.

14. Sangkomkamhang U, Lumbiganon P, Laopaiboon M, Progestogens or progestogen-releasing intrauterine systems for uterine fibroids. *Cochrane Database Syst Rev.* 2013;(2):CD008994.

15. Gupta S, Non-contraceptive benefits of the combined oral contraceptive pill. *TOG* 2013;15(2):138–139.

16. Donnez J, Hudecek R, Donnez O, *et al.* Efficacy and safety of repeated use of ulipristal acetate in uterine fibroids. *Fertil Steril* 2015;103(2):519–527.

17. Trefoux Bourdet A, Luton D, Koskas M, Clinical utility of ulipristal acetate for the treatment of uterine fibroids: current evidence. *Int J Women's Health* 2015;26;7:321–330.

18. Royal College of Obstetricians and Gynaecologists. Clinical recommendations of the use of uterine artery embolization (UAE) in the management of fibroids. 2013. www.rcog.org.uk/globalassets/documents/guidelines/23-12-2013_rcog_rcr_uae.pdf (accessed September 2016).

19. Pinto I, Chimeno P, Romo A, *et al.* Uterine fibroids: uterine artery embolization versus abdominal hysterectomy for treatment–a prospective, randomized, and controlled clinical trial. *Radiology* 2003;226(2):425–431.

20. Mara M, Maskova J, Fucikova Z, *et al.* Midterm clinical and first reproductive results of a randomized controlled trial comparing uterine fibroid embolization and myomectomy. *Cardiovasc Intervent Radiol* 2008;31(1):73–85.

21. Manyonda I, Bratby M, Horst J, *et al.* Uterine artery embolization versus myomectomy: impact on quality of life: Results of the FUME (Fibroids of the Uterus:

Myomectomy versus Embolization) Trial. *Cardiovasc Intervent Radiol* 2012;35(3):530–536.

22. Moss J, Cooper K, Khaund A, *et al.* Randomised comparison of uterine artery embolisation (UAE) with surgical treatment in patients with symptomatic

uterine fibroids (REST trial): 5-year results. *BJOG* 2011;118(8):936–944.

23. Homer H, Saridogan E, Uterine artery embolization for fibroids is associated with an increased risk of miscarriage. *Fertil Steril* 2010;94(1):324–330.

Chapter 29

Osteoporosis and Fracture Prevention in Primary Care

Pam Brown

Key Points

- Osteoporosis is important because of the fractures it causes. These are responsible for increased mortality and morbidity, and reduced mobility, independence and quality of life.
- All women (and men) with fragility fractures have increased future fracture risk and need further assessment (fracture liaison services (FLS) may assess and initiate treatment).
- Fracture risk increases with age; those over 80 are likely to have osteoporosis and be at high risk.
- Women treated with steroids or aromatase inhibitors are at risk of rapid bone loss. Treatment may be appropriate at higher bone mineral density (BMD).
- QFracture and FRAX risk assessment tools allow calculation of absolute 10-year fracture risk.
- SIGN guideline 142 summarizes the evidence base for bone-sparing drug treatments.
- Adherence and persistence with therapies are poor and benefit from regular review and support from primary care.

Osteoporosis is important because of the fractures it causes. These are responsible for increased mortality and morbidity, and reduced mobility, independence and quality of life.

Osteoporosis is a 'disease characterized by low bone mass and structural deterioration of bone tissue with increase in susceptibility to fragility fracture.' Fragility fractures are fractures which result from mechanical forces that would not normally cause a fracture, for example those caused by a fall from standing height or less, or by normal activities such as lifting a shopping bag or turning over in bed.

Osteoporosis is diagnosed using a dual energy x-ray absorptiometry (DXA) scan to measure bone mineral density (BMD) at the femoral neck and lumbar spine. A T score of ≤-2.5 standard deviations defines osteoporosis; a T score of -1 to -2.5 represents osteopenia or bone thinning, and a T score >-1 is normal.

Common sites for fragility fractures include the wrist, spine, hip and humerus, although any bone can be affected. Fractures of the hands, feet and skull are not included as fragility fractures.

In the UK each year there are around 300,000 fragility fractures including 70,000 hip fractures. Although fragility fractures are more likely in those with osteoporosis, around 70% actually occur in those without osteoporosis, mainly those with osteopenia. This makes it difficult to know where to target treatment to prevent first fractures. However, people who have sustained one fragility fracture are at increased risk of additional fractures. Although fragility fractures are more common in women, they also affect 1 in 12 men during their lifetime.

Getting Started on Fracture Prevention

The steps in diagnosing and managing osteoporosis and preventing fractures are:

- Identify who is at risk
- Quantify risk using risk-assessment tools
- Arrange DXA scan when appropriate
- Exclude underlying/secondary causes
- Decide who needs treatment
- Treat
- Ensure adherence and persistence with therapy
- Reassess after three to five years' treatment.

Women's Health in Primary Care, edited by Anne Connolly and Amanda Britton. Published by Cambridge University Press
© Cambridge University Press 2017

Identify Who is at Risk

Non-modifiable factors increasing fracture risk include: previous fracture, parental history of osteoporosis, early menopause (<45 years). Modifiable risk factors include: BMI <20, smoking, low bone density, alcohol intake, steroid or aromatase inhibitor treatment. Remember that those who fall are at increased risk of fractures – always ask about and code falls, and refer for full falls assessment, and gait and balance training if available.

NICE *Osteoporosis: assessing the risk of fragility fracture* guideline [1], the *Fragility fracture risk assessment pathway* [2] and NICE Clinical Knowledge Summary [3] segregate people by age and risk factors:

- Age <40 with major risk factors (multiple fragility fractures, major osteoporotic fracture (clinical vertebral, forearm, hip, shoulder), current or recent high-dose oral steroids (>7.5 mg prednisolone daily for three months or longer):
  - Use DXA to evaluate fracture risk
- Age 40–49 years with major risk factors:
  - consider risk assessment using FRAX/ Qfracture
- Women 50–64 (men 50–74) with risk factors (fragility fracture, oral steroids, falls, FH of hip fracture, secondary osteoporosis, BMI <18.5, smoker, alcohol >14 units per week):
  - consider risk assessment using FRAX/Qfracture
- Women ≥65 (men ≥75)
  - Consider risk assessment for all using FRAX/Qfracture.

NICE has issued a 'Do not do' recommendation: 'Do not routinely measure bone mineral density (BMD) to assess fracture risk without prior assessment using FRAX (without a BMD value) or Qfracture' (Figure 29.1).

SIGN 142 guideline [3] (Figure 29.2) recommends QFracture use and offers slightly different guidance from NICE for the following groups:

- People over 50 with a previous fragility fracture should be offered DXA scanning (NICE – fracture risk assessment first)
- Consider fracture risk assessment for people over 50 with:

  - parental history of osteoporosis, untreated early menopause, more than 3.5 units of alcohol daily, BMI <20, institutionalized people with epilepsy, neurological disease such as Alzheimer's, Parkinson's disease, MS and stroke, severe kidney disease (eGFR< 60), asthma, antidepressants especially SSRIs, proton pump inhibitors and pioglitazone

- Women over 50 taking aromatase inhibitors should undergo risk assessment (NICE – direct referral for DXA).

Quantify Risk

Two UK-validated fracture risk assessment tools, QFracture and the World Health Organisation's FRAX calculator (Figure 29.3), combine different risk factors to calculate individual absolute 10-year risk of hip or major osteoporotic (clinical vertebral, forearm, hip, shoulder) fracture, in the same way that QRisk calculates 10-year absolute risk of cardiovascular disease. These help target DXA scanning and drug treatment appropriately.

The link from the FRAX calculator to the National Osteoporosis Guideline Group (NOGG) guidance [4] graph (Figure 29.3) allows easy assessment of who needs DXA and who may benefit from treatment.

There are differences between QFracture and FRAX, summarized in Table 29.1.

When a decision is made to undertake a risk assessment using one of the tools:

- Estimate absolute 10-year fracture risk using FRAX without BMD, or Qfracture
- Consider factors that may affect accuracy (risk underestimated if multiple fractures, vertebral fracture, high-dose steroids or additional secondary causes)
- Undertake DXA if appropriate; recalculate 10-year risk using FRAX with BMD
- If no intervention required, recalculate fracture risk after two years, if risk factors change or if fracture occurs.

DXA Scan

When the FRAX calculator is used it links to the NOGG graphs where fracture risk is plotted against age. When using FRAX without BMD, the NOGG graph (see Figure 29.3) makes recommendations for

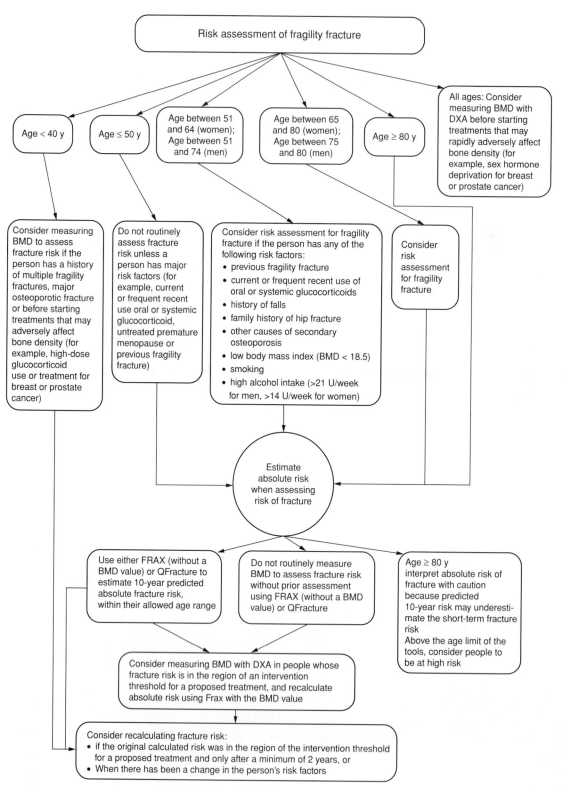

Figure 29.1 NICE Fragility fracture risk assessment algorithm.

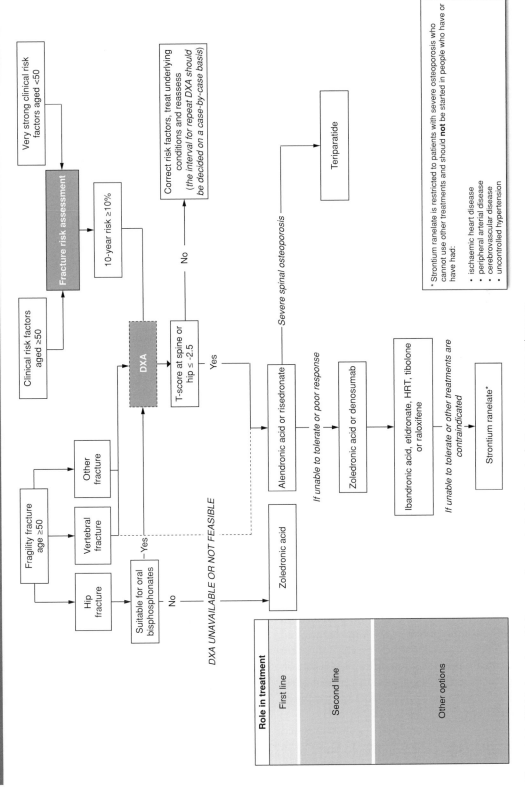

Figure 29.2 SIGN Pathway from risk factors to pharmacological treatment selection in postmenopausal women.

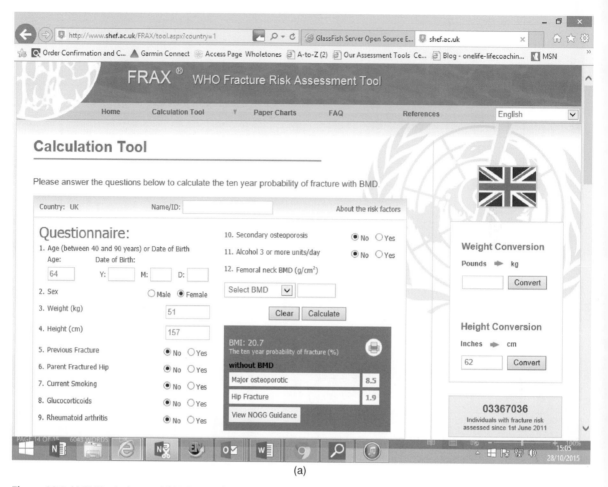

(a)

Figure 29.3 (a) FRAX calculator and (b) NOGG guidance graph.

lifestyle advice only, drug treatment or DXA to further quantify fracture risk.

When using Qfracture, SIGN and NICE propose undertaking DXA if the 10-year fracture risk is close to 10%. If DXA confirms osteoporosis (T ≤–2.5), then drug treatment should be considered.

Local DXA scanning units provide guidance on who should be scanned based on these guidelines, and recommend intervals for monitoring scans if these are available. Provide as much information as possible on the referral form, as this, together with a patient questionnaire, will inform the clinical report and treatment recommendations.

SIGN does not recommend starting therapy based on clinical risk factors alone, even in those >75, unless they have had vertebral fracture(s), while NICE suggests it may be appropriate to start therapy in

women >75 without DXA if there is a high risk of osteoporosis and the scan is inappropriate or impractical. SIGN recommends use of intravenous zoledronate in postmenopausal women (but not men) with hip fracture who are unable to take oral treatments, without a DXA scan if this is deemed to be inappropriate or impractical.

DXA scans are also required for some women who are reassessed after three to five years on treatment.

Exclude Secondary Causes

Conditions which may increase risk of osteoporosis and fractures include [3]:

- Endocrine – hypogonadism (untreated premature menopause), hypothyroidism, hyperparathyroidism, hyperprolactinaemia, Cushing's, diabetes

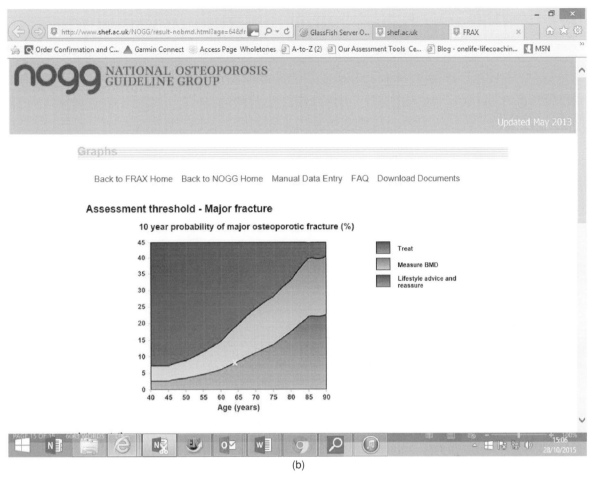

(b)

Figure 29.3 (*cont.*)

- Gastrointestinal – coeliac disease, inflammatory bowel disease, chronic liver disease, chronic pancreatitis, malabsorption
- Rheumatological – rheumatoid arthritis and inflammatory arthropathies
- Haematological – multiple myeloma, haemoglobinopathies, systemic mastocytosis
- Respiratory – cystic fibrosis, COPD
- Chronic renal disease
- Immobility.

Before starting osteoporosis treatment ensure untreated secondary causes of osteoporosis and fracture have been identified and treated. Investigations might include:

- FBC and C reactive protein
- Renal and hepatic function tests
- Bone profile

- Myeloma screen including protein electrophoresis and urine for Bence Jones protein
- Transglutaminase (TTG) for coeliac disease
- Testosterone or androgen profile if appropriate.

Around 50% of men with osteoporosis have a secondary cause. In people with vertebral fractures, it is important to exclude bony metastatic deposits and multiple myeloma – this may require further imaging, e.g. isotope bone scan.

Decide Who Needs Treatment and Treat [3,5,6]

When the FRAX calculator is used with femoral neck BMD added, the link to the NOGG graph provides recommendations for drug treatment or lifestyle advice only.

Table 29.1 QFracture and FRAX scores compared

	FRAX	QFracture
Availability	Open access web-based www.shef.ac.uk/FRAX/index.aspx data entry required	Calculation from practice clinical computer system
Age range	40–90 years	30–99 years
Risk factors	Age, sex, BMI, previous fracture, parental hip fracture, smoking, steroid use, RA, secondary osteoporosis (diabetes, osteogenesis imperfecta, untreated hyperthyroidism, hypogonadism, premature menopause, chronic malnutrition, malabsorption, chronic liver disease), three or more units/day alcohol intake	As for FRAX (except BMD) + quantity cigarettes and alcohol, ethnicity, anticonvulsants, CVD, falls, antidepressants, more secondary osteoporosis conditions, care/nursing home residence
Risks calculated	Hip fracture and other major osteoporotic fracture risk	Same
Time period	10 years	1 to 10 years
Interpretation	Link to NOGG website graph with guidance on DXA/treatment thresholds	SIGN threshold for DXA 10%; treatment less clear
DXA	Use with/without femoral neck BMD	Cannot incorporate BMD measurement
Assessment when on treatment	Validated	Not currently recommended
Additional comments	Recommended by NICE and NOGG May overestimate risk in younger women with fracture; may underestimate short-term risk in those >80. Underestimates vertebral fractures – many asymptomatic	Recommended by SIGN and NICE Validated extensively in UK. Underestimates vertebral fractures – many asymptomatic

Guidelines recommend drug therapy for those with osteoporosis (T score at hip or spine ≤−2.5) although the BMD threshold for treatment is higher in those on aromatase inhibitors for breast cancer (T ≤−2.0) and for those on oral steroids.

Non-Drug Therapies

SIGN recommendations are summarized in Table 29.2.

Drug Treatment

NICE published Technology Appraisals (TA) 160 and 161 in 2008 providing guidance on primary and secondary prevention of osteoporotic fragility fractures in post-menopausal women [5,6]. These are in the process of being updated. Since publication, use of strontium ranelate has been restricted by the European Medicine Agency guidance in 2011.

Alendronate or risedronate are recommended as first-line therapy for those with osteoporosis (T score ≤ −2.5) by UK guidelines. NICE TA 160/161 proposed that in those intolerant of alendronate or etidronate, other oral drugs (risedronate, raloxifene and strontium) should only be used at lower BMD levels and with increased risk factors. However, real-world use

differs. Having explained the need for treatment to prevent a first or subsequent fracture, it is not appropriate to deny treatment because of intolerance to first-line therapy.

SIGN Guideline 142 [3] provides a summary of the evidence for each management option and readers are advised to consult this for more detailed information on individual therapies. This section will focus on practical aspects of prescribing or managing people on bone-sparing therapies.

SIGN algorithm (Figure 29.2) includes:

- First-line – alendronic acid or risedronate; zoledronic acid if hip fracture and unsuitable for oral therapy.
- Second-line – zoledronic acid or denosumab if unable to tolerate or poor response to oral therapy. Teriparatide for severe spinal osteoporosis.
- Other options – ibandronate, etidronate or raloxifene (vertebral fracture prevention), tibolone (vertebral and non-vertebral fracture prevention) or HRT (vertebral, non-vertebral and hip fracture prevention). Strontium ranelate restricted to patients with severe osteoporosis without cardiovascular disease when other treatments unsuitable.

Table 29.2 SIGN recommendations on non-drug options for modifying risk factors and reducing fractures [3]

Non-drug options	Recommendation
Exercise	Combinations of exercise types to decrease fracture risk due to falls (balance, flexibility, stretching, strengthening, endurance exercise) Static weight-bearing exercise e.g. single leg standing to slow decline hip BMD Progressive resistance strength training +/− impact exercise to slow decline femoral neck BMD
Diet	Calcium intake 700 mg/day Consider 10 mcg (400 IU)/day vitamin D supplement if inadequate sunlight exposure Restrict consumption liver or liver products to once weekly; ensure diet and supplements provide <1500 mcg/day total retinol Adequate intake vitamin B can be achieved from diet 1 mcg/kg/day dietary vitamin K recommended but not high-dose supplements Insufficient evidence to make recommendations regarding protein, fatty acids or minerals such as potassium or magnesium. A balanced diet is recommended for bone health but dietary phyto-oestrogens or acid-balancing diets are not recommended to reduce fracture risk High coffee intake may be associated with increased fracture risk so restrict intakes to four cups daily particularly if low dietary calcium
Alcohol	If >3.5 units alcohol per day advise to reduce to recommended levels of <14 units per week (women) (<21 units per week for men)
Smoking	Advise smoking cessation
Weight	BMI< 20 – encourage to achieve and maintain BMI 20–25

Calcium and Vitamin D

These supplements should be considered:

- As adjunctive therapy in those receiving bone-sparing therapies unless calcium intake is adequate and they are vitamin D replete.
- As sole therapy in frail, institutionalized or housebound elderly without previous fracture to reduce hip fracture risk.

Controversy surrounds recommendations to increase dietary calcium intake or supplement with calcium and vitamin D3, but major fracture prevention studies included adjunctive calcium and vitamin D. SIGN recommends 700 mg dietary intake; calcium calculators are available online and as phone apps. Vitamin D increases absorption of intestinal calcium. Vitamin D deficiency (<30 nmol/L) and insufficiency (30–50 nmol/L) are common and may increase the risk of falls and fractures.

Several forms of calcium and vitamin D3 are available (chewable or effervescent tablets, swallowable caplets or liquid); patient choice may improve adherence and persistence. Vitamin D is available alone for those intolerant or unwilling to take calcium.

These should not be taken at the same time as bisphosphonates as they impair absorption. Calcium interacts with levothyroxine, fluoroquinolones, tetracyclines, levodopa and other commonly used drugs so timing of doses should be discussed carefully. Interacting drugs should be taken at least two, and ideally four, hours prior to calcium.

In those receiving IV zoledronic acid or subcutaneous denosumab, severe hypocalcaemia may occur at any stage during treatment, so it is important for patients to take supplements. Calcium levels should be checked prior to denosumab injections.

Oral Bisphosphonates

Updated NICE guidance on *Bisphosphonate use for preventing osteoporotic fractures* is in development, and will partially replace TA 160 and 161.

Once weekly alendronate is first-line therapy for prevention and treatment of osteoporotic fractures and steroid-induced osteoporosis due to cost effectiveness of weekly generic drugs.

Bisphosphonates are poorly absorbed orally and need to be taken exactly as directed to optimize bone-sparing effects and minimize upper gastrointestinal intolerance. They should be taken first thing in the morning, on an empty stomach, with a full glass of tap water, and no other food, drink or medication taken for *at least* 30 minutes (alendronate and risedronate) and at least 60 minutes with ibandronate. Patients should stay upright to ensure gravity assists the tablet in passing to the stomach, minimizing oesophageal damage. Alendronate effervescent tablets, dissolved in water to produce a buffered alendronate solution for once weekly treatment, have recently been launched in the UK. It is hoped these will allow more people to tolerate oral bisphosphonate therapy.

When starting treatment, patients should receive education regarding osteoporosis, how to take their medication, and be encouraged to report upper gastrointestinal symptoms. If these occur, bisphosphonate therapy should be stopped. Continuation of alendronate with ranitidine or a proton pump inhibitor is *not* recommended. Once symptoms have settled, a further trial of the same or a different oral bisphosphonate is appropriate, but if the patient remains intolerant they should be referred for initiation of intravenous or subcutaneous therapy.

In December 2014 the Medicines and Healthcare Products Regulatory Agency (MHRA) issued guidance on use and safety of bisphosphonates, discussing:

- Oesophageal reactions – minimize by avoiding use if stricture or achalasia. Ensure patients follow dosing instructions. Consider carefully before using with Barrett's oesophagus.
- Oesophageal cancer – small increased risk after five years' treatment in one study. Caution advised in those with Barrett's oesophagus.
- Osteonecrosis of the jaw – an area of exposed or dead bone in the jaw for >8 weeks in a patient who has had bisphosphonate. More common in those receiving intravenous bisphosphonates for cancer than with oral bisphosphonates for osteoporosis. If poor dental health or for intravenous bisphosphonates then dental examination recommended prior to treatment. Patients should maintain good oral hygiene, have regular dental review and report dental problems.
- Atrial fibrillation – small increased risk if treated with zoledronate or pamidronate; recent review suggests not with alendronate.
- Atypical femoral fractures – stress-type fractures of the femoral shaft after minimal or no trauma, often bilateral. Patients may have thigh pain for several weeks before the completed fracture occurs (they should be warned to report this and be referred for x-ray). Associated with long-term anti-resorptive therapy – all patients should be reviewed after five years' bisphosphonate use. Optimal duration of therapy to reduce risk of conventional fractures while minimizing atypical

fractures is unknown, as is the prevalence, therefore difficult to advise people (also occur with strontium ranelate or denosumab).

- Adverse effects on renal function – intravenous zoledronate. Patients should be well-hydrated prior to therapy and renal function monitored. Zoledronate not recommended if eGFR <35 mmol/L. (Alendronate is not recommended if eGFR <35 or risedronate if <30.)

Zoledronate is a potent bisphosphonate given annually by intravenous infusion. It reduces vertebral, non-vertebral and hip fractures and reduces mortality in post-hip-fracture patients. Around one-third of people develop a flu-like reaction within three days after the first infusion; this is much less common after subsequent infusions. One study demonstrated that AF was increased in those treated with zoledronate, with onset >30 days after infusion.

Subcutaneous Denosumab

Denosumab is a fully human monoclonal antibody to RANK ligand which is involved in differentiation and maturation of osteoclasts. Denosumab reduces hip, vertebral and non-vertebral fractures and effects are sustained while on treatment; 60 mg is given twice yearly by subcutaneous injection. Usually initiation occurs in specialist care with ongoing treatment in primary care under a shared care agreement. Treatment is associated with a small increase in infections, e.g. cellulitis and UTI.

NICE TA 204 recommends denosumab for secondary prevention in postmenopausal women at increased risk of osteoporotic fragility fractures who are unable to comply with the special instructions for taking oral alendronate and risedronate or etidronate, or are intolerant of these or have a contraindication. It can also be used for primary prevention in those who meet the NICE TA 204 criteria.

Selective Oestrogen Receptor Modulators

Raloxifene reduces the risk of vertebral fractures, but does not reduce hip fractures. It also reduces oestrogen-positive invasive breast cancers by almost half (absolute risk reduction 1.2 invasive breast cancers per 1000 women treated for one year). There is an increased risk of DVT or PE, and an increase in fatal stroke demonstrated in one study.

Hormone Replacement Therapy

HRT can be used to treat menopausal symptoms, and reduces the risk of hip and vertebral fractures by around one-third and significantly reduces non-vertebral fractures. Fracture reduction is similar with oestrogen only or combined HRT.

SIGN concludes that since HRT may increase the risk of cardiovascular disease and some cancers in older women and with long-term treatment, HRT may be considered for fracture prevention in younger post-menopausal women, but every woman should have their individual risk assessed prior to therapy and the 'lowest effective dose should be used for the shortest time'. Tibolone can also be considered to prevent vertebral and non-vertebral fractures in younger post-menopausal women.

Strontium Ranelate

This has a dual action increasing bone formation and decreasing resorption and reduces hip and vertebral fractures. It is a daily 2 g sachet made up in water and taken at least two hours after the last food and not with milky drinks. It is not associated with upper GI symptoms, but diarrhoea is common early in treatment. Previous DVT or VTE is a contraindication to use. Treatment has been associated with severe 'drug rash with eosinophila and systemic symptoms' (DRESS), therefore patients must be advised to stop treatment and seek medical attention if they develop a rash.

The European Medicines Agency (EMA) has advised that strontium is contraindicated in those with uncontrolled hypertension, current or past medical history of ischaemic heart disease, peripheral arterial disease or cerebrovascular disease, as it may increase risk of MI (with no increased mortality). Use is restricted to those with severe osteoporosis and high risk of fracture, when other therapies are unsuitable. Cardiovascular risk should be reviewed every 6–12 months.

Parathyroid Hormone

Daily subcutaneous injections of 20 mcg teriparatide for up to 18 months increase bone formation more than resorption particularly at spinal sites, resulting in significant reductions in vertebral and non-vertebral fractures.

NICE recommend referral for consideration of teriparatide in postmenopausal women [6, 7]:

- unable to take oral treatments or unsatisfactory response to oral bisphosphonates (fragility fracture despite adhering fully to treatment for one year and decline in BMD below pre-treatment baseline) AND
- ≥65 years with T score ≤–4.0, or T score ≤–3.5 plus > two fractures OR
- 55–64 years with T score ≤–4.0 plus > two fractures

Encourage Adherence and Persistence with Therapy

Adherence and persistence with oral osteoporosis therapies is poor. Many patients don't even request a second prescription (perhaps believing they have completed the 'course') and only 20–50% persist at one year. It is hypothesized that this is mainly due to upper GI symptoms and difficulties with dosing.

Persistence for at least three to five years is required to optimize fracture reduction. Reviewing tolerance and adherence three months after initiation may improve persistence. People should be encouraged to tell their doctor if considering discontinuing therapy for any reason.

SIGN [3] recommend considering repeat DXA scan at three years to assess benefit and that biochemical markers of bone turnover may also be used for monitoring if available.

Reassess After Three to Five Years

Due to the potential detrimental effects of bone-sparing treatments on normal bone repair, and risks of atypical subtrochanteric fractures and osteonecrosis of jaw, SIGN [3], NICE [3] and NOGG [4] have made recommendations regarding duration of therapy and 'drug holidays'. There is currently insufficient information about the prevalence of atypical subtrochanteric fractures to be able to accurately assess the relative risk of these versus conventional fragility fractures in individual patients. The guidance is therefore pragmatic and based on currently available evidence and is likely to change.

SIGN [3] recommends stopping zoledronate after three annual infusions and review after three years. People with vertebral fractures or pretreatment hip BMD ≤–2.5 will have increased vertebral fracture risk if treatment is stopped. Recommended maximum durations of therapy are shown in Table 29.3.

Table 29.3 SIGN recommended treatment durations [3]

Drug	SIGN treatment duration recommendations
Alendronic acid	Up to 10 years especially in those at high risk of vertebral fractures
Risedronate	Up to seven years if osteoporosis
Zoledronic acid	Three years and reassess fracture risk after three years without treatment
Strontium ranelate	Up to 10 years if severe osteoporosis and unsuitable for other treatments
Denosumab	Up to five years of treatment

Table 29.4 National Osteoporosis Guideline Group recommended continuation of treatment

Type of individual	Recommend continuation of treatment
High risk	≥75 years Previous hip or vertebral fracture Oral steroids ≥7.5 mg/day
Fracture on treatment	Exclude poor adherence or secondary causes
After DXA	Total hip or femoral BMD ≤−2.5

NOGG [4] recommend treatment review after five years on oral bisphosphonates and after 3 years on zoledronic acid. NOGG recommends some groups on oral therapy can continue without further assessment, as shown in Table 29.4. Other patients should have DXA and fracture risk reassessment using FRAX with femoral neck BMD to inform continuation of treatment or 'drug holiday'. In those where there is a recommendation to stop therapy, risk should be reassessed after two years or *immediately if there is a fracture at any time*.

The All Wales Medicine Strategy Group *Guidance to support the safe use of long-term oral bisphosphonate therapy* at www.awmsg.org includes patient information – a summary of the Cochrane review on alendronate efficacy and Newcastle upon Tyne Hospital NHS patient information leaflet on 'Drug holidays' which can be adapted for practice use.

Fracture Prevention and Special Groups

Steroid-Induced Osteoporosis

Oral or systemic steroid treatment increases bone loss, greatest in the first three months but continuing throughout treatment. When oral steroids are commenced and more than three months' use is likely, the need for prophylactic bone-sparing therapy should be considered and started as soon as possible.

The FRAX calculator can be used to estimate future fracture risk and calculates risk for those on an average steroid dose (2.5–7.5 mg daily). When the NOGG graph is displayed there are two crosses – one for 2.5–7.5 mg dose and one for high dose. Women with previous fracture or taking high-dose oral steroids should be considered for bone-sparing therapy.

Adequate calcium and vitamin D status should be maintained throughout steroid treatment even if bisphosphonate therapy is not required.

Vertebral Fractures

Women require analgesia after any fracture. After one or more vertebral fractures, long-term pain is common. In addition to analgesia, a trial of acupuncture, hydrotherapy or transcutaneous nerve stimulation (TENS) may be helpful.

It is important to ensure there is no underlying cause for vertebral fractures by undertaking a CRP and myeloma screen; additional imaging should be considered if there is a previous cancer diagnosis.

NICE has issued guidance on the use of vertebroplasty and kyphoplasty following vertebral fractures [8]. They state that these are:

'Recommended as options for treating osteoporotic vertebral compression fractures only in people:

- Who have severe ongoing pain after a recent, unhealed vertebral fracture despite optimal pain management and
- In whom the pain has been confirmed to be at the level of the fracture by physical examination and imaging.'

Although the decision to undertake these interventions will be made in secondary care, it is important that we know who provides these treatments and refer women urgently who may benefit.

Premenopausal Women

Premenopausal women requiring drug treatment for osteoporosis must avoid pregnancy during treatment and for at least three months afterwards as bisphosphonates may be teratogenic. Most premenopausal women with osteoporotic fractures will need initial specialist assessment.

Future Developments

Odanacatib, a once weekly selective cathepsin K inhibitor, is in late stage development and reduces bone resorption while maintaining bone formation, and has demonstrated significant fracture reduction. Intermittent nitrates, GLP-2 agonists and biological drugs such as romosozumab which blocks sclerostin function, are also in development.

The biggest challenges continue to be ensuring everyone at high fracture risk receives treatment, and improving adherence and persistence with therapy. It is hoped that further information regarding optimal duration of bisphosphonate and other treatment use will emerge, allowing us to optimize prevention of osteoporotic fractures without increasing ONJ and atypical subtrochanteric femoral fractures.

References

1. National Institute for Health and Care Excellence. Osteoporosis: assessing the risk of fragility fracture. 2012. www.nice.org.uk/guidance/cg146?unlid=1506419032015377531 (accessed September 2016).

2. National Institute for Health and Care Excellence. Fragility fracture risk assessment pathway. 2014. pathways.nice.org.uk/pathways/osteoporosis/fragility-fracture-risk-assessment (accessed September 2016).

3. National Institue for Health and Care Excellence. Clinical Knowledge Summary. Osteoporosis: Prevention of fragility fracture. 2016. cks.nice.org.uk/osteoporosis-prevention-of-fragility-fractures (accessed September 2016).

4. Scottish Intercollegiate Guidelines Network. SIGN 142 Management of osteoporosis and the prevention of fragility fractures. 2015. www.nos.org.uk/document.doc?id=1925&erid=0 (accessed September 2016).

5. National Osteoporosis Guideline Group. Osteoporosis Clinical Guideline for Prevention and Treatment. 2013. www.shef.ac.uk/NOGG/NOGG_Executive_Summary.pdf (accessed September 2016).

6. National Institute for Health and Clinical Excellence. TA 160 Alendronate, etidronate, risedronate and strontium ranelate for the primary prevention of osteoporotic fragility fractures in postmenopausal women. 2008. www.nice.org.uk/guidance/ta160?unlid=9383636202016224913 (accessed September 2016).

7. National Institute for Health and Clinical Excellence. TA 161 Alendronate, etidronate, risedronate, raloxifene, strontium ranelate and teriparatide for the secondary prevention of osteoporotic fragility fractures in postmenopausal women. 2008. www.nice.org.uk/guidance/ta161?unlid=13954958220169984914 (accessed September 2016).

8. National Institute for Health and Care Excellence. Percutaneous vertebroplasty and percutaneous balloon kyphoplasty for treating osteoporotic vertebral compression fractures. Technology Appraisal Guidance 279. 2013. www.nice.org.uk/guidance/ta279 (accessed September 2016).

Chapter 30

Management of the Patient with Benign and Malignant Breast Conditions in Primary Care

Jo Marsden and Robert A. Reichert

Key Points

- Most people overestimate significantly their risk of being diagnosed with and dying from breast cancer.
- Most breast symptoms are due to a benign breast condition and not cancer.
- Many women diagnosed with breast cancer have no known risk factors other than growing older and even with exposure to known lifestyle risk factors are never diagnosed.
- High risk Familial breast cancer accounts for <5% of cancers diagnosed annually in the UK.
- Most benign breast conditions are not associated with an increased risk of breast cancer diagnosis.
- Annually, screening prevents 1300 breast cancer deaths in the UK, but this at the expense of overdiagnosing 4000 cancers that would never have caused harm.
- Eight in ten women treated for breast cancer survive their disease for at least 10 years.
- Optimal breast cancer survivorship care requires incorporation of supportive needs into self-management pathways.

Case Scenario

Deborah, aged 52, came to the afternoon surgery yesterday as she has recently been diagnosed with a screen-detected right breast cancer. She is anxious previous exposure to hormonal contraception and current use of hormone replacement therapy 'caused' her cancer, especially as her mother was diagnosed with breast cancer in her 70s and that tests she had done for a right-sided breast lump six years ago 'missed' it. She has also asked about what side effects she may experience with treatment. What can you advise her?

Introduction

Breast cancer is the most commonly diagnosed female malignancy in the UK; in 2011 55,222 new cases were diagnosed, approximately a quarter via the NHS Breast Screening Programme (NHSBSP) (www.cancerresearchuk.org). The UK lifetime risk of diagnosis in women is one in eight, the corollary being that eight in nine women will not be diagnosed (www.cancerresearchuk.org). A full-time GP is likely to diagnose approximately one or two people with breast cancer annually, but will see many more women (and men) who present with troublesome breast symptoms, many of whom have misperception and unnecessary concern about their malignancy risk and associated mortality. Across all ages, UK deaths from breast cancer have fallen over the last 40 years by nearly 40% and survival continues to improve. Currently nearly eight in ten women diagnosed with breast cancer, with optimal treatment, will survive their disease for at least 10 years and two in three will survive their disease beyond 20 years (www.cancerresearchuk.org). To place this in context with all-cause mortality, breast cancer accounts for 3.7% of all female deaths in England and Wales, the commonest causes being due to Alzheimer's disease and dementia (15%), heart disease (9%) and stroke (7.5%) (www.ons.org.uk).

When should Symptomatic People be Referred to a Breast Clinic for Assessment?

In primary care GPs have an important role in determining whether symptoms are due to normal or benign change that does not necessitate referral or whether referral is indicated. Key recommendations

Women's Health in Primary Care, edited by Anne Connolly and Amanda Britton. Published by Cambridge University Press
© Cambridge University Press 2017

Table 30.1 NICE symptom referral recommendations

Refer women using a suspected breast cancer pathway referral (for an appointment within two weeks) if they are:
- Aged ≥ 30 with an unexplained breast lump +/− pain +/− an unexplained axillary lump
- Aged ≥ 50 with any of the following symptoms in one nipple only:
  · Discharge
  · Retraction
  · Other changes of concern
- With skin changes that suggest breast cancer (e.g. tethering, dimpling, peau d'orange)

Consider non-urgent referral in women aged under 30:
- With an unexplained breast lump with or without pain

Refer men with a breast lump for assessment if there is:
- Suspicion of malignancy (aged ≥ 50 with a unilateral lump +/− nipple discharge +/− skin and nipple changes as above). Male breast cancer is rare (349 cases were diagnosed in 2011 in the UK)
- A breast lump without a history of a physiological or drug cause
- Persistent pain and swelling
- Increased risk due to a family history
- Gynaecomastia is the commonest cause of a unilateral benign breast lump +/− pain, in men

from recently updated NICE guidance is summarised in Table 30.1 [1].

Breast pain (mastalgia) is usually due to fibrocystic change. It is common in premenopausal women, often (but not always) cyclical, variable in character and usually self-limiting. In the absence of other clinical concerns, it can be managed initially by primary care; simple analgesia and topical anti-inflammatories may help. There is no evidence dietary intervention or use of evening primrose oil has any more than a placebo effect. Non-cyclical breast pain is often musculoskeletal; costochondritis (Tietze's syndrome) is a particular variant. Referral for mastalgia is only recommended when initial treatment fails or with persistence of unexplained symptoms [2].

If referral is not indicated, GPs should provide appropriate written information and inform eligible women of the NHSBSP and not to wait for their next screening appointment if they develop further symptoms [3]. Any referring health professional needs to understand diagnostic procedures likely to be offered in order to align patient expectations. The diagnosis of breast symptoms involves triple assessment [4] and comprises:

- Clinical examination
- Imaging (i.e. mammography, ultrasound and on an individual basis, MRI) depends on clinical examination findings and the age of the patient

(mammography is not performed in women under 40).
- Tissue biopsy involves image-guided tissue sampling when a solid, discrete lump is confirmed on imaging (i.e. fine needle aspiration cytology, core biopsy); free hand core biopsy and nipple discharge cytology may be appropriate in some circumstances.

When triple assessment is negative for cancer, people are advised to seek advice from their GP if they remain concerned or if there is a change in symptoms or signs (they can be re-referred). If Deborah's previous breast lump was evaluated by triple assessment it is highly unlikely her cancer was 'missed'. Inadvertent, delayed diagnosis of breast cancer after false negative triple assessment is approximately 0.2% [3].

Breast Screening

Women registered with a GP aged 50 to 70 are eligible for participation in the NHSBSP and invited by their local screening centre for a screening mammogram every three years. In England a study is underway currently to assess the risks and benefits of extending the age when women are invited for screening to include those aged 47 to 73. Women over the upper age limit for automatic invitation are entitled to have screening three-yearly, but have to contact their local screening centre directly to request this (www.cancerscreening.nhs.uk).

The aim of screening mammography is to advance the timing of breast cancer diagnosis and thereby improve prognosis, the assumption being diagnosis at an earlier stage, before cancer becomes symptomatic, has a better survival and usually requires less complex treatment. However, significant debate about the benefits of screening persists. An independent UK review of evidence in 2012, which assessed efficacy in terms of breast cancer mortality, concluded of the 15,500 breast cancers diagnosed through the NHSBSP each year, about 1300 breast cancer deaths are prevented [4].

A major concern is overdiagnosis of cancers that would never have caused harm in a woman's lifetime. It is estimated annually that the UK NHSBSP results in the overdiagnosis of 4000 of such cancers. As it is not possible to determine reliably which cancers would never progress, some women will receive unnecessary treatment with the risk of side effects (99% will have surgery, 87% hormone therapy, 80% radiotherapy and 26% chemotherapy). For every breast cancer death

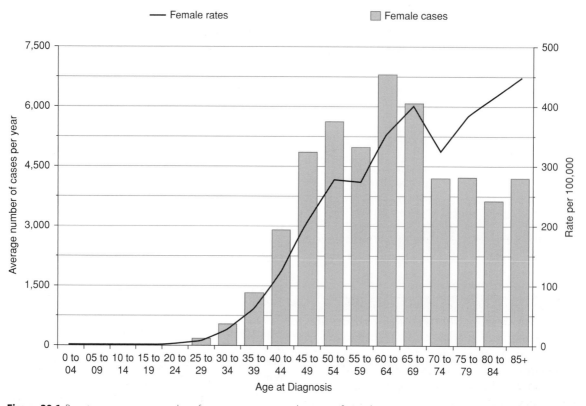

Figure 30.1 Breast cancer: average number of new cases per year and age-specific incidence rates per 100,000 population, females, UK. Prepared by Cancer Research UK – original data sources are available from www.cancerresearchuk.org/cancer-info/cancerstats (accessed September 2016). Reproduced with permission.

prevented by the NHSBSP, three women will be over-diagnosed and have unnecessary treatment [4].

Other possible harms of breast screening include:

- False positive results (i.e. anxiety due to recall for further investigation)
- False negative results (i.e. failure to diagnose a pre-existing cancer)
- Radiation exposure. It is estimated for every 10,000 women who have three-yearly mammograms between the age of 47 and 73 the radiation exposure will be associated with an excess diagnosis of three to six breast cancers.

Overall, the benefits from NHSBSP participation were concluded to outweigh the risks. Little is known about how much overdetection women would consider acceptable and whilst there is lack of consensus about how best to communicate this, it is important these issues are discussed, as appropriate, in primary care [5].

There is no evidence breast self-examination reduces breast cancer mortality by early detection;

however, it is encouraged to promote women's awareness of breast changes, hence presentation in primary care and reduce delayed diagnosis. In countries with screening mammography programmes, clinical breast examination by a health care professional does not reduce breast cancer mortality further [6].

Risk Factors for Breast Cancer

Little is known about the exact cause of the majority of breast cancers as the aetiology of this disease is complex. Genetic, reproductive and lifestyle factors are all associated with an increased risk of diagnosis, but by far the strongest risk factors are being female and increasing age. Most diagnoses (~80%) occur in women over the age of 50. The introduction of the NHSBSP in the late 1980s resulted in a steeper increase in diagnosis in women aged 50 to 64 as a prevalent pool of undiagnosed cancers was detected (www.cancerresearchuk.org) (Figure 30.1).

Most people diagnosed with breast cancer are at population risk. Only a minority have a higher than

Table 30.2 Subtypes of breast cancer

	Luminal A phenotype	Luminal B phenotype	HER2 type phenotype	Triple receptor negative phenotype
Oestrogen receptor: Positive (ER+ve) Negative (ER–ve)	ER+ve	ER+ve	ER-ve	ER-ve
Progesterone receptor: Positive (PR+ve) Negative (PR–ve)	+/– PR+ve	+/– PR+ve	Negative (PR-ve)	PR-ve
HER2/neu receptor: Positive (HER2+ve) Negative (HER2–ve)	HER2-ve	HER2+ve	HER2+ve	HER2-ve
Prevalence	40%	20%	10–15%	15–20%

expected baseline risk for developing breast cancer due to either an inherited genetic mutation or biopsy-proven high-risk breast lesions.

Lifestyle and Reproductive Factors

These are associated with either an increase or decrease in the risk of diagnosis and largely related to female sex hormone exposure, changes to sex hormone metabolism or a greater proportion of less differentiated breast epithelial cells, which are more susceptible to malignant transformation when exposed to carcinogens (e.g. nulliparity, late age at first full-term pregnancy, not breastfeeding). Overall lifestyle and reproductive risk factors confer a similar (small) degree of increased risk (i.e. risk ratio <2). As breast cancer is a heterogeneous condition with four phenotypic subtypes being identified to date (Table 30.2) population prevention strategies aimed at modifying endogenous or exogenous sex hormone exposure are only likely to impact on the diagnosis of oestrogen-receptor-positive disease [7].

Communicating risk using risk ratios and percentage changes can generate confusion and unnecessary anxiety. It is preferable (and least biased) to express risk as absolute numbers with positive and negative framing (Table 30.3). Deborah can be reassured her prior

Table 30.3 Risk of breast cancer diagnosis associated with lifestyle and reproductive risk factors

	Risk ratio	Percentage change in risk	Absolute change in risk per 1000 women aged 50 to 59 at population risk		
			Number of cancers diagnosed	Number of cancers not diagnosed	Excess risk
No exposure	1	–	12	988	–
Postmenopausal obesity or overweight	2.4	+ 140%	29	971	+17
Nulliparity (vs first live birth aged <20 years)	1.7	+70%	20	980	+8
Late age at first live birth (≥31 years)	1.35	+35%	16	984	+4
Alcohol (regular intake ≥6 g/day)	1.27	+27%	15	985	+3
Combined hormonal contraceptives	1.24	+24%	15	985	+3
Combined HRT	1.24	+24%	15	985	+3
Smoking (current smoker)	1.12	+12%	13	987	+1
Late age at menarche (≥ 15 years vs < 11 years)	0.84	−16%	11	989	−1
Unopposed oestrogen replacement	0.72	−27%	9	981	−3
Parity (≥ 4 live births vs 1)	0.64	−36%	7	993	−5
Physical activity (> 9 MET-h/wk)	0.57	−43%	7	995	−5

combined contraceptive and HRT use was unlikely to have resulted in her diagnosis; most women exposed are not diagnosed with breast cancer and accrue benefit from their other favourable outcomes [8].

Familial Breast Cancer

Mutations of DNA repair genes are necessary for the malignant transformation of normal breast epithelial cells, but only a minority (2% of breast cancer diagnosed annually [www.cancerresearchuk.org]) can be attributed to inherited mutations (i.e. familial breast cancer). Otherwise, genetic mutations are somatic and acquired during a person's lifetime (i.e. sporadic breast cancer).

A patient expressing concern about their personal risk due to a family history should have a history taken, as recommended by NICE, to determine whether referral for risk assessment is indicated [9]. If only one first-degree or second-degree relative has been diagnosed with breast cancer over the age of 40, they can be considered to be at population risk and managed in primary care [9].

Tertiary referral to specialist genetic services can only be undertaken from secondary care for people assessed to be at moderate or high increased risk compared to the general population.

- Women at moderate increased risk are eligible for secondary prevention by annual mammographic surveillance between the ages of 40 to 50 years, thereafter surveillance as part of the NHSBSP. Anti-oestrogenic chemoprevention may be discussed.
- Women confirmed or very likely to be at high risk due to an inherited high-risk-susceptibility gene may be recommended surveillance (mammography +/− MRI), prophylactic surgery (mastectomy, oophorectomy) or offered anti-oestrogenic chemoprevention as appropriate.

Deborah can be reassured her family history has not been causative of her breast cancer and if she has any daughters, her diagnosis at the age of 52 does not increase their individual risk.

Benign Breast Conditions and High-Risk Breast Lesions

Benign breast conditions due to fibrocystic change causes symptoms such as lumps, pain and nipple discharge. Most women at some stage will experience such symptoms, prompting at least 50% to seek advice from their GP [10].

- Most fibrocystic change arises due to variations of physiological change (i.e. cyclic changes in ovarian sex hormones during menstruation).
- After the menopause symptomatic benign conditions becomes less common although the use of hormone replacement therapy has been associated with an increased diagnosis [11].

In most women, symptoms and signs are transient and resolve, but if these persist or worsen referral for triple assessment is recommended.

The most widely recognized classification of fibrocystic change is histological, with categorization according the estimated risk of subsequent breast cancer diagnosis (Table 30.4) [12].

- For most benign breast lesions the associated risk of future cancer diagnosis is low and no treatment, follow-up or surveillance is indicated. Patients are reassured and discharged back to primary care.
- Only lesions with biopsy-proven atypia of breast epithelial cells are associated with a significant increased risk of a subsequent breast cancer diagnosis (Table 30.4). Atypia is currently considered a marker of future risk (this is equal in both breasts) rather than a precursor lesion and therefore managed by annual surveillance mammograms for five years.
- Histological classification does *not* correlate with symptoms.

In Situ Carcinoma of the Breast

With *in situ* change abnormal cells are confined to the breast ducts or lobules and do not grow into the surrounding breast tissue. There are two categories of *in situ* disease (Table 30.4) [12]:

1. Lobular carcinoma *in situ* (LCIS) (Figure 30.2a). The abnormal cells are not malignant and as with epithelial atypia, their presence is considered a marker of increased risk and managed by annual mammographic surveillance.
2. Ductal carcinoma *in situ* (DCIS) (Figure 30.2b). This is also called preinvasive cancer, as if untreated it may progress to invasive disease. Treatment is aimed at removing the affected breast tissue and minimizing the risk of local recurrence (i.e. surgery +/− radiotherapy). Risk is greatest with high-grade DCIS, but there is

Table 30.4 Benign and high risk breast conditions

Histological classification	Pathology	Common symptoms	Relative risk of breast cancer	Absolute change in risk in women aged 50 to 59 over 10 years		
				Number of cancers diagnosed	Number of cancers not diagnosed	Excess risk
No benign change	Normal breast tissue	–	1.0	12	988	–
Non-proliferative change	Fibroadenoma Duct ectasia Solitary cysts	Breast lump (usually in younger women) Multiduct nipple discharge, nipple inversion Lump (+/− pain), peak incidence in 40s	1.2	15	985	+3
Proliferative disease without atypia	Multiple cysts Ducal papilloma (solitary or multiple) Sclerosing adenosis	Lump (+/− pain), peak incidence in 40s Lump or single duct nipple discharge (serous, blood-stained) Lump/lumpiness	1.8	23	977	+11
Atypical hyperplasia	Atypical ductal or lobular hyperplasia	Usually an incidental biopsy finding	4.3	52	948	+40
LCIS	–	None. Usually an incidental finding in 0.5% to 3.8% of benign breast biopsies	10	120	880	+108
DCIS	–	Can be an incidental finding or associated with mammographic micro-calcification	≥10	≥120	≥880	≥108

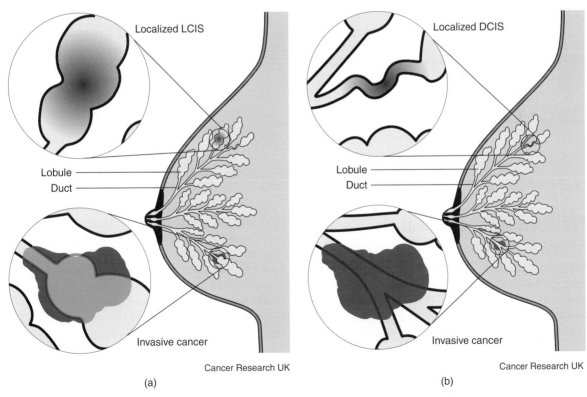

Localized LCIS

Lobule
Duct

Invasive cancer

Cancer Research UK

(a)

Localized DCIS

Lobule
Duct

Invasive cancer

Cancer Research UK

(b)

Figure 30.2 *In situ* carcinoma (LCIS 2a, DCIS 2b) is restricted to the breast ducts and lobules in contrast with invasive breast cancer, where malignant cells invade through the duct wall into the surrounding breast tissue. *Source:* www.cancerresearchuk.org/about-cancer/type/breast-cancer/about/types/lcis-lobular-carcinoma-in-situ and www.cancerresearchuk.org/about-cancer/type/breast-cancer/about/types/dcis-ductal-carcinoma-in-situ (accessed September 2016). Reproduced with permission.

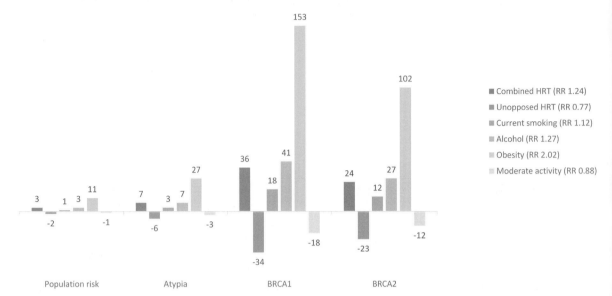

Figure 30.3 The impact of lifestyle risk factors is determined by baseline breast cancer risk and increases as individual baseline risk increases. The risk conferred by lifestyle factors is unchanged (absolute risk = baseline relative risk x lifestyle factor relative risk).

uncertainty whether low or intermediate grade DCIS if left would progress; the UK LORIS trial is comparing local treatment with mammographic surveillance (www.cancerresearchuk.org).

In women at an elevated individual risk due to a family history or personal history of epithelial atypia or LCIS, there is no evidence for an additive effect of lifestyle and reproductive risk factors [13,14]. Instead their impact is determined by individual baseline risk (Figure 30.3).

Principles of Management of Breast Malignancy

When malignancy is confirmed by triple assessment, management is agreed and co-ordinated by the breast unit multidisciplinary team (MDT) [3,15]. Invasive breast cancer is considered to be a systemic condition from the outset, as malignant epithelial cells have acquired the ability to invade surrounding breast tissue and potentially metastasize (Figure 30.2).

The majority of patients present without detectable systemic disease and have 'early' breast cancer, but management is based on the assumption there are undetectable, occult systemic micrometastases. The aim of treatment is twofold.

1. Local control treatments (i.e. surgery, radiotherapy) are used to prevent complications such as skin ulceration and reduce the risk of recurrence in the breast and ipsilateral axillary glands.

2. Adjuvant therapies (i.e. chemotherapy, anti-oestrogenic endocrine therapy, immunotherapy such as herceptin) are used to prevent the development of distant metastases by eradicating occult micro-metastases. The increase in breast cancer survival observed since the early 1990s is attributed in part to the introduction of the NHSBSP, but mostly due to the more widespread use of adjuvant therapy [16]. Selection of adjuvant therapy is based on;

a. Assessment of the breast cancer oestrogen receptor (ER) and human epidermal growth factor 2 (HER2) receptor status. Most breast cancers are ER positive, but only a minority are HER2 positive when tested. Anti-oestrogenic, endocrine therapy is

Table 30.5 Signs and symptoms of breast cancer recurrence

Symptoms and signs around a scar, or in the breast or chest area that could indicate local recurrence	Symptoms and signs that do not improve over a few weeks and for which there is no obvious cause that could indicate systemic recurrence
• A change in shape and size of the breast • A new breast lump or thickening • Skin puckering, dimpling, redness or rash • Swelling in the arm • Pain • Nipple discharge • Change in nipple shape or inversion • Axillary or supraclavicular lymphadenopathy	• Pain in the back or hips • Unexplained weight loss and loss of appetite • Nausea • Abdominal discomfort or swelling • Unexplained tiredness • A persistent dry cough and shortness of breath • Severe headaches especially if worse in the mornings • Scans and blood tests are only done at the advent of systemic symptoms. Investigations in asymptomatic patients do not reduce breast cancer mortality and impair quality of life [15]

prescribed for cancer that is ER+ve and herceptin for cancer that is HER2 positive.

b. Assessment of individual risk of systemic recurrence using prognostic factors is used to inform decisions about the use of chemotherapy (axillary nodal status, tumour size, grade, lympho-vascular invasion, HER2 receptor status). Predictive factors such as genomic tests, which analyze activity of genes that can affect cancer behaviour and response to treatment, e.g. Oncotype DX, can also be used.

3. Routine staging investigations for distant metastatic disease are not performed at diagnosis in the absence of symptoms.

Overall 5, 10 and greater than 20-year survival rates for breast cancer are 87%, 78% and 65% respectively. Survival is affected by stage at diagnosis; for women with stage I disease, five-year survival is 90%, but this falls to 15% for those presenting with advanced (stage IV) breast cancer. Advanced breast cancer is incurable and can only be palliated [15].

Supporting Breast Cancer Patients in Primary Care

The aim of follow-up for early-stage breast cancer is:

- To detect recurrence of a previous breast cancer or a new primary breast cancer
- Manage physical and psychological health problems induced by breast cancer diagnosis and treatment.

Currently the UK follow-up pathway is being changed (www.ncsi.org.uk). There is a move away from routine, outpatient-based appointments (including regular clinical breast examination), as evidence this reduces breast cancer mortality and meets patients' supportive needs is lacking. Instead mammographic surveillance and self-management is being promoted at the completion of 'active' treatment. 'Active' treatment refers to surgery, chemotherapy, herceptin and radiotherapy and may include some or all of these modalities. Anti-oestrogenic adjuvant systemic therapy is recommended for five to ten years if a breast cancer is ER+ve. No further therapy is indicated if a cancer is ER–ve [15].

- Surveillance entails annual mammograms following diagnosis until patients reach the NHSBSP screening age or for patients over screening age, annual mammograms for five years [16]. Thereafter NHSBSP screening frequency is stratified in line with individual risk category.

- Self-management involves breast units issuing patients individual, written follow-up care plans with information about their treatment and named specialist contact details in the event of concerns about recurrence or side effects (www.ncsi.org.uk). Primary care contacts need to be familiar with the latter as inevitably some patients will seek advice from them (Tables 30.5 and 30.6). Primary care also has an important role in promoting physical activity after diagnosis as this improves overall morbidity (physical and psychological) and mortality (www.ncsi.org.uk).

Conclusion

Health professionals in primary care have a key role in aligning patient expectations surrounding the diagnosis and management of benign and malignant

Table 30.6 Side effects of breast cancer treatments

Problems due to lack of oestrogen	Problems due to fatigue	Problems due to change in emotional wellbeing
• Hot flushes • Night sweats • Vaginal dryness • Urinary frequency • Discomfort during intercourse • Decreased interest in sex • Small joint pain or discomfort • Skin dryness • Hair thinning or dryness • Brittle Nails • Premature menopause • Change of mood • Feeling anxious • Feeling low • Poor memory and concentration	• Persistent or recurring tiredness • Poor memory and concentration • Un-refreshing sleep • Tiredness more than 24 hours after exercise **Problems due to lymphoedema** • Arm and/or hand swelling on the side of lymph node surgery	• Change of mood • Feeling anxious or low • Poor memory and concentration • Worrying about cancer recurrence **Problems due to previous surgery or chemotherapy** • Reduced arm or shoulder movement on the side of breast cancer surgery • Leg weakness **Problems due to pain** • Discomfort or pain in the operated breast or axilla • Pain affecting the hands or feet or lower limbs

breast conditions. This can be achieved by supporting patients' information needs, clear communication of risk, providing reassurance as needed and for those with breast malignancy directing appropriate contact with specialist breast services during treatment through to survivorship.

References

1. National Institute for Health and Care Excellence. Suspected cancer: recognition and referral. NICE guidelines NG12.2015. www.nice.org.uk/guidance/ng12 (accessed September 2016).

2. Iddon J, Dixon JM. Mastalgia, *BMJ* 2013;347: bmj.f3288.

3. Willett AM, Michell MJ, Lee MJR, Best practice diagnostic guidelines for patients presenting with breast symptoms. 2010. www.associationofbreastsurgery.org.uk/media/4585/best_practice_diagnostic_guidelines_for_patients_presenting_with_breast_symptoms.pdf (accessed September 2016).

4. Independent UK Panel on Breast Cancer Screening. The benefits and harms of breast cancer screening: an independent review. *Lancet* 2012;380:1778–1786.

5. Waller J, Whitaker KL, Winstanley K, Power E, Wardle J, A survey study of women's responses to information about overdiagnosis in breast cancer screening in Britain. *Br J Cancer* 2014,28;111:1831–1835

6. Nelson HD, Tyne K, Naik A, *et al.* Screening for breast cancer: systematic evidence review update for the US Preventive Services Task Force *Ann Intern Med* 2009;151(10):727–W242.

7. Anderson KN, Schwab RB, Martinez ME, Reproductive risk factors and breast cancer subtypes: a review of the literature. *Breast Cancer Res Treat* 2014;144:1–10.

8. Bassuk SS, Manson JE, Oral contraceptives and menopausal hormone therapy: relative and attributable risks of cardiovascular disease, cancer, and other health outcomes. *Ann Epidemiol* 2015;25;193–200.

9. NICE. Familial breast cancer: Classification and care of people at risk of familial breast cancer and management of breast cancer and related risks in people with a family history of breast cancer. NICE guidelines CG164. 2013. www.nice.org.uk/Guidance/CG164 (accessed September 2016).

10. Seltzer MH, Breast complaints, biopsies, and cancer correlated with age in 10,000 consecutive new surgical referrals. *Breast J* 2004;10:111–117.

11. Santen RJ, Mansel R, Benign breast disorders. *N Engl J Med* 2005;353:275–285.

12. Morrow M, Schnitt SJ, Norton L, Current management of lesions associated with an increased risk of breast cancer. *Nat Rev Clin Oncol* 2015;12:227–238.

13. Pan H, He Z, Ling L, *et al.* Reproductive factors and breast cancer risk among BRCA1 or BRCA2 mutation carriers: results from ten studies. *Cancer Epidemiol* 2014;38:1–8.

14. Kabat GC, Jones JG, Olson N, *et al.* Risk factors for breast cancer in women biopsied for benign breast disease: a nested case-control study. *Cancer Epidemiol* 2010;34:34–39.

15. NICE. Early and locally advanced breast cancer: Diagnosis and treatment. NICE guidelines CG80. 2009. www.nice.org.uk/guidance/cg80 (accessed September 2016).

16. Gøtzsche PC, Jørgensen KJ, Screening for breast cancer with mammography. *Cochrane Database Syst Rev.* 2013;(4):CD001877.

Index